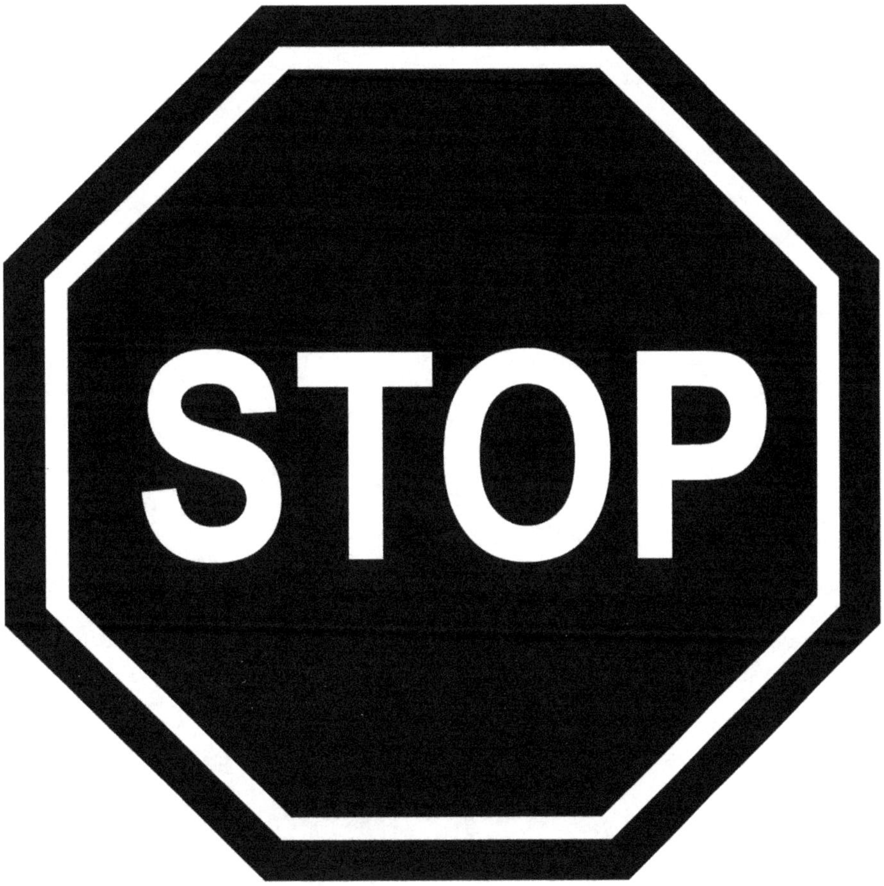

FREE Test Taking Tips DVD Offer

To help us better serve you, we have developed a Test Taking Tips DVD that we would like to give you for FREE. **This DVD covers world-class test taking tips that you can use to be even more successful when you are taking your test.**

All that we ask is that you email us your feedback about your study guide. Please let us know what you thought about it – whether that is good, bad or indifferent.

To get your **FREE Test Taking Tips DVD**, email freedvd@studyguideteam.com with “FREE DVD” in the subject line and the following information in the body of the email:

a. The title of your study guide.

b. Your product rating on a scale of 1-5, with 5 being the highest rating.

c. Your feedback about the study guide. What did you think of it?

d. Your full name and shipping address to send your free DVD.

If you have any questions or concerns, please don’t hesitate to contact us at freedvd@studyguideteam.com.

Thanks again!

Med Surg Study Guide

CMSRN Review Book and Medical Surgical Nursing Certification Prep (RN-BC) with Practice Test Questions [4th Edition]

TPB Publishing

Written and edited by TPB Publishing.

ISBN 13: 9781628456684
ISBN 10: 162845668X

Table of Contents

Quick Overview

As you draw closer to taking your exam, effective preparation becomes more and more important. Thankfully, you have this study guide to help you get ready. Use this guide to help keep your studying on track and refer to it often.

This study guide contains several key sections that will help you be successful on your exam. The guide contains tips for what you should do the night before and the day of the test. Also included are test-taking tips. Knowing the right information is not always enough. Many well-prepared test takers struggle with exams. These tips will help equip you to accurately read, assess, and answer test questions.

A large part of the guide is devoted to showing you what content to expect on the exam and to helping you better understand that content. In this guide are practice test questions so that you can see how well you have grasped the content. Then, answer explanations are provided so that you can understand why you missed certain questions.

Don't try to cram the night before you take your exam. This is not a wise strategy for a few reasons. First, your retention of the information will be low. Your time would be better used by reviewing information you already know rather than trying to learn a lot of new information. Second, you will likely become stressed as you try to gain a large amount of knowledge in a short amount of time. Third, you will be depriving yourself of sleep. So be sure to go to bed at a reasonable time the night before. Being well-rested helps you focus and remain calm.

Be sure to eat a substantial breakfast the morning of the exam. If you are taking the exam in the afternoon, be sure to have a good lunch as well. Being hungry is distracting and can make it difficult to focus. You have hopefully spent lots of time preparing for the exam. Don't let an empty stomach get in the way of success!

When travelling to the testing center, leave earlier than needed. That way, you have a buffer in case you experience any delays. This will help you remain calm and will keep you from missing your appointment time at the testing center.

Be sure to pace yourself during the exam. Don't try to rush through the exam. There is no need to risk performing poorly on the exam just so you can leave the testing center early. Allow yourself to use all of the allotted time if needed.

Remain positive while taking the exam even if you feel like you are performing poorly. Thinking about the content you should have mastered will not help you perform better on the exam.

Once the exam is complete, take some time to relax. Even if you feel that you need to take the exam again, you will be well served by some down time before you begin studying again. It's often easier to convince yourself to study if you know that it will come with a reward!

Test-Taking Strategies

1. Predicting the Answer

When you feel confident in your preparation for a multiple-choice test, try predicting the answer before reading the answer choices. This is especially useful on questions that test objective factual knowledge. By predicting the answer before reading the available choices, you eliminate the possibility that you will be distracted or led astray by an incorrect answer choice. You will feel more confident in your selection if you read the question, predict the answer, and then find your prediction among the answer choices. After using this strategy, be sure to still read all of the answer choices carefully and completely. If you feel unprepared, you should not attempt to predict the answers. This would be a waste of time and an opportunity for your mind to wander in the wrong direction.

2. Reading the Whole Question

Too often, test takers scan a multiple-choice question, recognize a few familiar words, and immediately jump to the answer choices. Test authors are aware of this common impatience, and they will sometimes prey upon it. For instance, a test author might subtly turn the question into a negative, or he or she might redirect the focus of the question right at the end. The only way to avoid falling into these traps is to read the entirety of the question carefully before reading the answer choices.

3. Looking for Wrong Answers

Long and complicated multiple-choice questions can be intimidating. One way to simplify a difficult multiple-choice question is to eliminate all of the answer choices that are clearly wrong. In most sets of answers, there will be at least one selection that can be dismissed right away. If the test is administered on paper, the test taker could draw a line through it to indicate that it may be ignored; otherwise, the test taker will have to perform this operation mentally or on scratch paper. In either case, once the obviously incorrect answers have been eliminated, the remaining choices may be considered. Sometimes identifying the clearly wrong answers will give the test taker some information about the correct answer. For instance, if one of the remaining answer choices is a direct opposite of one of the eliminated answer choices, it may well be the correct answer. The opposite of obviously wrong is obviously right! Of course, this is not always the case. Some answers are obviously incorrect simply because they are irrelevant to the question being asked. Still, identifying and eliminating some incorrect answer choices is a good way to simplify a multiple-choice question.

4. Don't Overanalyze

Anxious test takers often overanalyze questions. When you are nervous, your brain will often run wild, causing you to make associations and discover clues that don't actually exist. If you feel that this may be a problem for you, do whatever you can to slow down during the test. Try taking a deep breath or counting to ten. As you read and consider the question, restrict yourself to the particular words used by the author. Avoid thought tangents about what the author *really* meant, or what he or she was *trying* to say. The only things that matter on a multiple-choice test are the words that are actually in the question. You must avoid reading too much into a multiple-choice question, or supposing that the writer meant something other than what he or she wrote.

5. No Need for Panic

It is wise to learn as many strategies as possible before taking a multiple-choice test, but it is likely that you will come across a few questions for which you simply don't know the answer. In this situation, avoid panicking. Because most multiple-choice tests include dozens of questions, the relative value of a single wrong answer is small. As much as possible, you should compartmentalize each question on a multiple-choice test. In other words, you should not allow your feelings about one question to affect your success on the others. When you find a question that you either don't understand or don't know how to answer, just take a deep breath and do your best. Read the entire question slowly and carefully. Try rephrasing the question a couple of different ways. Then, read all of the answer choices carefully. After eliminating obviously wrong answers, make a selection and move on to the next question.

6. Confusing Answer Choices

When working on a difficult multiple-choice question, there may be a tendency to focus on the answer choices that are the easiest to understand. Many people, whether consciously or not, gravitate to the answer choices that require the least concentration, knowledge, and memory. This is a mistake. When you come across an answer choice that is confusing, you should give it extra attention. A question might be confusing because you do not know the subject matter to which it refers. If this is the case, don't eliminate the answer before you have affirmatively settled on another. When you come across an answer choice of this type, set it aside as you look at the remaining choices. If you can confidently assert that one of the other choices is correct, you can leave the confusing answer aside. Otherwise, you will need to take a moment to try to better understand the confusing answer choice. Rephrasing is one way to tease out the sense of a confusing answer choice.

7. Your First Instinct

Many people struggle with multiple-choice tests because they overthink the questions. If you have studied sufficiently for the test, you should be prepared to trust your first instinct once you have carefully and completely read the question and all of the answer choices. There is a great deal of research suggesting that the mind can come to the correct conclusion very quickly once it has obtained all of the relevant information. At times, it may seem to you as if your intuition is working faster even than your reasoning mind. This may in fact be true. The knowledge you obtain while studying may be retrieved from your subconscious before you have a chance to work out the associations that support it. Verify your instinct by working out the reasons that it should be trusted.

8. Key Words

Many test takers struggle with multiple-choice questions because they have poor reading comprehension skills. Quickly reading and understanding a multiple-choice question requires a mixture of skill and experience. To help with this, try jotting down a few key words and phrases on a piece of scrap paper. Doing this concentrates the process of reading and forces the mind to weigh the relative importance of the question's parts. In selecting words and phrases to write down, the test taker thinks about the question more deeply and carefully. This is especially true for multiple-choice questions that are preceded by a long prompt.

9. Subtle Negatives

One of the oldest tricks in the multiple-choice test writer's book is to subtly reverse the meaning of a question with a word like *not* or *except*. If you are not paying attention to each word in the question, you can easily be led astray by this trick. For instance, a common question format is, "Which of the following is...?" Obviously, if the question instead is, "Which of the following is not...?," then the answer will be quite different. Even worse, the test makers are aware of the potential for this mistake and will include one answer choice that would be correct if the question were not negated or reversed. A test taker who misses the reversal will find what he or she believes to be a correct answer and will be so confident that he or she will fail to reread the question and discover the original error. The only way to avoid this is to practice a wide variety of multiple-choice questions and to pay close attention to each and every word.

10. Reading Every Answer Choice

It may seem obvious, but you should always read every one of the answer choices! Too many test takers fall into the habit of scanning the question and assuming that they understand the question because they recognize a few key words. From there, they pick the first answer choice that answers the question they believe they have read. Test takers who read all of the answer choices might discover that one of the latter answer choices is actually *more* correct. Moreover, reading all of the answer choices can remind you of facts related to the question that can help you arrive at the correct answer. Sometimes, a misstatement or incorrect detail in one of the latter answer choices will trigger your memory of the subject and will enable you to find the right answer. Failing to read all of the answer choices is like not reading all of the items on a restaurant menu: you might miss out on the perfect choice.

11. Spot the Hedges

One of the keys to success on multiple-choice tests is paying close attention to every word. This is never truer than with words like almost, most, some, and sometimes. These words are called "hedges" because they indicate that a statement is not totally true or not true in every place and time. An absolute statement will contain no hedges, but in many subjects, the answers are not always straightforward or absolute. There are always exceptions to the rules in these subjects. For this reason, you should favor those multiple-choice questions that contain hedging language. The presence of qualifying words indicates that the author is taking special care with his or her words, which is certainly important when composing the right answer. After all, there are many ways to be wrong, but there is only one way to be right! For this reason, it is wise to avoid answers that are absolute when taking a multiple-choice test. An absolute answer is one that says things are either all one way or all another. They often include words like *every*, *always*, *best*, and *never*. If you are taking a multiple-choice test in a subject that doesn't lend itself to absolute answers, be on your guard if you see any of these words.

12. Long Answers

In many subject areas, the answers are not simple. As already mentioned, the right answer often requires hedges. Another common feature of the answers to a complex or subjective question are qualifying clauses, which are groups of words that subtly modify the meaning of the sentence. If the question or answer choice describes a rule to which there are exceptions or the subject matter is complicated, ambiguous, or confusing, the correct answer will require many words in order to be expressed clearly and accurately. In essence, you should not be deterred by answer choices that seem excessively long. Oftentimes, the author of the text will not be able to write the correct answer without offering some qualifications and modifications. Your job is to read the answer choices thoroughly and completely and to select the one that most accurately and precisely answers the question.

13. Restating to Understand

Sometimes, a question on a multiple-choice test is difficult not because of what it asks but because of how it is written. If this is the case, restate the question or answer choice in different words. This process serves a couple of important purposes. First, it forces you to concentrate on the core of the question. In order to rephrase the question accurately, you have to understand it well. Rephrasing the question will concentrate your mind on the key words and ideas. Second, it will present the information to your mind in a fresh way. This process may trigger your memory and render some useful scrap of information picked up while studying.

14. True Statements

Sometimes an answer choice will be true in itself, but it does not answer the question. This is one of the main reasons why it is essential to read the question carefully and completely before proceeding to the answer choices. Too often, test takers skip ahead to the answer choices and look for true statements. Having found one of these, they are content to select it without reference to the question above. Obviously, this provides an easy way for test makers to play tricks. The savvy test taker will always read the entire question before turning to the answer choices. Then, having settled on a correct answer choice, he or she will refer to the original question and ensure that the selected answer is relevant. The mistake of choosing a correct-but-irrelevant answer choice is especially common on questions related to specific pieces of objective knowledge. A prepared test taker will have a wealth of factual knowledge at his or her disposal, and should not be careless in its application.

15. No Patterns

One of the more dangerous ideas that circulates about multiple-choice tests is that the correct answers tend to fall into patterns. These erroneous ideas range from a belief that B and C are the most common right answers, to the idea that an unprepared test-taker should answer "A-B-A-C-A-D-A-B-A." It cannot be emphasized enough that pattern-seeking of this type is exactly the WRONG way to approach a multiple-choice test. To begin with, it is highly unlikely that the test maker will plot the correct answers according to some predetermined pattern. The questions are scrambled and delivered in a random order. Furthermore, even if the test maker was following a pattern in the assignation of correct answers, there is no reason why the test taker would know which pattern he or she was using. Any attempt to discern a pattern in the answer choices is a waste of time and a distraction from the real work of taking the test. A test taker would be much better served by extra preparation before the test than by reliance on a pattern in the answers.

FREE DVD OFFER

Don't forget that doing well on your exam includes both understanding the test content and understanding how to use what you know to do well on the test. We offer a completely FREE Test Taking Tips DVD that covers world class test taking tips that you can use to be even more successful when you are taking your test.

All that we ask is that you email us your feedback about your study guide. To get your **FREE Test Taking Tips DVD**, email freedvd@studyguideteam.com with "FREE DVD" in the subject line and the following information in the body of the email:

- The title of your study guide.
- Your product rating on a scale of 1-5, with 5 being the highest rating.
- Your feedback about the study guide. What did you think of it?
- Your full name and shipping address to send your free DVD.

Introduction to the Medical-Surgical Exams

About this Guide

This study guide is intended for preparation for the following two exams:

- Certified Medical-Surgical Registered Nurse (CMSRN) Exam produced by the Medical-Surgical Nursing Certification Board (MSNCB)
- The Medical-Surgical Nursing Certification (RN-BC) produced by the American Nurses Credentialing Center (ANCC)

The CMSRN and RN-BC outlines are structured differently but cover very similar material. The CMSRN outline is structured around knowledge topics (Gastrointestinal, Pulmonary, Cardiovascular/Hematological, etc.). The RN-BC outline is structured around skill topics such as Assessment and Diagnosis. The two outline structures are complementary as nursing knowledge and nursing skills must be paired together, and both are covered on each exam.

The developers of this guide have chosen to follow the CMSRN outline heading structure, so each chapter title is that of a knowledge topic. The skill content, as emphasized in the RN-BC outline, is then integrated into each concept that is discussed. Because the exams test such similar content, the two practice tests at the end can be used to prepare for either exam.

In summary, whether you are preparing for the CMSRN or the RN-BC, this the guide for you. It will educate you on the topics you need to know and then provide an opportunity to thoroughly test your knowledge. Be sure to take advantage of the detailed answer explanations as well.

We wish you the best on your exam!

Certified Medical-Surgical Registered Nurse (CMSRN)

Function of the Test

The Certified Medical-Surgical Registered Nurse (CMSRN) Exam is a test given by the Medical-Surgical Nursing Certification Board (MSNCB) to those who hold a license as a registered nurse (RN), have accrued at least 2,000 hours of practice within the past three years, and have practiced two years as an RN in a medical-surgical setting.

The CMSRN gives nurses the credential they need to work as Medical-Surgical Nurses. The CMSRN certification is accredited by the Accreditation Board for Specialty Nursing Certification (ABSNC) and recognized for Magnet status. In 2018, the CMSRN exam had 7,004 test takers. Out of that number, 5,648 passed, making the overall pass rate 81%.

Test Administration

The CMSRN is offered in computer and paper-based format. For the computer-based exam, more than 230 sites in the U.S. are available for test taking. Within five weeks of applying to take the exam, test takers will receive a permit from the testing agency, C-NET, which specifies the test taking accommodations in the area.

Test takers who do not pass the exam have the option of taking the exam again for a one-time discount, but only if it is considered their first retake. This is offered up to four months after the exam date. Those who require accommodations for a disability may submit an application form to MSNCB, then send the appropriate documentation to C-NET. Test takers must bring a valid government ID with a photo and signature to their testing appointment.

Test Format

The CMSRN is broken into six different patient problems: Gastrointestinal, Pulmonary, Cardiovascular/Hematological, Diabetes/Endocrine/Immunological, Urological/Renal, and Musculoskeletal/Neurological/Integumentary. The table below breaks down the percentages of the content:

Patient Problem	Percentage
Gastrointestinal	16–18%
Pulmonary	15–17%
Cardiovascular/Hematological	16–18%
Diabetes/Other Endocrine/Immunological	18–20%
Urological/Renal	14–16%
Musculoskeletal/Neurological/Integumentary	15–17%

Scoring

To pass the CMSRN, a standard score of 95, or 71% correct, is required. Test takers' scores are not compared to each other, but rather are based on the Angoff procedure.

A scaled score for the CMSRN will be given at the end of the exam. For those who do not pass the exam, a total score with subscores will be given to highlight the areas that need work. For those who pass the exam, a total score is given.

Recent Developments

The blueprint for the CMSRN changed for the 2019 year, so please see the previous table or the recent blueprint on the website to get up-do-date information on the exam.

The Medical-Surgical Nursing Certification (RN-BC)

Function of the Test

The American Nurse Credential Center's Medical-Surgical Nursing Certification [Registered Nurse-Board Certified (RN-BC)] exam is a competency-based exam for entry-level registered nurses in the medical-surgical specialty to demonstrate their clinical knowledge and skills. Successfully passing the exam earns the test taker the RN-BC credential, which is then valid for five years. After this time, the credential can be maintained by keeping nursing license active and satisfying the requirements for renewal.

Candidates must meet eligibility criteria in order to register and sit for the exam. They must hold a current, active RN license. This license must be either from a state or territory of the United States or what is considered to be the legally-recognized, professional equivalent in another country. Candidates must have a minimum of two years of full-time professional experience as a registered nurse. Within the three years immediately prior to sitting for the exam, a candidate must have accrued at least 2,000 hours of clinical practice specifically in the area of medical-surgical nursing, and completed 30 hours of continuing education in this specialty area.

Test Administration

The RN-BC exam is administered via computer year round at Prometric testing sites throughout the United States. Candidates must apply to take the test and provide proof of satisfying the eligibility requirements. Test takers are permitted to retake the exam after 60 days if they do not pass. However, within a 12-month period, only three test attempts are permitted. Accommodations are available for test takers with documented disabilities. Candidates seeking accommodations must submit supporting paperwork and wait for confirmation or approval of the requested accommodations prior to registering for the exam.

Test Format

The exam includes 150 multiple-choice questions, of which 125 are scored. The other 25 are considered pretest questions, and are used by the ANCC to assess their validity and utility as scored questions for future exams. Test takers have three hours to complete the exam. The major content areas and the number of questions and percentage of the test comprised by each is listed in the table below:

Content Area	**Number of Questions**	**Percentage of Test**
Assessment and Diagnosis	52	42%
Planning, Implementation, and Evaluation	58	46%
Professional Role	15	12%

Scoring

The RN-BC exam is a pass-fail exam. Test takers must meet the minimum passing score to receive passing status and the RN-BC credential. A test taker's raw score is determined by the number of questions answered correctly. Incorrect responses are not penalized, so test takers should guess, or complete all questions, if possible. The raw score is then converted to a scaled score from 0–500. The passing score is 350. Test takers earning at least 350 will receive the passing status. Those who score lower than 350 will receive their scaled score, the "fail" status, and diagnostic feedback pertaining to each of the three content areas on the exam.

Gastrointestinal

Acute Abdomen Peritonitis and Appendicitis

An **acute abdomen** is defined as the presence of manifestations associated with nontraumatic intra-abdominal pathology that often requires surgical intervention.

Peritonitis

Peritonitis is an inflammatory process affecting the peritoneum, which is the serosal membrane that lines the abdominal cavity. The normally sterile environment of the peritoneum can become infected by a pathogen, irritated by bile from a perforated gallbladder or lacerated liver, or from secretions from the perforation of the stomach. The onset, severity, and course of the condition vary according to the precipitating event. Presenting manifestations may include abdominal pain, nausea and vomiting, diarrhea, fever and chills, altered peristalsis, abdominal distention, and possible encephalopathy. Diagnosis is based on the patient's history, in addition to the results of routine lab studies and blood cultures; ultrasound, computerized tomography (CT), and x-ray studies of the abdomen; and paracentesis. Emergency care of peritonitis is focused on eliminating the source of infection or irritation, controlling the infection and inflammatory process with aggressive antibiotic therapy as appropriate to prevent progression to generalized sepsis, and maintaining organ function of the abdominal organs.

Appendicitis

Appendicitis is defined as the inflammation of the vermiform appendix, which extends from the cecum at the terminal end of the ileum. The inflammation results from the obstruction of the lumen of the appendix by accumulated fecaliths, bacteria, or parasites. The condition presents a surgical emergency due to the risk of perforation of the wall of the structure with resulting peritonitis and sepsis. The classic presenting symptoms are anorexia and periumbilical pain that evolves to the right lower quadrant, followed by vomiting. The diagnosis is made by the results of the physical examination, routine lab studies, pregnancy testing to rule out ectopic pregnancy, and ultrasound imaging. Emergency care includes antibiotic therapy and appendectomy.

Bleeding

Gastrointestinal (GI) bleeding is defined according to the area of the defect. Upper GI bleeding occurs superiorly to the junction of the duodenum and jejunum. Lower GI bleeding occurs in the large and small intestine. Conditions associated with upper GI bleeding include esophageal varices, gastric and duodenal ulcers, cancer, and Mallory-Weiss tears. Risk factors include age, history of gastroesophageal reflux disorder (GERD), use of nonsteroidal anti-inflammatory drugs (NSAIDs) and steroids, and alcoholism. Acute presenting manifestations include hematemesis, melena, hematochezia, and lightheadedness or fainting. Hematemesis, or bloody vomit, will appear with either a coffee ground (older blood) or bright red (new blood) appearance. The diagnosis is made by the patient's history and physical examination, routine lab studies including complete blood count (CBC) and coagulation tests, endoscopy, and chest films. Treatment is specific to the cause; e.g., peptic ulcer disease will be treated with the appropriate antibiotic and a proton-pump inhibitor (PPI).

Causative factors for GI bleeding of the lower intestine include anatomical defects such as diverticulosis, ischemic events of the vasculature related to radiation therapy or other embolic events, cancer, and infectious or noninfectious inflammatory conditions. Manifestations that are specific to the cause and location of the hemorrhage include melena, maroon stools or bright red blood, fever, dehydration, possible abdominal pain or distention, and hematochezia. Common diagnostic studies include routine lab studies, endoscopy, radionucleotide studies, and angiography. Treatment is focused on the identification and resolution of the source of the bleeding and correction of any hematologic deficits that resulted from the hemorrhage. Emergency providers are aware that orthostatic hypotension defined as a decrease in diastolic blood pressure (BP) of 10 millimeters of mercury or more is associated with a blood loss of approximately 1000 milliliters. Therefore, the emergency care of massive GI bleeding requires aggressive fluid volume replacement with isotonic crystalloids while the exact source of the bleeding is being confirmed.

Cholecystitis

Cholecystitis is defined as an inflammation of the gallbladder. It is most often due to blockage of the cystic duct by gallstones. The condition may be complicated by the presence of perforation or gangrene of the gallbladder. Common risk factors include increasing age, female gender, obesity or rapid weight loss, and pregnancy. Symptoms include colicky epigastric pain that radiates to the right upper quadrant that may become constant and a palpable gallbladder, jaundice, nausea, vomiting, and fever. Emergency providers understand that the elderly and chronically ill children may present with atypical manifestations of cholecystitis. Presenting symptoms in elderly patients may be limited to vague complaints of localized tenderness; however, the condition can rapidly progress to a more complicated form of cholecystitis due to infection, leading to gangrene or perforation of the gallbladder. This risk is increased in elderly patients with diabetes. Children with sickle cell disease, congenital biliary defects, or chronic illness requiring total parenteral nutrition (TPN) therapy may present with generalized abdominal pain and jaundice.

Diagnostic studies include routine lab tests, liver function tests, and abdominal ultrasounds. Additional imaging studies may be required; however, ultrasound is very sensitive for cholecystitis, does not expose the patient to radiation, and is readily available in the emergency care setting. Treatment options depend on the severity of symptoms. Acalculous cholecystitis may progress quickly to perforation and gangrene of the gallbladder requiring emergency intervention, while uncomplicated cases of acute cholecystitis can be treated with bowel rest, intravenous (IV) fluids, and short-term antibiotic therapy. Emergency providers understand that elective laparoscopic cholecystectomy is the procedure of choice, with the rate of conversion to open cholecystectomy at 5 percent; however, emergency laparoscopic cholecystectomy is associated with a 30 percent conversion rate.

Early recognition and intervention are required due to the rapid progression of acute acalculous cholecystitis to gangrene and perforation.

Cirrhosis

Cirrhosis of the liver is characterized by fibrotic changes that eventually accumulate as scar tissue that replaces functioning liver cells. The manifestations and onset of the disease, which may be gradual or rapid, depend on the exact etiology. Chronic hepatitis due to the hepatitis C virus has replaced alcoholic liver disease as the most common cause of cirrhosis in the United States. Although there are several additional conditions that are associated with the development of cirrhosis as noted below, nonalcoholic fatty liver disease (NAFLD), which is common in patients with diabetes, obesity, and elevated triglyceride levels and is estimated to affect 33 percent of all individuals in the United States, is a growing concern for providers. Cirrhosis is characterized by the abnormal retention of lipids in the cells that worsens as the process of hepatic fibrosis progresses. Other contributing conditions to the development of cirrhosis include sarcoidosis, primary biliary cirrhosis, chronic right-sided heart failure, tricuspid regurgitation, autoimmune hepatitis, and alpha 1 antitrypsin deficiency.

Common symptoms include ascites; abdominal pain; portal hypertension; hepatic encephalopathy with the deterioration of the level of consciousness from normal to somnolence, drowsiness, and coma; hepatorenal disease; fever; anorexia; weight loss; spider angiomas; jaundice; and coagulopathy. Treatment is initially focused on preventing the progression of the precipitating conditions. Hepatitis C is treated with antiviral agents; cardiac conditions are treated with diuretics, beta-blockers, and digoxin; and autoimmune disorders are treated with immunosuppressant agents. Once the fibrotic changes have occurred, symptomatic interventions include treatment of pruritus, zinc deficiency, and osteoporosis. Patients with advanced cirrhosis may be candidates for a liver transplantation. The Model for End-Stage Liver Disease (MELD), which is used to allocate donor organs in the United States, calculates the projected patient survival rate following a liver transplant based on patient's age, serum bilirubin, creatinine, pro time international normalized ratio (INR), sodium level, and a history of current or recent renal dialysis.

Diverticulitis

Diverticulitis is the inflammation of the diverticula, which are described as outpouchings or defects in the wall, most commonly located in the rectosigmoid segment of the large intestine. The diverticula are common in people over fifty years old, due to the increased pressure in the lumen of the bowel during defecation; however, most people do not experience diverticulitis. Inflammation of the diverticula occurs when fecaliths and other cellular debris become impacted in the outpouchings, initiating the changes in the mucous lining of the intestine.

Common manifestations of an acute episode include lower left quadrant pain, nausea, vomiting, chills, fever, and tachycardia. The condition must be differentiated from other inflammatory bowel diseases (IBDs), including Crohn's disease and ulcerative colitis, because the underlying pathology and treatment are different. Severe or prolonged manifestations will be treated with bowel rest, IV fluids, antibiotic therapy, and assessment of routine lab studies, including coagulation assay, blood cultures, and nasogastric decompression. More commonly, progressing from a clear liquid diet to a low-fiber diet until symptoms subside, followed by progression to a high-fiber diet is successful in treating the disorder. Repeated episodes with increasingly severe manifestations are associated with possible thinning of the intestinal wall, which increases the risk of perforation of the bowel, resulting in hemorrhage and peritonitis.

Decisions related to surgical intervention may be based on the Hinchey classification criteria, which stage the disease according to the extent of inflammatory changes and the integrity of the bowel wall. Surgical interventions may include colectomy, which is the resection of the diseased segment with anastomosis of the normal bowel segments, or the placement of a temporary or permanent colostomy depending on the dimensions of the damage. Postoperative risks include hemorrhage, altered fluid volume status, infection, delayed wound healing, impaired self-image, and repeated inflammatory attacks.

Diverticulosis and Diverticulitis

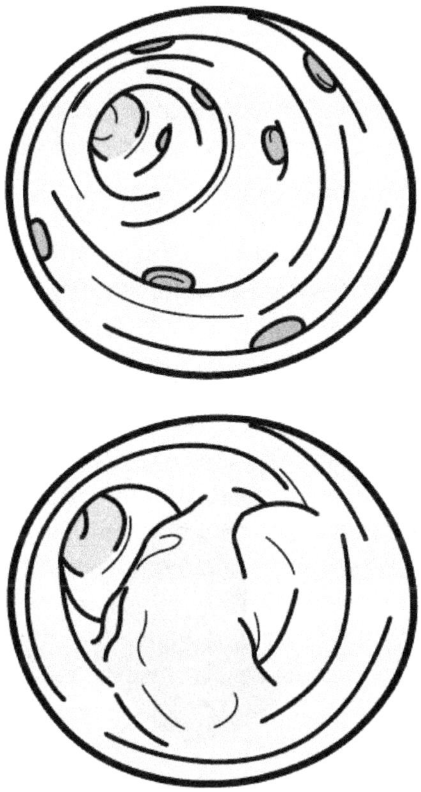

Esophageal Varices

Esophageal varices develop as a compensatory mechanism for the portal hypertension that occurs in liver disease. The superficial veins of the esophagus and the stomach function as a collateral circulation by diverting blood from the portal system to reduce pressure in the vasculature of the liver. Approximately 60 percent of patients with severe cirrhosis will develop esophageal varices at some point because portal hypertension is progressive in these patients. There may be no indication of the presence of esophageal varices until the vessels rupture, which means that all patients with cirrhosis require annual endoscopic screening for the assessment of the presence of varices.

Prophylactic treatment is recommended for varices that are 5 millimeters or more in diameter and/or exhibit longitudinal red streaks or wales along the varices, due to the significant risk of rupture and hemorrhage associated with these findings. Additional risk factors for hemorrhage include a patient history of constipation, vomiting, severe coughing, and alcohol abuse. Beta-blocker therapy is indicated for the prevention of hemorrhage; however, the medications are not effective in delaying the initial formation of the varices. The therapy is aimed at maintaining the heart at fifty-five beats per minute, and the therapy must be continued indefinitely because the risk of hemorrhage returns if the medication is stopped. Research indicates that as many as one-third of patients with esophageal varices will not respond to this therapy and instead, report fatigue, dyspnea, and bradycardia.

Up to one-third of all patients with esophageal varices will suffer a hemorrhagic episode. The emergency care of this life-threatening condition includes endoscopy with ligation of the varices, vasopressin, placement of a transjugular intrahepatic shunt, and surgery, in addition to aggressive crystalloid and colloid fluid replacement.

Esophagitis

Esophagitis is defined as the inflammation of the mucosal lining of the esophagus that may be caused by chronic GERD, infectious agents such as Candida, cytomegalovirus (CMV), human immunodeficiency virus (HIV), herpes, or as the result of chemotherapy or radiation therapy. The condition may be asymptomatic or associated with common manifestations that include heartburn, dyspepsia, dysphagia, hoarseness, and retrosternal chest pain. Symptoms associated with infection may also include nausea, vomiting, fever, and sepsis. Diagnostic tests include CBC to identify signs of neutropenia or alterations in the hematocrit and hemoglobin, fecal occult blood exam, barium studies and endoscopy, ECG to rule out cardiac disease as the cause of the chest discomfort, and testing for autoimmune conditions.

Complications may include anorexia and weight loss, Barrett's esophagus, and rarely, perforation. With Barrett's esophagus, the cells that have been irritated by reflux disease undergo metaplastic transformation and exhibit an increased risk for the development of esophageal adenocarcinoma. Interventions include resolution of the causative agent or condition, pain management, histamine 2 receptor antagonists, PPIs, coating agents, blood component replacement as necessary, and lifestyle changes to alleviate the manifestations of chronic GERD. Corticosteroids may be necessary for esophagitis due to IBD or eosinophilic conditions. Emergency care of this condition involves treatment of bleeding or perforation and elimination of acute cardiac disease as the source of any reported chest pain.

Foreign Bodies

When a foreign body is swallowed accidentally or intentionally, the progress of that object through the GI system is largely dependent on the size of the object. Objects may become lodged in the oropharynx and are either expelled with coughing or advance to the esophagus. Commonly, if an object does not become lodged in the esophagus and reaches the stomach, it will continue through the system and be passed out of the body. Coins may become trapped in the small intestine, objects more than 2 centimeters long may become trapped in the pylorus, and objects more than 6 centimeters long may become lodged in the duodenum. Disc-like or button batteries require emergency care because they cause necrosis of the intestinal wall within 2 hours of contact. Small spherical magnets, which were previously used in some toys that have since been removed from the market, also can adhere to one another with intestinal tissue lodged between them, resulting in ischemia and necrosis of the tissue.

The incidence of intentional or accidental swallowing of foreign bodies is higher in children from eighteen to forty-eight months of age, patients who use dentures, psychiatric patients, and prisoners. The identification of the swallowed object is critical for appropriate treatment and prevention of complications and is often difficult in young children. Radiographs of the entire GI tract are used initially to locate the object and estimate the size. Ultrasound is essential if the patient has respiratory distress and is also preferred if the swallowed object is nonradiopaque or sharp. Treatment is dependent upon the characteristics of the swallowed object and the patient's resulting condition. The administration of promotility medications and positioning the patient with respiratory manifestations in high Fowler's position are the primary interventions unless there is an apparent need for immediate surgical intervention. Possible complications include gagging, dysphagia, respiratory distress, and possible abdominal symptoms such as gas and bloating. Emergency treatment for the ingestion of button batteries is focused on prevention of complications that may include necrosis, perforation, infection, obstruction, and volvulus.

Gastroenteritis

Gastroenteritis is a general term used to describe GI tract alterations. The characteristic manifestation is diarrhea; however, the exact characteristics of this manifestation are specific to the causative agent. These conditions may be related to osmotic, inflammatory, secretory, or motility alterations. The villi of the small intestine are most commonly affected by these alterations, resulting in fluid loss. Presenting symptoms may be mild to life-threatening, and outbreaks of these infectious conditions can rapidly reach epidemic proportions in susceptible populations. Prolonged diarrhea and vomiting result in severe fluid and electrolyte deficits, which may be associated with hypovolemic shock in high-risk individuals, including children and the elderly.

The norovirus is the causative agent for 50 to 70 percent of all cases of gastroenteritis. The virus is easily transmitted from person to person and is resistant to common cleaning agents. The attacks, manifested by diarrhea, fever, chills, and headache, usually last 36 hours. The rotavirus species may cause severe illness in children. The food-borne Salmonella infection is the second most common cause of gastroenteritis and is associated with fever, in addition to abdominal pain, nausea, vomiting, and diarrhea. Infection caused by *C. difficile* is the leading cause of hospital-acquired GI disease. The elderly population is more commonly affected; however, all patients are susceptible to this infection.

The organism exists in the feces and is spread by contact with contaminated surfaces. This condition is commonly associated with broad-spectrum antibiotic therapy that reduces the normal flora of the GI tract. Common manifestations include diarrhea, nausea, vomiting, and abdominal pain. This infection may be complicated by pseudomembranous colitis, toxic megacolon, perforation of the colon, and sepsis. Treatment is aimed at the agent-specific antibiotic therapy, supportive treatment of all manifestations, and possible surgical excision of compromised bowel segments. Emergency care requires restoration of fluid volume and electrolyte homeostasis.

Gastritis

Gastritis may be acute or chronic, and acute gastritis is further differentiated as erosive or nonerosive. Involvement of the entire stomach lining is termed pangastritis, while regional involvement is termed antral gastritis. Acute gastritis may be asymptomatic or may present with nonspecific abdominal pain, nausea, vomiting, anorexia, belching, and bloating. The most common causes of acute gastritis include use of NSAIDs and corticosteroids and infection by the *H. pylori* bacteria. Acute gastritis may also be associated with alcohol abuse. Double-contrast barium studies, endoscopy, and histological examination of biopsy samples most often confirm the diagnosis and the causative agent. Treatment includes normalization of fluid and electrolyte balance, discontinuance of causative agents such as NSAIDs, and corticosteroids, H^2 blockers, PPIs, and appropriate antibiotic therapy in the event of *H. pylori* infection.

Chronic gastritis is an inflammatory state that has not responded to therapy for acute gastritis. Chronic *H. pylori* infection is associated with the development of peptic ulcers, gastric adenocarcinoma, and mucosal-related lymphoid tissue (MALT) lymphoma. In addition to endoscopy and barium studies, gastric biopsy for assessment of antibiotic sensitivity is done because the initial antibiotic therapy was unsuccessful in eradicating the organism. Autoimmune gastritis is related to vitamin B-12 deficiency due to intrinsic factor deficiency and is associated with megaloblastic anemia and thrombocytopenia. Chemical or reactive gastritis is due to chronic NSAID and steroid use and is manifested by mucosal epithelial erosion, ulcer formation, and mucosal edema and possible hemorrhage. Chronic gastritis is diagnosed by endoscopy, biopsy, and histological studies. Treatment is specific to the causative agent, and in the instance of *H. pylori* infection, a course of three antibiotics will be administered. *H. pylori* infection also requires long-term surveillance for reoccurrence of infection. Emergency care of the patient with acute or chronic gastritis is focused on the assessment for hemorrhage or other potential complications, restoration of fluid volume status, and pain management.

Hepatitis

Hepatitis is an inflammatory condition of the liver, which is further categorized as infectious or noninfectious. Causative infectious agents for hepatitis may be viral, fungal, or bacterial, while noninfectious causes include autoimmune disease, prescription and recreational drugs, alcohol abuse, and metabolic disorders. More than 50 percent of the cases of acute hepatitis in the United States are caused by a virus. Transmission routes include fecal-oral, parenteral, sexual contact, and perinatal transmission. There are four phases of the course of viral hepatitis. During phase 1, which is asymptomatic, the host is infected, and the virus replicates; the onset of mild symptoms occurs in phase 2; progressive symptoms of liver dysfunction appear in phase 3; and recovery from the infection occurs in phase 4. These phases are specific to the causative agent and the individual.

The most common viral agents are hepatitis A (HAV), hepatitis B (HBV), and hepatitis C (HCV). Less commonly, hepatitis D (HDV), hepatitis E (HEV), CMV, Epstein-Barr virus, and adenovirus may cause hepatitis. HAV and HBV often present with nausea, jaundice, anorexia, right upper quadrant pain, fatigue, and malaise. HCV may be asymptomatic or, alternatively, may present with similar symptoms. Approximately 20 percent of acute infections with HBV and HCV result in chronic hepatitis, which is a risk factor for the development of cirrhosis and liver failure. The care of the patient with acute hepatitis due to HAV and HCV is focused on symptom relief, while the antiviral treatment for HBV is effective in decreasing the incidence of adenocarcinoma.

Chronic hepatitis is a complication of acute hepatitis and frequently progresses to hepatic failure, which is associated with deteriorating coagulation status and the onset of hepatic encephalopathy due to alterations in the blood-brain barrier that result in brain cell edema. Emergency care of the patient with hepatic failure is focused on fluid volume, homeostasis, and reduction of encephalopathy.

Hernia

A **hernia** is manifested by the displacement or protrusion of a segment of the bowel through an area of weakness in the abdominal wall. This weakness may be an anatomical site, such as the umbilicus, or acquired due to a surgical incision. Hernias are also defined as reversible or irreversible, depending on whether the protruding bowel segment can be repositioned with gentle pressure. An irreversible hernia may become incarcerated or strangulated if the blood supply is compromised for any period of time. Either of these conditions represents a surgical emergency and may be associated with necrosis and perforation of the bowel loop and possible intestinal obstruction.

Manifestations include possible visible protrusion or fullness at the site that increases with any increase in intrabdominal pressure and diffuse pain radiating to the site. Risk factors include male gender, advanced age, increased intra-abdominal pressure related to pregnancy and obesity, and genetic defects. Inguinal hernias in the male account for 75 percent of the 800,000 hernia repairs performed annually in the United States.

CT scans and ultrasonography may be used to identify hernias that are not readily identified by the physical examination. A flat plate of the abdomen is useful for identifying free air that may result from bowel perforation secondary to a strangulated hernia. Conservative management of reducible hernias includes modified activity such as no lifting or straining and prevention of constipation. If the manifestations worsen or the protrusion becomes irreversible, surgery is required to prevent incarceration and/or strangulation. Emergency care of the patient with a strangulated hernia is focused on restoration of the blood segment to the bowel segment and prevention of perforation and obstruction.

Inflammatory Bowel Disease

Inflammatory bowel disease (IBD) is an idiopathic disease that results from a harmful immune response to normal intestinal flora. Two types of IBD include Crohn's disease and ulcerative colitis (UC). Crohn's disease is characterized by inflammatory changes in all layers of the bowel. Although the entire length of the GI tract may be involved, the ileum and colon are affected most often. The inflamed areas are commonly interrupted by segments of normal bowel. Endoscopic views reveal the cobblestone appearance of these affected segments. UC is characterized by inflammatory changes of the mucosa and submucosa of the bowel that affect only the colon. There is a genetic predisposition for Crohn's disease, and there is also an increased incidence of cancer in patients with either form of IBD. Additional risk factors include a family history of IBD or colorectal cancer, NSAID and antibiotic use, smoking, and psychiatric disorders. IBD is diagnosed by a patient's history, including details of any recent foreign travel or hospitalization to rule out tuberculosis or *C. difficile* as the precipitating cause, in addition to endoscopy, CT and magnetic resonance imaging (MRI), serum and stool studies, and histologic studies.

Manifestations are nonspecific and are most often associated with the affected bowel segment. Common manifestations of IBD include diarrhea with blood and mucus and possible incontinence; constipation primarily with UC that is associated with progression to obstipation and bowel obstruction; rectal pain with associated urgency and tenesmus; and abdominal pain and cramping in the right lower quadrant with Crohn's disease, and in the umbilical area or left lower quadrant with UC. In addition, anemia, fatigue, and arthritis may be present.

The treatment of IBD focuses on attaining periods of remission and preventing recurrent attacks by modifying the inflammatory response. The stepwise treatment protocol begins with aminosalicylates and progresses to antibiotics, corticosteroids, and immunomodulators. Emergency care of the patient with IBD is focused on assessment and treatment of possible hemorrhage, megacolon, or bowel obstruction.

Intussusception

Intussusception is the abnormal movement of one portion of the bowel that is folded back into the subsequent segment. The condition is most common in infants and appears to be due to altered peristalsis that results in decreased lymphatic and venous drainage, which leads to ischemia and necrosis of the affected bowel segment. Left untreated, the condition is fatal in two to five days. The condition often presents with a history of recent upper respiratory infection, in addition to lethargy, vomiting, colicky abdominal pain that may be severe or intermittent, a palpable abdominal mass, and diarrhea that contains blood and mucus, which is often the initial manifestation of the intussusception.

The contrast enema is used most often to confirm the diagnosis. The treatment is specific to the age of the patient and the precipitating cause. The cause of the condition in infants and children up to three years of age is most often idiopathic, while adhesions, tumor formation, effects of bariatric surgery, and inflammatory changes due to IBD are possible causes of intussusception in older children and adults. Nonoperative reduction with therapeutic enemas is the treatment of choice in infants and young children. Barium, water-based contrast material or air insufflation may be used as the reducing agent. The two contraindications to the nonoperative approach include the presence of peritonitis or perforation of the bowel. The surgical treatment is appropriate for older children, adults, and infants in whom the nonoperative reduction was unsuccessful. A laparoscopic approach is used to manually reduce the intussusception. If reduction is not possible or if there is additional bowel damage such as perforation present, surgical resection and anastomosis of the affected bowel segment are necessary. Emergency care is focused on the identification and immediate intervention of the condition.

Obstructions

There are three anatomical areas of the GI system that are prone to obstruction, including the gastric outlet at the pylorus, the small intestine, and the bowel. The small intestine is the most commonly affected site, and adhesions are responsible for more than 60 percent of all obstructions. These conditions may also be categorized as mechanical or nonmechanical depending on the cause, where mechanical obstructions are due to some extrinsic source such as adhesions, tumor formation, intussusception, or hernias, and nonmechanical obstructions are due to decreased peristalsis, neurogenic disorders, vascular insufficiency, or electrolyte imbalance. The mechanical obstruction of the biliary tract is due to effects of cirrhosis and hepatitis.

The manifestations are specific to the anatomical site of obstruction. The gastric outlet obstruction occurs most commonly in the pylorus and is associated with upper abdominal distention, nausea, vomiting, weight loss, and anorexia. Diagnostic tests include endoscopy and assessment of nutritional deficits, in addition to testing to eliminate *H. pylori* or diabetic gastric paresis as the cause. Obstruction of the small bowel is associated with severe fluid and electrolyte losses, metabolic acidosis, nausea and vomiting, fever, and tachycardia, and may lead to strangulation of the affected bowel segment. Bowel obstruction, most frequently due to tumor formation or stricture resulting from diverticular disease, is manifested by lower abdominal distention, possible metabolic acidosis, cramping abdominal pain, and minimal fluid and electrolyte losses. Common diagnostic studies include endoscopy, common lab studies, flat plate of the abdomen to assess for free air, and CT imaging.

Treatments are specific to the cause and may include tumor excision, antibiotic therapy for *H. pylori*, colectomy to remove the affected bowel segment, and/or colostomy placement. Although some obstructions may be treated with gastric or enteric decompression, bowel rest, and fluids, emergency intervention is usually necessary to prevent complications such as peritonitis and hemorrhage.

Pancreatitis

Pancreatitis has a rapid onset and progression to a critical illness, which is manifested by characteristic abdominal pain, nausea, vomiting, and diarrhea. In addition, fever, tachycardia, hypotension, and abdominal distention and rebound tenderness may be present. The exocrine function of the pancreas is the production and secretion of digestive enzymes. Pancreatitis exists when one of the causative agents inhibits the homeostatic suppression of the enzyme secretion, resulting in excessive amounts of the enzymes in the pancreas.

This excess of enzymes precipitates the inflammatory response, which results in increased pancreatic vascular permeability, which, in turn, leads to edema, hemorrhage, and eventual necrosis of the pancreas. The inflammatory mediators can result in systemic complications that may include sepsis, respiratory distress syndrome, renal failure, and GI hemorrhage. Chronic alcoholism and biliary tract obstruction are the most common causes of pancreatitis; however, as many as 35 percent of the cases of pancreatitis are idiopathic. Pancreatitis can also occur after endoscopic retrograde cholangiopancreatography (ERCP) due to defects in the sphincter of Oddi. Aggressive pre-procedure hydration and rectal indomethacin post procedure are employed to prevent this complication. Less common causes include some antibiotics and chemotherapy agents.

Diagnosis is based on the patient's presenting history and routine lab studies that include amylase P, lipase, metabolic panel, liver panel, C-reactive protein, CBC, and arterial blood gases (ABGs). Imaging studies may be used if the diagnosis is unclear to rule out gallbladder disease. Nonsurgical treatment includes bowel rest with nasogastric decompression, analgesics, and IV fluid administration. Surgical procedures may be open or minimally invasive and are aimed at removing diseased tissue to limit the progression to systemic complications, to repair the pancreatic duct, or to repair defects in the biliary tree. The emergency care of pancreatitis focuses on prompt diagnosis, aggressive fluid management, and treatment of the cause because the disease is associated with the rapid onset of systemic complications.

Trauma

The GI system may be traumatized by blunt or penetrating forces. Penetrating trauma is most commonly due to gunshot or stabbing injuries and usually results in a predictable pattern of injury; however, careful assessment for occult injuries is necessary to prevent catastrophic damage. Presenting manifestations depend on the degree of penetration and the site of the damage but commonly include visible hemorrhage, alterations in level of consciousness, tachycardia, and hypotension. Diagnosis requires a detailed inquiry into all of the facts of the incident, including a description of the weapon, the number of times the patient was stabbed, and an estimation of blood loss at the scene, in addition to the progression of the patient's manifestations during resuscitation and transport. Treatment is aimed at restoring and maintaining fluid volume status with colloids and crystalloids, assessment for and treatment of hemorrhage, prevention of infection, and surgical repair of the damaged structures.

GI injuries due to blunt force trauma often are not immediately apparent, which means that assessment for progression of the original insult is ongoing. Abdominal pain and tenderness and hypotension may be the only signs of massive internal injuries. Trauma related to automobile accidents may present with a characteristic seatbelt or steering wheel pattern, Cullen's sign due to periumbilical trauma, or an abdominal bruit that may be associated with comorbid vascular disease or acute vascular trauma. Domestic violence must be considered in the event of abdominal blunt force trauma. Diagnosis is based on the history of the event, routine lab studies, ultrasound and CT scanning, peritoneal lavage, and possible exploratory laparotomy. The goals of treatment for blunt trauma are similar to penetrating trauma and include restoring and maintaining fluid volume status with colloids and crystalloids, assessment for and treatment of hemorrhage, prevention of infection, and surgical repair of the damaged structures.

Ulcers

Ulcers of the GI tract are categorized as to the anatomical site of injury. Gastric ulcers are located in the body of the stomach, and peptic ulcers are located in the duodenum. The presenting symptom is abdominal pain 2 to 4 hours after eating for duodenal ulcers, in addition to hematemesis and melena. The defect is due to erosion of the mucosal lining by infectious agents, most commonly *H. pylori*; extreme systemic stress such as burns or head trauma; ETOH abuse; chronic kidney and respiratory disease; and psychological stress. Untreated, the mucosal erosion can progress to perforation, hemorrhage, and peritonitis.

Laboratory studies include examination of endoscopic tissue samples for the presence of the *H. pylori* organism, urea breath test, CBC, stool samples, and metabolic panel. Endoscopy (which is used to obtain tissue samples and achieve hemostasis) and double barium imaging studies may be obtained. The treatment depends on the extent of the erosion and will be focused on healing the ulcerated tissue and preventing additional damage. The treatment protocol for *H. pylori* infection includes the use of a PPI, amoxicillin, and clarithromycin for a minimum of seven to fourteen days. Subsequent testing will be necessary to ensure that the organism has been eradicated. Patients infected with *H. pylori* also must discontinue the use of NSAIDs or continue the long-term use of PPIs. Surgery may be indicated for significant areas of hemorrhage that were not successfully treated by ultrasound, and the procedure will be specific to the anatomical area of ulceration. Emergency care is focused on prompt management of bleeding and identification of the causative agent to guide treatment.

Pulmonary

Aspiration

There are four types of respiratory aspiration that can result in aspiration pneumonitis, pneumonia, or an acute respiratory emergency. The aspiration of gastric contents often causes a chemical pneumonitis. Infective organisms from the oropharynx can result in aspiration pneumonia. Depending on its size and composition, the aspiration of a foreign body can result in a respiratory emergency or bacterial pneumonia. Rarely, aspiration of mineral or vegetable oil can cause an exogenous lipoid pneumonia.

Aspiration Pneumonitis/Pneumonia

Respiratory aspiration is the abnormal entry of foreign substances (such as food, drink, saliva, or vomitus) into the lungs as a person swallows. This is normally prevented by the epiglottis, a flap of cartilage that pulls forward and forces substances into the esophagus and digestive tract. If inoculum is inhaled into the lungs, it can (depending on the amount) lead to aspiration pneumonitis/pneumonia. Aspiration pneumonia often results from a primary bacterial infection, while aspiration pneumonitis (which is non-infectious) results from aspiration of the acidic gastric contents.

Risk factors for aspiration pneumonitis/pneumonia are altered or reduced consciousness and a poor gag reflex. These risk factors are associated with the following conditions:

- Excessive alcohol and/or drugs
- Stroke
- Seizures
- Dysphagia
- Head trauma
- General anesthesia
- Critical illness
- Dementia
- Intracranial mass lesion
- Multiple sclerosis
- Pseudobulbar palsy
- Myasthenia gravis
- Gastroesophageal reflux disease (GERD)
- Use of H_2 agonists, H_2 blockers, or proton pump inhibitors
- Bronchoscopy
- Endotracheal intubation
- Tracheostomy
- Upper endoscopy
- Nasogastric (NG) tube
- Feeding tubes

Signs and symptoms of aspiration pneumonitis/pneumonia include:

- Fever
- Cyanosis
- Wheezing
- Dyspnea
- Tachypnea
- Tachycardia
- Rales
- Hypoxia
- Altered mental status
- Hypotension
- Decreased breath sounds
- Fatigue
- Cough with discolored phlegm
- Chest pain
- Hypothermia (possible in older patients)
- Pleuritic chest pain

The diagnosis of aspiration pneumonitis/pneumonia is based upon a chest X-ray revealing pulmonary infiltrates; an arterial blood gas (ABG) analysis consistent with hypoxemia; a complete blood count (CBC) with an elevated white blood cell count (WBC) with neutrophils predominating; and other clinical findings. Infiltrates are most commonly found in the right, lower lobe of the lung, but can be found in other lobes, depending on an individual's position at the time of aspiration. If possible, a sputum specimen for culture, sensitivity, and gram stain should be collected before beginning antibiotic therapy. In addition, blood cultures should be obtained, as indicated.

Treatment of aspiration pneumonitis/pneumonia includes:

- Suctioning of the upper airway as needed to remove the aspirate
- Oxygen supplementation
- Pulse oximetry
- Cardiac monitoring
- Antibiotics (only if symptoms fail to resolve within 48 hours)
- Supportive care with intravenous fluids (IVFs) and electrolyte replacement
- For those with severe respiratory distress, possible intubation and mechanical ventilation
- NG drainage to avoid gastric distention (in the ventilated patient)

Foreign Body Aspiration

Foreign body aspiration is a respiratory emergency. A foreign body can lodge in the larynx or trachea causing varying degrees of airway obstruction. Complete airway obstruction can quickly lead to asphyxia and death. The most commonly aspirated object is food. Other frequently aspirated objects include nuts, nails, seeds, coins, pins, small toys, needles, bone fragments, and dental appliances. In children and adolescents, aspirated foreign bodies are found with equal frequency on either side of the lungs. In adults, they are most often found in the right lung because of the acute angle of the right mainstem bronchus.

Signs and symptoms of foreign body aspiration include:

- Coughing
- Wheezing
- Decreased breath sounds
- Dyspnea
- Choking
- Cyanosis
- Hemoptysis
- Chest pain
- Asphyxia (with complete airway obstruction)
- Inability to speak (with complete airway obstruction)

As more time elapses, local inflammation and edema can worsen the airway obstruction. This also makes removing the foreign body more difficult and the lung more likely to bleed with manipulation.

Foreign body aspiration can be diagnosed using a chest x-ray or a computed tomography (CT) scan. Less than 20% of all aspirated foreign bodies are radiopaque. A CT scan can provide information about the anatomic location, composition, shape, size, and extent of edema associated with the aspirated foreign body. ABG analysis can reveal hypoxemia. Bronchoscopy (rigid or flexible) can be diagnostic as well as therapeutic.

Treatment of foreign body aspiration can include:

- Heimlich maneuver for acute choking with total airway obstruction by foreign body
- Foreign body extraction via bronchoscopy (rigid or flexible)
- Surgical bronchotomy or segmental lung resection (rarely required)
- Antibiotics for secondary pneumonia or other respiratory infection
- Oxygen supplementation
- Symptomatic respiratory support

Since the likelihood of complications increases after 24 to 48 hours, prompt extraction of the foreign body is critical. Complications can include mediastinitis, atelectasis, pneumonia, tracheoesophageal fistulas, or bronchiectasis.

Asthma

Status Asthmaticus

Status asthmaticus is an acute episode of worsening asthma that's unresponsive to treatment with bronchodilators. Even after increasing their bronchodilator use to every few minutes, individuals still experience no relief. Status asthmaticus represents a respiratory emergency that can lead to respiratory failure. Airway inflammation, bronchospasm, and mucus plugging highlight the condition. Common triggers include exposure to an allergen or irritant, viral respiratory illness, and exercise in cold weather. Status asthmaticus is more common among individuals of low socioeconomic status, regardless of race.

The main symptoms of status asthmaticus are wheezing, cough, and dyspnea; however, severe airway obstruction can result in a "silent chest" without audible wheezes. This can be a sign of impending respiratory failure. Other signs and symptoms of status asthmaticus include:

- Chest tightness or pain
- Tachypnea
- Tachycardia
- Cyanosis
- Use of accessory respiratory muscles
- Inability to speak more than one or two words at a time
- Altered mental status
- Pulsus paradoxus >20mm Hg
- Syncope
- Hypoxemia
- Hypercapnia
- Retractions and the use of abdominal muscles to breathe
- Hypertension
- Seizures (late sign)
- Bradycardia (late sign)
- Hypotension (late sign)
- Agitation (late sign)

Useful tests for the diagnosis of status asthmaticus include:

- Chest x-ray (for the exclusion of pneumonia, pneumothorax, and CHF)

- ABG analysis can be diagnostic as well as therapeutic (tracking response to treatment measures). Assess cost/benefit for children due to pain associated with ABG sampling.

- CBC with differential can reveal an elevated WBC count with left shift (possible indication of a microbial infection)

- Peak flow measurement can be diagnostic as well as therapeutic (tracking response to treatment measures)

- Pulse oximetry provides continuous measurement of O_2 saturation. Reading is affected by decreased peripheral perfusion, anemia, and movement.

- Blood glucose levels, stress, and therapeutic medications can lead to hyperglycemia. Younger children may exhibit hypoglycemia.

- Blood electrolyte levels (therapeutic medications can lead to hypokalemia)

Intubation and mechanical ventilation should be used with extreme caution in individuals with status asthmaticus. It's usually considered a therapy of last resort due to its inherent dangers: air trapping leading to an increased risk for barotrauma (especially pneumothorax); decreased cardiac output; and increasing bronchospasm. Mechanical ventilation of individuals with status asthmaticus often requires controlled hypoventilation with low tidal volumes, prolonged exhalation times, low respiratory rates, and tolerance of permissive hypercapnia. The majority of individuals needing mechanical ventilation can be extubated within 72 hours.

Supportive Treatment

- O_2 therapy to maintain O_2 saturation > 92%; non-rebreathing mask can deliver 98% O_2
- Hydration
- Correction of electrolyte abnormalities
- Antibiotics only with evidence of concurrent infective process

Pharmacological Agents Used for Acute Asthma

Various classes of pharmacological agents are used for the treatment and control of status asthmaticus. The following discussion concentrates on pharmacological agents to treat and control acute asthma rather than chronic asthma. Urgent care of asthma can include the following:

Beta-2 Adrenergic Agonists (Beta-2 Agonists)

Short-acting preparations of Beta-2 agonists are the first line of therapy for the treatment of status asthmaticus. These medications relax the muscles in the airways, resulting in bronchodilation (expanding of the bronchial air passages) and increased airflow to the lungs. It is important to remember that one of the underlying factors in asthma is bronchoconstriction. Albuterol is the most commonly used short-acting Beta-2 agonist. Dosing for acute asthma is 2.5 mg to 5 mg once, then 2.5 mg every twenty minutes for 3 doses via nebulizer, and finally 2.5 mg to 10 mg every one to four hours as needed. Adverse effects of albuterol include tachycardia, tremors, and anxiety. Another short-acting Beta-2 agonist used to treat acute asthma is levalbuterol (Xopenex™). This medication is related to albuterol and has the same result, but without the adverse effects. Dosage for acute asthma is 1.25 mg to 2.5 mg every twenty minutes for 3 doses, then 1.25 mg to 5 mg every one to four hours as needed. However, it must be noted that the frequent use of adrenergic agents prior to receiving emergency care can decrease a patient's response to these medications in a hospital setting.

Anticholinergics

These medications block the action of the neurotransmitter acetylcholine which, in turn, causes bronchodilation. Anticholinergics can also increase the bronchodilating effects of short-acting Beta-2 agonists. The most commonly used anticholinergic is ipatroprium (Atrovent ™), which is used in combination with short-acting Beta-2 agonists for the treatment of status asthmaticus. Dosing for acute asthma is 2.5 mL (500 mcg) every twenty minutes for 3 doses via nebulizer, then as needed. Adverse effects can include dry mouth, blurred vision, and constipation.

Corticosteroids

Corticosteroids are potent anti-inflammatory medications that fight the inflammation accompanying asthma. Corticosteroids commonly used in the treatment of status asthmaticus include prednisone, prednisolone, and methylprednisolone. Methylprednisolone (Solu-Medrol™) is administered once in doses of 60 mg to 125 mg intravenously (IV) in cases of status asthmaticus and then followed by a taper of oral prednisone over seven to ten days. The intravenous administration of corticosteroids is equal in effectiveness to oral corticosteroid administration. Corticosteroids have numerous adverse effects, and they should not be used for more than two weeks. Adverse effects of long-term corticosteroid use can include weight gain, osteoporosis, thinning of skin, cataracts, easy bruising, and diabetes. Therefore, it is necessary to monitor blood glucose routinely and use regular insulin on a sliding scale. Electrolytes (particularly potassium) must also be monitored.

Methylxanthines

These medications are used as bronchodilators and as adjuncts to Beta-2 agonists and corticosteroids in treating status asthmaticus. The primary methylxanthines are theophylline and aminophylline. At therapeutic doses, methylxanthines are much weaker bronchodilators than Beta-2 agonists. The adverse effects of methylxanthines can include nausea, vomiting, tachycardia, headaches, and seizures. As a result, therapeutic monitoring is mandatory. Therapeutic levels of theophylline range from 10 mcg/mL to 20 mcg/mL. Dosing of theophylline is a loading dose of 6 mg/kg, followed by a maintenance dose of 1 mg/kg/h IV. Methylxanthines aren't frequently used to treat status asthmaticus because of their possible adverse effects and the need for close monitoring of drug blood levels.

Magnesium Sulfate

Magnesium sulfate is a calcium antagonist that relaxes smooth muscle in the lung passages leading to bronchodilation. Clinical studies indicate it can be used as an adjunct to Beta-2 agonist therapy during status asthmaticus. A dose of 30 mg/kg to 70 mg/kg is administered by IV over 20 to 30 minutes. It is given slowly to prevent adverse effects such as bradycardia and hypotension. The use of magnesium sulfate is controversial.

Leukotriene Inhibitors

These medications target inflammation related to asthma. Typically used for the long-term control of asthma, a minority of individuals with status asthmaticus may respond to this class of medication. The primary leukotriene inhibitors used in the treatment of asthma are zafirlukast (Accolate™) and zileuton (Zyflo™). Zafirlukast can be administered orally in doses of 10 mg to 20 mg twice daily. Zileuton can be administered in a dose of 600 mg four times daily. Adverse effects of leukotriene inhibitors include headache, rash, fatigue, dizziness, and abdominal pain.

Heliox

Heliox, administered via face mask, is a mixture of helium and oxygen that can help relieve airway obstruction associated with status asthmaticus. Benefits of heliox include decreased work of breathing, decreased carbon dioxide production, and decreased muscle fatigue. It can only be used in individuals able to take a deep breath or while on mechanical ventilation. The 80/20 mixture of helium to oxygen has been the most effective in clinical trials. One limitation to using heliox is the amount of supplemental oxygen required by an individual suffering from status asthmaticus. Heliox loses its clinical efficacy when the fraction of inspired oxygen (FiO_2) is greater than 40%. No significant adverse effects have been reported with heliox.

Chronic Obstructive Pulmonary Disease (COPD)

Chronic Obstructive Pulmonary Disease (COPD) is characterized by an airflow obstruction that's not fully reversible. It's usually progressive and is associated with an abnormal inflammatory response in the lungs. The primary cause of COPD is exposure to tobacco smoke and is one of the leading causes of death in the United States. COPD includes chronic bronchitis, emphysema, or a combination of both. Though asthma is part of the classic triad of obstructive lung diseases, it is not part of COPD. However, someone with COPD can have an asthma component to their disease. Chronic bronchitis is described as a chronic productive cough for three or more months during each of two consecutive years. Emphysema is the abnormal enlargement of alveoli (air sacs) with accompanying destruction of their walls. Signs and symptoms of COPD can include:

- Dyspnea
- Wheezing
- Cough (usually worse in the morning and that produces sputum/phlegm)
- Cyanosis
- Chest tightness
- Fever
- Tachypnea
- Orthopnea
- Use of accessory respiratory muscles
- Elevated jugular venous pressure (JVP)
- Barrel chest
- Pursed lip breathing
- Altered mental status

A diagnosis of COPD can be made through pulmonary function tests (PFTs), a chest x-ray, blood chemistries, ABG analysis, or a CT scan. A formal diagnosis of COPD can be made through a PFT known as spirometry, which measures lung function. PFTs measure the ratio of forced expiratory volume in one second over forced vital capacity (FEV_1/FVC) and should normally be between 60% and 90%. Values below 60% usually indicate a problem. The other diagnostic tests mentioned are useful in determining the acuity and severity of exacerbations of the disease. In acute exacerbations of COPD, ABG analysis can reveal respiratory acidosis, hypoxemia, and hypercapnia. Generally, a pH less than 7.3 indicates acute respiratory compromise. Compensatory metabolic alkalosis may develop in response to chronic respiratory acidosis. A chest x-ray can show flattening of the diaphragm and increased retrosternal air space (both indicative of hyperinflation), cardiomegaly, and increased bronchovascular markings. Blood chemistries can suggest sodium retention or hypokalemia. A CT scan is more sensitive and specific than a standard chest x-ray for diagnosing emphysema.

Treatment for acute exacerbations of COPD can include oxygen supplementation, short acting Beta-2 agonists, anticholinergics, corticosteroids, and antibiotics. Oxygen should be titrated to achieve an oxygen saturation of at least 90%. Short-acting Beta-2 agonists (albuterol or levalbuterol) administered via nebulizer can improve dyspnea associated with COPD. The anticholinergic medication ipratroprium, administered via nebulizer, can be added as an adjunct to Beta-2 agonists. Short courses of corticosteroids can be given orally or intravenously. In clinical trials, the administration of oral corticosteroids in the early stage of a COPD exacerbation decreased the need for hospitalization. Also in clinical trials, the use of antibiotics was found to decrease the risk of treatment failure and death in individuals with a moderate to severe exacerbation of COPD.

Infections

Bronchiolitis

Bronchiolitis is inflammation of the bronchioles (the small airways in the lungs) and is most commonly caused by respiratory syncytial virus (RSV). It typically affects children under the age of two, with a peak onset of three to six months of age. The disease is spread through direct contact with respiratory droplets. Bronchiolitis results in hospitalization of approximately 2% of children, the majority of which are under six months of age. Criteria for hospitalization can include prematurity, under three months of age, diagnosis of a congenital heart defect, respiratory rate >70-80 bpm, inability to maintain oral hydration, and cyanosis.

Signs and symptoms of bronchiolitis include:

- Difficulty feeding
- Fever
- Congestion
- Cough
- Dyspnea
- Tachypnea
- Nasal flaring
- Tachycardia
- Wheezing
- Fine rales
- Hypoxia
- Retractions
- Apnea

A diagnosis of bronchiolitis is usually established through a clinical examination. The most common diagnostic tests for the disease are: a rapid, viral antigen test of nasopharyngeal secretions for RSV; white blood cell (WBC) count with differential; ABG analysis; a chest x-ray; and a test of C-reactive protein (a marker of inflammation).

Although highly contagious, the disease is self-limiting and typically resolves without complication in one to two weeks. Treatment of bronchiolitis is supportive and can include oxygen supplementation, maintenance of hydration, fever reducers, nasal and oral suctioning, and intubation and mechanical ventilation.

Croup and Other Infections

Acute Laryngotracheobronchitis

Acute laryngotracheobronchitis, or classic croup, is a common viral illness in children. It results in inflammation of the larynx, trachea, and occasionally the bronchi. As a result, croup can be life-threatening in some children. Croup is primarily a disease of infants and toddlers, peaking between the ages of six months and three years. It rarely occurs after age six. The most common cause of croup is the parainfluenza viruses (types 1, 2, and 3), accounting for approximately 80% of the diagnosed cases. Other viral causes include adenovirus, rhinovirus, RSV, enterovirus, coronavirus, echovirus, and influenza A and B.

Croup is the most common pediatric ailment that causes stridor, an abnormal, high-pitched breath sound indicating partial or complete airway obstruction. Other signs and symptoms of the disease can include:

- Barking cough
- Pharyngitis
- Rhinorrhea
- Wheezing
- Tachypnea
- Tachycardia
- Fever
- Cyanosis
- Agitation
- Hypoxemia
- Respiratory failure

Croup is primarily a clinical diagnosis that relies on clues from the patient history and physical examination. In children, a chest x-ray occasionally reveals the "steeple sign," which indicates airway narrowing at the level of the glottis.

Treatment of croup can include:

- Corticosteroids, especially dexamethasone administered intravenously (IV), intramuscularly (IM), or orally (PO)

- Nebulized racemic epinephrine (typically reserved for hospital use; effects last only one and a half to two hours and require observation for at least three hours after dose)

- Cool mist (once the mainstay of treatment, but little evidence supports its clinical utility)

- Intubation and mechanical ventilation (for severe cases)

Acute Epiglottitis

Acute epiglottitis (also known as supraglottitis) is inflammation of the epiglottis. The epiglottis is the small piece of cartilage that's pulled forward to cover the windpipe when a person swallows. The cause of the condition is usually bacterial, with *Haemophilus influenzae* type B being the most common. Other bacterial causes include *Streptococcus pneumoniae*, *Streptococcus* groups A, B, and C, and non-typeable *Haemophilus influenzae*. The disease is most commonly diagnosed in children but can be seen in adolescents and adults. A decline in the number of cases of acute epiglottitis has been noted since the introduction of the *Haemophilus influenzae* type B (Hib) vaccine in the 1980s.

Acute epiglottitis is usually accompanied by the classic triad of symptoms: dysphagia, drooling, and respiratory distress. Other signs and symptoms can include:

- Fever
- Sore throat
- Inability to lay flat
- Voice changes (can be muffled or hoarse)
- Tripod breathing position (a position said to optimize the mechanics of breathing where an individual sits up on their hands, head leaning forward, and tongue protruding)
- Tachypnea
- Hypoxia
- Agitation
- Cyanosis

Direct visualization of the epiglottis via a nasopharyngoscopy/laryngoscopy is the gold standard for diagnosing acute epiglottitis since an infected epiglottis has a cherry red appearance.

Acute epiglottitis is a potentially life-threatening medical emergency and should be treated promptly. It can quickly progress to total obstruction of the airway and death. Treatment of the condition can include:

- IV antibiotics (after blood and epiglottic cultures have been obtained)

- Analgesic-antipyretic agents such as aspirin, acetaminophen, and nonsteroidal anti-inflammatory drugs (NSAIDs), such as ibuprofen

- Intubation with mechanical ventilation, tracheostomy, or needle-jet insufflation (options for immediate airway management, if needed)

- Racemic epinephrine, corticosteroids, and Beta-2 agonists are also sometimes used; however, they have yet to be proven as useful treatments

Acute Tracheitis

A rare condition, **acute tracheitis**, is the inflammation and infection of the trachea (windpipe). The majority of cases occur in children under the age of sixteen. The etiology of acute tracheitis is predominantly bacterial, with Staphylococcus aureus being the leading cause. Community-associated, methicillin-resistant Staphylococcus aureus (CA-MRSA) has recently emerged as an important causative agent. Other bacterial causes of acute tracheitis include Streptococcus pneumoniae, Haemophilus influenzae, and Moraxella catarrhalis.

Acute tracheitis is often preceded by an upper respiratory infection (URI). Signs and symptoms of acute tracheitis can include:

- Bark-like cough
- Dyspnea
- Fever
- Tachypnea
- Respiratory distress
- Stridor
- Wheezing
- Hoarseness
- Nasal flaring
- Cyanosis

The only definitive means of diagnosis is the use of a laryngotracheobronchoscopy to directly visualize mucopurulent membranes lining the mucosa of the trachea. Additional tests can include pulse oximetry, blood cultures, nasopharyngeal and tracheal cultures, and neck x-rays.

Treatment of acute tracheitis should be prompt because of the increased likelihood of complete airway obstruction leading to respiratory arrest and death. Treatment can include:

- IV antibiotics (if living in an area with high or increasing rates of CA-MRSA, the addition of vancomycin should be considered)

- Intubation and mechanical ventilation or tracheostomy (rarely needed) are options if immediate airway management is needed

- Fever reducers

Viral Pneumonia

Viral pneumonia is more common at the extremes of age (young children and the elderly). It accounts for the majority of cases of childhood pneumonia. Cases of viral pneumonia have been increasing over the past decade, mostly as a result of immunosuppression (weakened immune system). Common causes of viral pneumonia in children, the elderly, and the immunocompromised are the influenza viruses (most common), RSV, parainfluenza virus, and adenovirus.

Signs and symptoms of viral pneumonia largely overlap those of bacterial pneumonia and can include:

- Cough (nonproductive)
- Fever/chills
- Myalgias
- Fatigue
- Headache
- Dyspnea
- Tachypnea
- Tachycardia
- Wheezing
- Cyanosis
- Hypoxia

- Decreased breath sounds
- Respiratory distress

Viral pneumonia is diagnosed via a chest x-ray and viral cultures. The chest x-ray usually reveals bilateral lung infiltrates, instead of the lobar involvement commonly seen in bacterial causes. Viral cultures can take up to two weeks to confirm the diagnosis. Rapid antigen testing and gene amplification via polymerase chain reaction (PCR) have been recently incorporated into the diagnostic mix to shorten the diagnosis lag.

Treatment of viral pneumonia is usually supportive and can include:

- Supplemental oxygen
- Rest
- Antipyretics
- Analgesics
- Intravenous fluids
- Parenteral nutrition
- Intubation and mechanical ventilation

Specific causes of viral pneumonia can benefit from treatment with antiviral medications. Influenza pneumonia can be treated with oseltamivir (Tamiflu®) or zanamivir (Relenza®). Ribavirin® is the only effective antiviral agent for the treatment of RSV pneumonia.

Acute Respiratory Tract Infections

Acute Bronchitis

Acute bronchitis is inflammation of the bronchial tubes (bronchi), which extend from the trachea to the lungs. It is one of the top five reasons for visits to healthcare providers and can take from ten days to three weeks to resolve. Common causes of acute bronchitis include respiratory viruses (such as influenza A and B), RSV, parainfluenza, adenovirus, rhinovirus, and coronavirus. Bacterial causes include Mycoplasma species, Streptococcus pneumoniae, Chlamydia pneumoniae, Haemophilus influenzae, and Moraxella catarrhalis. Other causes of acute bronchitis are irritants such as chemicals, pollution, and tobacco smoke.

Signs and symptoms of acute bronchitis can include:

- Cough (most common symptom) with or without sputum
- Fever
- Sore throat
- Headache
- Nasal congestion
- Rhinorrhea
- Dyspnea
- Fatigue
- Myalgia
- Chest pain
- Wheezing

Acute bronchitis is typically diagnosed by exclusion, which means tests are used to exclude more serious conditions such as pneumonia, epiglottitis, or COPD. Useful diagnostic tests include a CBC with differential, a chest x-ray, respiratory and blood cultures, PFTs, bronchoscopy, laryngoscopy, and a procalcitonin (PCT) test to determine if the infection is bacterial.

Treatment of acute bronchitis is primarily supportive and can include:

- Bedrest
- Cough suppressants, such as codeine or dextromethorphan
- Beta-2 agonists, such as albuterol for wheezing
- Nonsteroidal anti-inflammatory drugs (NSAIDs) for pain
- Expectorants, such as guaifenesin

Although acute bronchitis should not be routinely treated with antibiotics, there are exceptions to this rule. It's reasonable to use an antibiotic when an existing medical condition poses a risk of serious complications. Antibiotic use is also reasonable for treating acute bronchitis in elderly patients who have been hospitalized in the past year, have been diagnosed with congestive heart failure (CHF) or diabetes, or are currently being treated with a steroid.

Pneumonia

Pneumonia is an infection that affects the functional tissue of the lung. Microscopically, it is characterized by consolidating lung tissue with exudate, fibrin, and inflammatory cells filling the alveoli (air sacs). Pneumonia can represent a primary disease or a secondary disease (e.g., post-obstructive pneumonia due to lung cancer), and the most common causes of pneumonia are bacteria and viruses. Other causes of pneumonia include fungi and parasites.

Pneumonia can be categorized according to its anatomic distribution on a chest x-ray or the setting in which it is acquired. Pneumonia categorized according to its anatomic distribution on chest x-ray can be:

- Lobar: Limited to one lobe of the lungs. It can affect more than one lobe on the same side (multilobar pneumonia) or bilateral lobes ("double" pneumonia).

- Bronchopneumonia: Scattered diffusely throughout the lungs

- Interstitial: Involving areas between the alveoli

Pneumonia categorized according to the setting in which it is acquired can be:

- Community-Acquired Pneumonia (CAP): Pneumonia in an individual who hasn't been recently hospitalized, or its occurrence in less than 48 hours after admission to a hospital.

- Hospital-Acquired (Nosocomial) Pneumonia: Pneumonia acquired during or after hospitalization for another ailment with onset at least 48 hours or more after admission.

- Aspiration Pneumonia: Pneumonia resulting from the inhalation of gastric or oropharyngeal secretions.

Community-Acquired Pneumonia (CAP)

Common causes of community-acquired pneumonia (CAP) include:

- Streptococcus pneumoniae
- Haemophilus influenzae
- Moraxella catarrhalis
- Atypical organisms (such as Legionella species, Mycoplasma pneumoniae, and Chlamydia pneumonia)
- Staphylococcus aureus
- Respiratory viruses

Streptococcus Pneumoniae

Streptococcus pneumonia (also known as S. pneumonia or pneumococcus) is a gram-positive bacterium and the most common cause of CAP. Due to the introduction of a pneumococcal vaccine in 2000, cases of pneumococcal pneumonia have decreased. However, medical providers should be aware there is now evidence of emerging, antibiotic-resistant strains of the organism. Signs and symptoms of pneumococcal pneumonia can include:

- Cough productive of rust-colored sputum (mucus)
- Fever with or without chills
- Dyspnea
- Wheezing
- Chest pain
- Tachypnea
- Altered mental status
- Tachycardia
- Rales over involved lung
- Increase in tactile fremitus
- E to A change
- Hypotension
- Lung consolidation

Diagnosis of pneumococcal pneumonia can include:

- CBC with differential
- Chest x-ray
- CT scan (if underlying lung cancer is suspected)
- Sputum gram stain and/or culture
- Blood cultures
- Procalcitonin and C-reactive protein blood level tests
- Sputum, serum, and/or urinary antigen tests
- Immunoglobulin studies
- Bronchoscopy with bronchoalveolar lavage (BAL)

Treatment of pneumococcal pneumonia can include:

- Antibiotics, such as ceftriaxone plus doxycycline, or azithromycin
- Respiratory quinolones, such as levofloxacin (Levaquin®), moxifloxacin (Avelox®), or Gemifloxacin (Factive®)
- Supplemental oxygen
- Beta-2 agonists, such as albuterol via nebulizer or metered-dose inhaler (MDI), as needed for wheezing
- Analgesics and antipyretics
- Chest physiotherapy
- Active suctioning of respiratory secretions
- Intubation and mechanical ventilation

Mycoplasma Pneumoniae

Mycoplasma pneumonia, also known as M. pneumoniae, is a bacterium that causes atypical CAP. It is one of the most common causes of CAP in healthy individuals under the age of forty. The most common symptom of mycoplasmal pneumonia is a dry, nonproductive cough. Other signs and symptoms can include diarrhea, earache, fever (usually $\leq$ 102 °F), sore throat, myalgias, nasal congestion, skin rash, and general malaise. Chest x-rays of individuals with mycoplasmal pneumonia reveal a pattern of bronchopneumonia. Cold agglutinin titers in the blood can be significantly elevated (> 1:64). Polymerase chain reaction (PCR) is becoming the standard confirmatory test for mycoplasmal pneumonia, though currently it is not used in most clinical settings. Other diagnostic tests for M. pneumoniae are usually nonspecific and therefore do not aid in its diagnosis.

Treatments for mycoplasmal pneumonia are no different than for CAP, except for antibiotic choices, which include:

- Macrolide antibiotics, such as erythromycin, azithromycin (Zithromax®), clarithromycin (Biaxin®, Biaxin XL®)
- Doxycycline (a tetracycline antibiotic derivative)

Methicillin-Resistant Staphylococcus Aureus

Community-Acquired Methicillin-Resistant Staphylococcus Aureus (CA-MRSA) has emerged as a significant cause of CAP over the past twenty years. It also remains a significant cause of hospital-acquired pneumonia. The majority (up to 75%) of those diagnosed with CA-MRSA pneumonia are young, previously healthy individuals with influenza as a preceding illness. Symptoms are usually identical to those seen with other causes of CAP. Chest x-ray typically reveals multilobar involvement with or without cavitation/necrosis. Gram staining of sputum and/or blood can reveal gram-positive bacteria in clusters. Other diagnostic tests are nonspecific and do not aid in the diagnosis of CA-MRSA pneumonia.

Treatment of CA-MRSA should be prompt as it has a high mortality rate. Supportive measures are needed as in other cases of CAP. CA-MRSA is notoriously resistant to most antibiotics with the exception of the following:

- Vancomycin: The mainstay and only treatment for CA-MRSA pneumonia for many years (unfortunately with a disappointing cure rate). A loading dose of 25 mg/kg (max 2,000 mg) is needed with a maintenance dose based on creatinine clearance and body weight (in kg). Vancomycin trough should be drawn prior to fourth dose with a target goal of 15-20 mcg/mL (mg/L).

- Linezolid: An alternative to vancomycin and quickly becoming the agent of choice for the treatment of CA-MRSA pneumonia. It is administered 600 mg PO/IV every twelve hours.

Inhalation Injuries

Gases and vapors are the most common causes of lung inhalation injuries. This is because inhaled substances cause direct injury to respiratory epithelium. Exposure to accidental chemical spills, fires, and explosions can all lead to lung inhalation injuries. Some of the more common pulmonary irritants and gases include smoke, ozone, chlorine (Cl_2), hydrogen chloride (HCl), ammonia (NH_3), hydrogen fluoride (HF), sulfur dioxide (SO_2), and nitrogen oxides. The degree of inhalation injury is dependent on such factors as:

- Specific gas or substance inhaled
- Presence of soot
- Degree of exposure
- Presence of underlying lung disease
- Inability to flee the area

Inhalation injuries can even occur when there are no skin burns or other visible, external signs of exposure. Therefore, medical professionals should maintain a high level of suspicion when it comes to inhalation injuries, watching for signs and symptoms that can include:

- Tachypnea
- Dyspnea
- Facial burns
- Cough productive of carbonaceous sputum
- Wheezing
- Rhinitis
- Retractions
- Decreased breath sounds
- Hoarseness
- Blistering or swelling involving the mouth
- Singed nasal hairs
- Headache
- Vomiting
- Dizziness
- Change in mental status
- Coma

The best diagnostic tools for inhalation injuries are clinical presentation and findings from a bronchoscopy (the gold standard for diagnosing inhalation injuries). Other useful tests include:

- Chest x-ray
- CT scan
- Pulse oximetry
- ABG analysis
- Blood carboxyhemoglobin levels (for all fire and explosion victims)
- Pulmonary function tests (PFTs)

Inhalation injuries have an excellent prognosis since more than 90% of those affected make complete recoveries with no long-term pulmonary complications. However, depending on the injury source, medical providers should be aware that respiratory function can deteriorate up to 36 hours post-injury. Treatment of inhalation injuries is largely supportive care, which can include:

- Supplemental oxygen (usually 100% humidified oxygen)
- IV fluids, especially in individuals with burns
- Inhaled bronchdilators for bronchospasm, such as albuterol
- Gentle respiratory suctioning
- Close observation of developing edema around the head and neck
- Mucolytic agents such as N-acetylcysteine (NAC)
- Hyperbaric oxygen therapy (specifically for carbon monoxide poisoning)
- Hydroxocobalamin (Cyanokit®) (preferred agent), sodium thiosulfate, or sodium nitrite for hydrogen cyanide (HCN) poisoning/toxicity
- Intubation and mechanical ventilation, tidal volume of 6 mL/kg recommended to reduce likelihood of barotrauma
- Monitoring for the onset of secondary pneumonia (commonly caused by Staphylococcus aureus and Pseudomonas aeruginosa)

Obstruction

Obstruction is a blockage in any part of the respiratory tract. The upper respiratory tract consists of the nose, paranasal sinuses, throat, and larynx. The lower respiratory tract consists of the trachea, bronchi, and lungs. Obstructions can be categorized as upper airway obstructions or lower airway obstructions. Obstructions can be partial (allowing some air to pass) or complete (not allowing any air to pass), and they can also be acute or chronic. This discussion focuses on acute upper airway obstruction.

The most common causes of acute upper airway obstruction are anaphylaxis, croup, epiglottitis, and foreign objects. These are all considered respiratory emergencies. Anaphylaxis is a severe allergic reaction usually occurring within minutes of exposure to an allergen. During anaphylaxis, the airways swell and become blocked. Bee stings, penicillin (an antibiotic), and peanuts are the most common allergens that cause anaphylaxis.

Signs and symptoms of acute upper airway obstruction can include:

- Dyspnea
- Agitation/panic
- Wheezing
- Cyanosis
- Drooling
- Decreased breath sounds
- Tachypnea
- Tachycardia
- Swelling of the face and tongue
- Choking
- Confusion
- Unconsciousness

Diagnosis of acute upper airway obstruction can entail imaging studies (x-rays of the neck and chest; CT scans of the head, neck, or chest), pulse oximetry, blood tests and cultures, and bronchoscopy/laryngoscopy. Treatment depends on the etiology of the obstruction and can include:

- Heimlich maneuver (if choking on a foreign object)
- Epinephrine, antihistamines, and anti-inflammatory medications (if anaphylaxis)
- Supplemental oxygen
- Tracheostomy or cricothyrotomy (to bypass a total obstruction)
- CPR (if unconsciousness and unable to breathe)

Pleural Effusion

A **pleural effusion** is an abnormal accumulation of fluid in the pleural space. The pleural space is located between the parietal and visceral pleurae of each lung. The parietal pleura covers the inner surface of the chest cavity, while the visceral pleura surrounds the lungs. Approximately 10 milliliters of pleural fluid is maintained by oncotic and hydrostatic pressures and lymphatic drainage and is necessary for normal respiratory function. Pleural effusions can be categorized as transudates or exudates. Transudates result from an imbalance between oncotic and hydrostatic pressures, so they are characterized by low protein content. The transudates are often the result of congestive heart failure (CHF), cirrhosis, low albumin blood levels, nephrotic syndrome, and peritoneal dialysis. Exudates result from decreased lymphatic drainage or inflammation of the pleura, so they are characterized by high protein content. The exudates are often the result of malignancy, pancreatitis, pulmonary embolism, uremia, infection, and certain medications.

The main symptoms of a pleural effusion include dyspnea, cough, and chest pain. Diagnosis of a pleural effusion can include chest x-ray, chest CT scan, ultrasonography, and thoracentesis. Thoracentesis can provide pleural fluid for analysis such as LDH, glucose, pH, cell count and differential, culture, and cytology. Pleural fluid should be distinguished as either transudate or exudate. Exudative pleural effusions are characterized by:

- Ratio of pleural fluid to serum protein > 0.5
- Ratio of pleural fluid to serum LDH > 0.6
- Pleural fluid LDH > 2/3 of the upper limit of normal blood value

Treatment of a pleural effusion is usually dictated by the underlying etiology; however, the treatment of a very large pleural effusion can include:

- Thoracentesis
- Chest tube (also known as tube thoracostomy)
- Pleurodesis (instillation of an irritant to cause inflammation and subsequent fibrosis to obliterate the pleural space)
- Indwelling tunneled pleural catheters

Pneumothorax

Pneumothorax is the abnormal presence of air in the pleural cavity, which is the space between the parietal and visceral pleurae. Pneumothorax can be categorized as:

- Spontaneous Pneumothorax: This can be classified as either primary or secondary. Primary spontaneous pneumothorax (PSP) occurs in individuals with no history of lung disease or inciting event. Those at risk for PSP are typically eighteen to forty years old, tall, thin, and smokers. There's also a familial tendency for primary spontaneous pneumothorax. Secondary spontaneous pneumothorax occurs in individuals with an underlying lung disease such as COPD, cystic fibrosis, asthma, tuberculosis (TB), or lung cancer.
- Traumatic Pneumothorax: This occurs as a result of blunt or penetrating trauma to the chest wall. The trauma disrupts the parietal and/or visceral pleura(e). Examples of inciting events include gunshot or stab wounds; air bag deployment in a motor vehicle accident; acute respiratory distress syndrome (ARDS); and medical procedures such as mechanical ventilation, lung biopsy, thoracentesis, needle biopsy, and chest surgery.
- Tension Pneumothorax: This is the trapping of air in the pleural space under positive pressure. It causes a mediastinal shift toward the unaffected lung and a depression of the hemidiaphragm on the side of the affected lung. Shortly after, the event is followed by severe cardiopulmonary compromise. Tension pneumothorax can result from any of the conditions or procedures listed for Spontaneous and Traumatic Pneumothorax.

Signs and symptoms of pneumothorax depend on the degree of lung collapse (partial or total) and can include:

- Chest pain
- Dyspnea
- Cyanosis
- Tachypnea
- Tachycardia
- Hypotension
- Hypoxia
- Anxiety
- Adventitious breath sounds
- Unilateral distant or absent breath sounds
- Jugular venous distention (JVD)
- Tracheal deviation away from the affected side (with tension pneumothorax)

Diagnosis of pneumothorax is primarily clinical (based on signs and symptoms), but can involve an upright posteroanterior chest x-ray, chest CT scan (the most reliable imaging for diagnosis), ABG analysis, and ultrasonography of the chest. Treatment of a pneumothorax depends on the severity of the condition and can include:

- Supplemental oxygen
- The standard of treatment for all large, symptomatic pneumothoraces is a tube thoracostomy (chest tube).
- Observation (a reasonable option for small asymptomatic pneumothorax; multiple series of chest X-rays are needed until resolution)
- Simple needle aspiration (an option for small, primary spontaneous pneumothorax)
- Because they can quickly cause life-threatening cardiopulmonary compromise, the standard of treatment for all tension pneumothoraces is an emergent needle thoracostomy.

Pulmonary Edema, Noncardiogenic

Pulmonary edema can be categorized as cardiogenic or noncardiogenic in origin. Cardiogenic pulmonary edema is the most common type, while noncardiogenic pulmonary edema is the least common. This discussion focuses on noncardiogenic pulmonary edema. Direct injury to the lungs, followed by subsequent inflammation, leads to the development of noncardiogenic pulmonary edema. The inflammation causes lung capillaries in the alveoli to leak and fill with fluid, resulting in impaired oxygenation. Common causes of noncardiogenic pulmonary edema include:

- Acute respiratory distress syndrome (ARDS)
- High altitudes
- Nervous system conditions (especially head trauma, seizures, or subarachnoid hemorrhage)
- Pulmonary embolism
- Kidney failure
- Illicit drug use (especially cocaine and heroin)
- Medication side effects (such as aspirin overdose or chemotherapy)
- Inhaled toxins (such as ammonia, chlorine, or smoke)
- Pneumonia
- Near drowning

Signs and symptoms of noncardiogenic pulmonary edema can include:

- Dyspnea (most common symptom)
- Wheezing
- Respiratory distress
- Cough
- Anxiety
- Hypoxia
- Tachypnea
- Altered mental status
- Fatigue
- Lung crackles
- Headache
- Cyanosis

There is no single test to determine whether the cause of the pulmonary edema is cardiogenic or noncardiogenic. Diagnosis of noncardiogenic pulmonary edema can include chest x-ray, blood tests, pulse oximetry, ABG analysis, electrocardiogram (ECG), echocardiogram, cardiac catheterization with coronary angiogram, and pulmonary artery catheterization. For pulmonary artery catheterization, a pulmonary artery wedge pressure <18 mmHg is consistent with pulmonary edema of noncardiogenic origin. Most of these tests help to differentiate between cardiogenic and noncardiogenic causes of pulmonary edema.

Treatment of noncardiogenic pulmonary edema is directed toward its underlying cause and can include:

- Supplemental oxygen (first-line treatment)
- Hyperbaric oxygen chamber
- Intubation and mechanical ventilation
- Morphine (can be used to allay anxiety)

Pulmonary Embolism

A **pulmonary embolism** (PE) is the abnormal presence of a blood clot, or thrombus, causing a blockage in one of the lungs' pulmonary arteries. It is not a specific disease, but rather a complication due to thrombus formation in the venous system of one of the lower extremities, which is termed *deep venous thrombosis* (DVT). Other rarer causes of PEs are thrombi arising in the veins of the kidneys, pelvis, upper extremities, or the right atrium of the heart. Occasionally, other matter besides blood clots can cause pulmonary emboli, such as fat, air, and septic (infected with bacteria) emboli. PE is a common and potentially fatal condition.

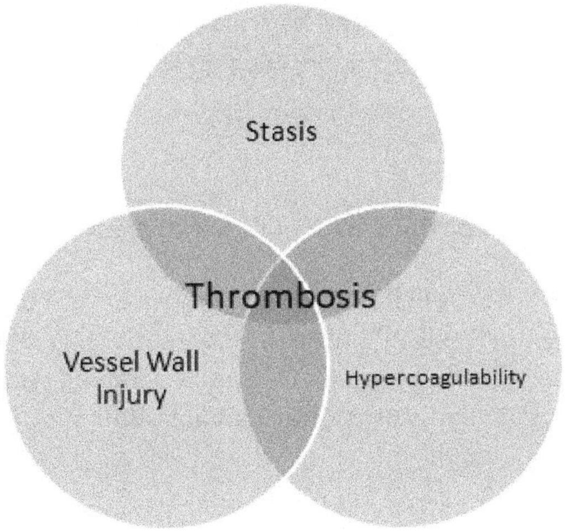

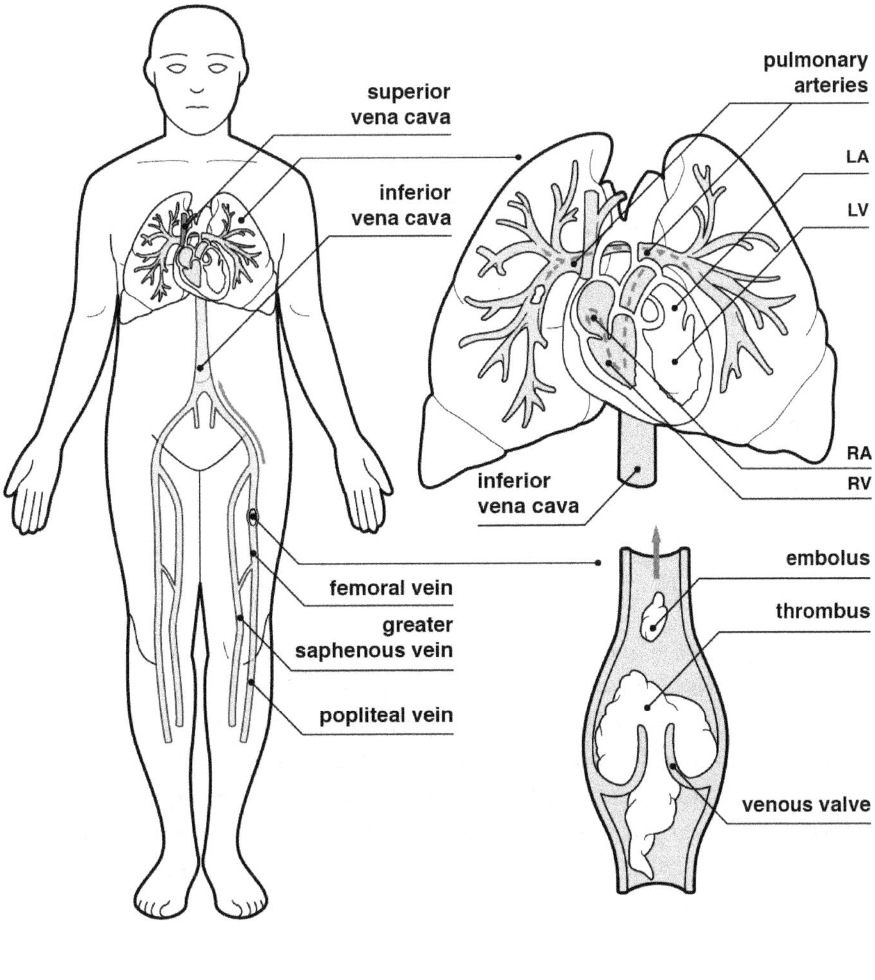

The primary influences on the development of DVT and PE are shown in Virchow's triad: blood hypercoagulability, endothelial injury/dysfunction, and stasis of blood. Risk factors for DVT and PE include:

- Cancer
- Heart disease, especially congestive heart failure (CHF)
- Prolonged immobility (such as prolonged bedrest or lengthy trips in planes or cars)
- Surgery (one of the leading risk factors, accounting for up to 15% of all postoperative deaths)
- Overweight/obesity
- Smoking
- Pregnancy
- Supplemental estrogen from birth control pills or estrogen replacement therapy (ERT)

The signs and symptoms of PE are nonspecific, which often presents a diagnostic dilemma and a delay in diagnosis. Nearly half of all individuals with PE are asymptomatic. The signs and symptoms of PE can vary greatly depending on the size of the blood clots, how much lung tissue is involved, and an individual's overall health. Signs and symptoms of PE can include:

- Pleuritic chest pain
- Dyspnea
- Cough
- Tachypnea
- Hypoxia
- Fever
- Diaphoresis
- Rales
- Cyanosis
- Unilateral lower extremity edema (symptom of DVT)

The diagnosis of PE can be a difficult task. Many clinicians support determining the clinical probability of PE before proceeding with diagnostic testing. This process involves assessing the presence or absence of the following manifestations:

- Pulmonary Signs: Tachypnea, rales, and cyanosis

- Cardiac Signs: Tachycardia, S_3 - S_4 gallop, attenuated second heart sound, and cardiac murmur

- Constitutional Signs: Fever, diaphoresis, signs and symptoms of thrombophlebitis, and lower extremity edema

Once the clinical probability of PE has been determined, diagnostic testing ensues. Duplex ultrasonography is the standard for diagnosing a DVT. A spiral computed tomography (CT) scan with or without contrast has replaced pulmonary angiography as the standard for diagnosing a PE. If spiral CT scanning is unavailable or if individuals have a contraindication to the administration of intravenous contrast material, ventilation-perfusion (V/Q) scanning is often selected. Magnetic resonance imaging (MRI) is usually reserved for pregnant women and individuals with a contraindication to the administration of intravenous contrast material. A D-dimer blood test is most useful for individuals with a low or moderate pretest probability of PE, since levels are typically elevated with PE. Arterial blood gas (ABG) analysis usually reveals hypoxemia, hypocapnia, and respiratory alkalosis.

A chest x-ray, though not diagnostic for PE since its findings are typically nonspecific, can exclude diseases that mimic PE, as can an echocardiography. Electrocardiography is also useful because it can assess right ventricular heart function and be prognostic, since there's a 10% death rate from PE with right ventricular dysfunction. Lastly, transesophageal echocardiography (TEE) can reveal central PE.

Treatment of PE should begin immediately to prevent complications or death. PE treatment is focused on preventing an increase in size of the current blood clots and the formation of new blood clots. Supportive care treatment of PE can include:

- Supplemental oxygen to ease hypoxia/hypoxemia
- Dopamine (Inotropin®) or dobutamine (Dobutrex®) administered via IV for related hypotension
- Cardiac monitoring in the case of associated arrhythmias or right ventricular dysfunction
- Intubation and mechanical ventilation

Medications involved in treatment can include: thrombolytics or clot dissolvers (such as tissue plasminogen activator (tPA), alteplase, urokinase, streptokinase, or reteplase). These medications are reserved for individuals with a diagnosis of acute PE and associated hypotension (systolic BP < 90 mm Hg). They are not given concurrently with anticoagulants. Anticoagulants or blood thinners may also be used. The historical standard for the initial treatment of PE was unfractionated heparin (UFH) administered via IV or subcutaneous (SC) injection, which requires frequent blood monitoring. Current treatment guidelines recommend low-molecular weight heparin (LMWH) administered via SC injection over UFH IV or SC as it has greater bioavailability than UFH and blood monitoring is not necessary. Fondaparinux (Arixtra®) administered via SC injection is also recommended over UFH IV or SC; blood monitoring is not necessary.

Warfarin (Coumadin®), an oral anticoagulant was the historical standard for the outpatient prevention and treatment of PE. It is initiated the same day as treatment with UFH, LMWH, or fondaparinux. It is recommended INR of 2-3 with frequent blood monitoring, at which time IV or SC anticoagulant is discontinued. Alternatives to Warfarin include oral factor Xa inhibitor anticoagulants such as apixaban (Eliquis®), rivaroxaban (Xarelto®), and edoxaban (Savaysa®), or dabigatran (Pradaxa®), an oral direct thrombin inhibitor anticoagulant. Blood monitoring is not necessary with these medications. The most significant adverse effect of both thrombolytics and anticoagulants is bleeding.

An embolectomy (removal of emboli via catheter or surgery) is reserved for individuals with a massive PE and contraindications to thrombolytics or anticoagulants. Vena cava filters (also called inferior vena cava (IVC) filters or Greenfield filters) are only indicated in individuals with an absolute contraindication to anticoagulants, a massive PE who have survived and for whom recurrent PE will be fatal, or documented recurrent PE.

Respiratory Distress Syndrome

Acute respiratory distress syndrome (ARDS) is the widespread inflammation of the lungs and capillaries of the alveoli and results in the rapid development of pulmonary system failure. It can occur in both adults and children and is considered the most severe form of acute lung injury. Presence of the syndrome is determined by:

- Timing: Onset of symptoms within one week of inciting incident
- Chest X-ray: Bilateral lung infiltrates not explained by consolidation, atelectasis, or effusions
- Origin of Edema: Not explained by heart failure or fluid overload
- Severity of Hypoxemia

It should be noted that the severity of hypoxemia is based on PaO_2/FiO_2 ratio while on 5 cm of continuous positive airway pressure (CPAP). PaO_2 is the partial pressure of oxygen, while FiO_2 is the fraction of inspired oxygen. Categories are:

- Mild (PaO_2/FiO_2 = 200-300)
- Moderate (PaO_2/FiO_2 = 100-200)
- Severe ($PaO_2/FiO_2 \leq 100$)

ARDS has a high mortality rate (30–40%), which increases with advancing age. It also leads to significant morbidity because of its association with extended hospital stays, frequent nosocomial (hospital-acquired) infections, muscle weakness, significant weight loss, and functional impairment. The most common cause of ARDS is sepsis, a life-threatening bacterial infection of the blood. Other common causes include:

- Severe pneumonia
- Inhalation of toxic fumes
- Trauma (such as falls, bone fractures, motor vehicle accidents, near drowning, and burns)
- Massive blood transfusion

It should also be noted that, for one in five patients with ARDS, there will be no identifiable risk factors. Therefore, the cause of ARDS may not be evident.

The onset of ARDS symptoms is fairly rapid, occurring 12 to 48 hours after the inciting incident. Many of the signs and symptoms of ARDS are nonspecific. Signs and symptoms of ARDS can include:

- Dyspnea (initially with exertion, but rapidly progressing to occurring even at rest)
- Hypoxia
- Tachypnea
- Tachycardia
- Fever
- Bilateral rales
- Cyanosis
- Hypotension
- Fatigue

The diagnosis of ARDS is clinical since there's no specific test for the condition. Diagnosing ARDS is done by exclusion, ruling out other diseases that mimic its signs and symptoms. Tests used to diagnose ARDS can include:

- Chest x-ray, which, by definition, should reveal bilateral lung infiltrates
- ABG analysis (usually reveals extreme hypoxemia and respiratory alkalosis or metabolic acidosis)
- CBC with differential (can reveal leukocytosis, leukopenia, and/or thrombocytopenia)
- Plasma *B*-type natriuretic peptide (BNP), a level < 100 pg/mL favors ARDS rather than CHF
- CT scan
- Echocardiography, which is helpful in excluding CHF (cardiogenic pulmonary edema)
- Bronchoscopy with bronchoalveolar lavage (BAL), which is helpful in excluding lung infections

Numerous medications, such as corticosteroids, synthetic surfactant, antibody to endotoxin, ketoconazole, simvastatin, ibuprofen, and inhaled nitric oxide, have been used for the treatment of ARDS, but none have proven effective. Therefore, treating the underlying symptoms of ARDS and providing supportive care are the most crucial components of therapy. The only therapy found to improve survival in ARDS is intubation and mechanical ventilation using low tidal volumes (6 mL/kg of ideal body weight). Because sepsis, an infection, is the most common etiology of ARDS, early administration of a broad-spectrum antibiotic is crucial.

Treatment also includes fluid management and nutritional support. For individuals with shock secondary to sepsis, initial aggressive fluid resuscitation is administered, followed by a conservative fluid management strategy. It is best to institute nutritional support within 48 to 72 hours of initiation of mechanical ventilation.

Important preventative measures include DVT prophylaxis with enoxaparin, stress ulcer prophylaxis with sucralfate or omeprazole, turning and skin care to prevent decubitus ulcers, and elevating the head of the bed and using a subglottic suction device to help prevent ventilator-associated pneumonia.

Trauma

Chest trauma is a significant factor in all trauma deaths. There are two general categories of chest traumas: blunt chest traumas and penetrating chest traumas.

Pulmonary Contusion

A **pulmonary contusion** is a deep bruise of the lung secondary to chest trauma. Associated swelling and blood collecting in the alveoli of the lung lead to loss of structure and function. It is estimated that 50% to 60% of individuals with pulmonary contusions develop ARDS. Motor vehicle accidents, sports injuries, explosive blast injuries, work injuries, serious falls, or crush injuries can cause blunt chest trauma. Signs and symptoms of a pulmonary contusion typically develop 24 to 48 hours after the inciting event. Signs and symptoms can include:

- Dyspnea
- Hypoxia
- Cyanosis
- Tachypnea

- Tachycardia
- Hemoptysis
- Chest pain
- Hypotension

Diagnosis of a pulmonary contusion relies on physical examination and diagnostic tests. A chest x-ray is useful in the diagnosis of most significant pulmonary contusions; however, it often underestimates the extent of the injury, which is sometimes not apparent for 24 to 48 hours after event. CT scans are more accurate than chest x-rays for identifying of a pulmonary contusion; they can also accurately assess and reflect the extent of lung injury. ABG analysis is used to assess the extent of hypoxemia, and pulse oximetry is used to assess the extent of hypoxia.

Treatment for a pulmonary contusion is primarily supportive, and no treatment is known to accelerate its resolution. These treatments can include:

- Supplemental oxygen to relieve hypoxia
- Analgesics (as needed for pain)
- Conservative fluid management to reduce the likelihood of fluid overload and PE
- Aggressive suction of pulmonary secretions to reduce likelihood of pneumonia
- Incentive spirometry to reduce the likelihood of atelectasis, which can lead to pneumonia
- Intubation and mechanical ventilation (in severe cases)

Hemothorax

Hemothorax, the presence of blood in the pleural space, is most commonly the result of blunt or penetrating chest trauma. The pleural space lies between the parietal pleura of the chest wall and the visceral pleura of the lungs. A large accumulation of blood in the pleural space can restrict normal lung movement and lead to hemodynamic compromise. Common signs and symptoms of hemothorax include chest pain, dyspnea, and tachypnea. When there is substantial systemic blood loss, tachycardia and hypotension can also be present.

Diagnosis of hemothorax primarily involves a chest x-ray, which reveals blunting at the costophrenic angle on the affected side of the lung. A helical CT scan has a complementary role in the management of hemothorax, and it can localize and quantify the retention of blood or clots within the pleural space.

Small hemothoraces usually require no treatment but need close observation to ensure resolution. Tube thoracostomy drainage is the mainstay of treatment for significant hemothoraces. Needle aspiration has no place in the management of hemothorax. Blood transfusions can be necessary for those with significant blood loss or hemodynamic compromise. Complications from hemothorax can include empyema (secondary bacterial infection of a retained clot) or fibrothorax (fibrosis of the pleural space which can trap lung tissue and lead to decreased pulmonary function).

Flail Chest

Flail chest is clinically defined as the paradoxical movement of a segment of the chest wall caused by at least two fractures per rib (usually anteriorly and posteriorly) in three or more ribs while breathing. The ribs are then free to float away from the chest wall and produce paradoxical breathing, which is the flail area contracting on inspiration and relaxing on expiration. The flail area of the chest disrupts the normal mechanics of breathing. Variations include anterior flail segments, posterior flail segments, and flail affecting the sternum and fractures of the ribs bilaterally. Flail chest requires a tremendous amount of blunt force trauma to the thorax in order to fracture multiple ribs in multiple places. This type of trauma can be produced by motor vehicle accidents, serious falls, crush injuries, rollover injuries, and physical assaults.

The diagnosis of flail chest is visual. It is seen in individuals with a history of blunt chest trauma by the presence of paradoxical chest wall motion while spontaneously breathing. The rib fractures can be verified with chest x-ray. A CT scan of the chest provides very little additional information and isn't usually indicated in the initial assessment of a chest wall injury. In flail chest, the lungs cannot expand properly, which can lead to varying degrees of respiratory compromise. Treatment of flail chest can include:

- Supplemental oxygen (to relieve hypoxia, if present)
- Analgesia (for relief of pain secondary to multiple rib fractures, usually via patient-controlled administration (PCA) or continuous epidural infusion)
- External fixation and stabilization of rib fractures (once the historical standard for treatment, it has been replaced by intubation and mechanical ventilation)
- Intubation and mechanical ventilation (usually needed for the treatment of an underlying disease such as pulmonary contusion; addition of positive pressure provides stabilization of the chest wall and helps improve oxygenation and ventilation)
- Operative fixation of ribs (reserved for individuals requiring a thoracotomy for underlying lung injuries)

Common complications of flail chest include hemothorax, pneumothorax, pulmonary contusion, and pneumonia. Hemothorax or pneumothorax would require concomitant tube thoracostomy drainage. Chest physiotherapy and aggressive pulmonary hygiene should be implemented to reduce the likelihood of complicating pneumonia.

Fractured Ribs

A **fracture** is a crack or splinter in a bone. Simple rib fractures are the most common injury after sustaining blunt chest trauma. Only 10% of individuals admitted with a diagnosis of blunt chest trauma have multiple rib fractures. Causes of rib fractures include falls from an elevation or from standing (most common in the elderly), motor vehicle accidents (most common in adults), and recreational and athletic activities (most common in children). Rib fractures can also be pathologic or related to cancers that have undergone metastasis such as prostate, renal, and breast.

Ribs four through nine (4–9) are the most commonly fractured ribs. Other rib fractures and possible underlying injuries are:

- Ribs 1–2: Tracheal, bronchus, or great vessels can be injured
- Right-sided $\geq$ rib 8: Liver trauma
- Left-sided $\geq$ rib 8: Spleen trauma

Common signs and symptoms of rib fractures include tenderness on palpation, chest wall deformities, and crepitus. Other signs and symptoms can include cyanosis, dyspnea, tachycardia, agitation, tachypnea, retractions, and use of accessory respiratory muscles.

Laboratory blood tests are of no use in the diagnosis of fractured ribs. A chest x-ray can be used to diagnose rib fractures and other underlying injuries such as hemothorax, lung contusion, pneumothorax, atelectasis, and pneumonia. A chest CT scan is more sensitive than a chest x-ray for the detection of rib fractures. A bone scan of the chest wall is the preferred diagnostic imaging study for the diagnosis of rib stress fractures.

The treatment of rib fractures is primarily supportive. Younger individuals with rib fractures have a better prognosis than older individuals (age $\geq$ 65 years) who have higher rates of serious lung complications. Therapies for rib fractures can include:

- Supplemental oxygen
- Incentive spirometry (to avoid complications such as atelectasis and pneumonia)
- Pain control, which is essential and usually provided by NSAIDs and/or other analgesics

Tracheal Perforation/Injury

Tracheal perforation/injury is a tear in the trachea or bronchial tubes, which are major airways leading to the lungs. Common causes of tracheal perforation/injury include trauma (gunshot wounds and motor vehicle accidents), infections, and ulcerations secondary to foreign objects. Common signs and symptoms of tracheal perforation/injury can include hemoptysis, dyspnea, subcutaneous emphysema, and respiratory distress. Diagnosis may include chest x-rays, a chest CT scan, and MRI. A CT scan is the preferred imaging method for diagnosing a tracheal perforation/injury. Treatment should be prompt and depends on the etiology and the extent of the damage to the area. Surgical repair of the tear is often needed, and other measures to manage a tracheal perforation/injury include:

- Intubation and mechanical ventilation
- Tube thoracostomy drainage
- Rigid or fiberoptic bronchoscopy (to extract foreign objects)
- Antibiotics (as indicated)

Ruptured Diaphragm

The diaphragm separates the thoracic (chest) cavity and the abdominal cavity. Rupture of the diaphragm is rare and usually the result of a blunt or penetrating trauma. The majority of blunt traumas causing ruptures of the diaphragm are the result of motor vehicle accidents. Gunshot and knife injuries are the most common causes of a traumatic diaphragmatic rupture. A ruptured diaphragm can lead to significant ventilatory compromise, and difficulty breathing is a common symptom. A chest x-ray is the most important diagnostic tool in diagnosing a ruptured diaphragm. It can reveal elevation of a hemidiaphragm, a nasogastric (NG) tube being present in chest (rather than in the abdomen), or the abnormal presence of bowel in the chest. Abnormalities such as widening of the mediastinum can also be observed on a chest x-ray. Treatment of a ruptured diaphragm requires surgical repair. The prognosis is excellent with the emergent repair of the diaphragmatic rupture.

Cardiovascular/Hematological

Cardiovascular emergencies are life-threatening conditions. Any condition that impedes circulation has the potential to damage the myocardium, or heart muscle. A damaged myocardium may be unable to meet the oxygen demands of the body. It is important to quickly identify any patient exhibiting symptoms indicative of such emergencies so that they can receive prompt treatment to prevent further cardiovascular injury or death. Every patient presenting to the emergency department with possible cardiovascular symptoms should immediately be given a focused assessment followed by a history and physical. Simultaneously, an intravenous (IV) line should be established and an electrocardiogram (ECG) and laboratory and radiographic studies should be performed. The triage, assessment, diagnostics, and treatment of such patients must be prioritized to preserve cardiac function and, ultimately, life.

Acute Coronary Syndrome

Acute coronary syndrome (ACS) is the term used to describe the clinical symptoms caused by the sudden reduction in blood flow to the heart, but it is also known as **acute myocardial ischemia**. The causes of the ischemia include stable and unstable angina (UA), non-ST elevation myocardial infarction (NSTEMI), and ST elevation myocardial infarction (STEMI), which are shown in the figure below.

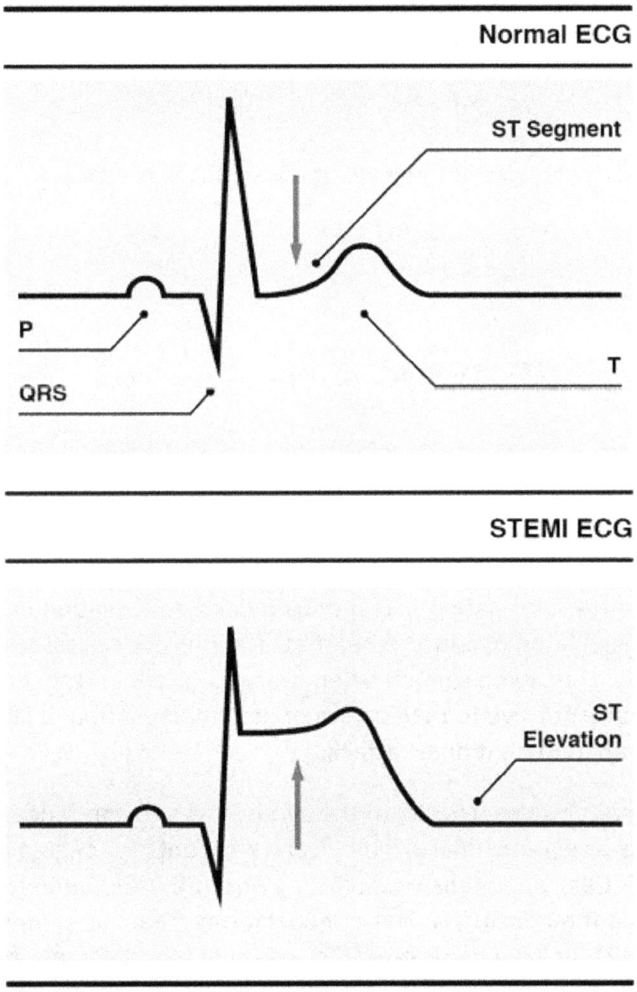

Common symptoms of a patient presenting with ACS include:

- Chest pain or discomfort in the upper body that radiates to the arms, back, neck, jaw, or stomach, as shown in the image below

Typical Pain Radiation Patterns of Acute Coronary Syndrome

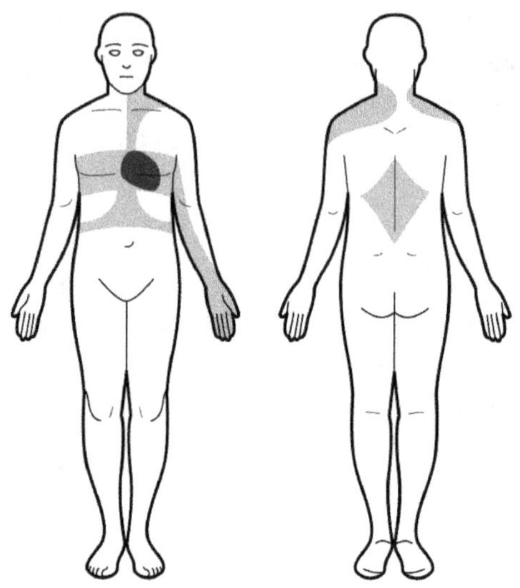

- Dizziness, syncope, or changes in the level of consciousness (LOC)
- Nausea or vomiting
- Palpitations or tachycardia
- Shortness of breath (SOB) or dyspnea
- Unusual fatigue

Angina

Angina is the term used to describe chest pain caused by decreased blood flow to the myocardium. The two primary categories of angina are stable or unstable, with stable angina being more common. It presents in a predictable pattern for patients, responds quickly to cessation or exertion or medication, and while it increases the likelihood of a future heart attack, it is not necessarily indicative of such an event occurring imminently. Unstable angina is often more frequent and severe. It may occur without physical exertion and be unresponsive to medication or activity cessation. It should be treated as an emergency and can signal an imminent heart attack.

Treatment for angina depends on the severity of the symptoms and can range from lifestyle modifications to surgical intervention. Pharmacological treatments for angina include beta-blockers, calcium channel blockers (CCBs), angiotensin-converting enzyme (ACE) inhibitors, statins, and antiplatelet and anticoagulant medications. These medications treat the symptoms related to angina by lowering blood pressure (BP), slowing heart rate (HR), relaxing blood vessels, reducing strain on the heart, lowering cholesterol levels, and preventing blood clot formation. Generally, the risk factors for the development of angina include:

- Diabetes
- Dietary deficiency (fruits and vegetables)
- Excessive alcohol consumption
- Family history of early coronary heart disease
- Hypertension (HTN)
- High LDL (low-density lipoprotein)
- Low HDL (high-density lipoprotein)
- Males
- Obesity
- Old age
- Sedentary lifestyle
- Smoking

Stable Angina

Atherosclerotic buildup generally occurs slowly over time. Because the buildup is gradual, the heart can usually continue to meet the body's oxygen demands despite the narrowing lumen of the vessel. However, in situations with increased oxygen demand, such as exercise or stress, the myocardium may not be able to meet the increased demands, thereby causing angina. The angina subsides with rest. Stable angina is predictable; it occurs in association with stress or certain activities. It does not increase in intensity or worsen over time. Nitroglycerine is effective in the treatment of stable angina because it dilates the blood vessels, reducing the resistance to blood flow, which decreases the demand on the myocardium. Lifestyle modifications such as smoking cessation and a regular exercise program are needed to slow atherosclerotic buildup.

Unstable Angina

Unstable angina (UA) is a more severe form of heart disease than stable angina. The angina associated with UA is generally related to small pieces of atherosclerotic plaque that break off and cause occlusions. The occlusions suddenly decrease blood flow to the myocardium, resulting in angina, without causing an actual MI. The pain symptomatic of UA occurs suddenly without a direct cause, worsens over a short period of time, and may last 15 to 20 minutes. Dyspnea (shortness of breath) and decreased blood pressure are also common. Because the angina is related to an acute decrease in blood flow, rest does not alleviate symptoms. Generally, UA does not respond to the vasodilatory effect of nitroglycerine. Laboratory values are typically negative for cardiac enzymes related to cardiac damage, but they can be slightly elevated. Therefore, a comprehensive history and physical exam that properly identify pertinent risk factors are critical for early diagnosis and treatment.

Depending on the severity of symptom presentation, pharmacological treatment for UA will include one or more antiplatelet medications and a cholesterol medication. In addition, medications to treat hypertension, arrhythmias, and anxiety may be necessary. The recommended intervention is angioplasty with coronary artery stenting. A coronary artery bypass grafting (CABG) surgery may be necessary in the case of extensive occlusion of one or more of the coronary arteries.

NSTEMI

The **NSTEMI** does not produce changes in the ST segment of the EKG cycle. However, troponin levels are positive. Patients with a confirmed NSTEMI are hospitalized. Morphine, oxygen, nitroglycerin, and aspirin (MONA protocol) is administered. Additional pharmacological agents for treatment are beta-blockers, ACE inhibitors, statins, and antiplatelet medications. Coronary angiography and revascularization may be necessary.

The primary difference between UA and an NSTEMI is whether the ischemia is severe enough to damage the myocardium to the extent that cardiac markers indicative of injury are released and detectable through laboratory analysis. A patient is diagnosed with an NSTEMI when the ischemia is severe enough to cause myocardial damage and the release of a myocardial necrosis biomarker into the circulation (usually cardiac-specific troponins T or I). In contrast, a patient is diagnosed with UA if such a biomarker is undetectable in his or her bloodstream hours after the ischemic chest pain's initial onset.

STEMI

The **STEMI** is the most serious form of MI. It occurs when a coronary artery is completely blocked and unable to receive blood flow. Emergent revascularization is needed either through angioplasty or a thrombolytic medication.

UA and NSTEMIs generally indicate a partial-thickness injury to the myocardium, but a STEMI indicates injury across the full thickness of the myocardium, as shown in the image below. The etiology behind ischemia is partial or full occlusion of coronary arteries.

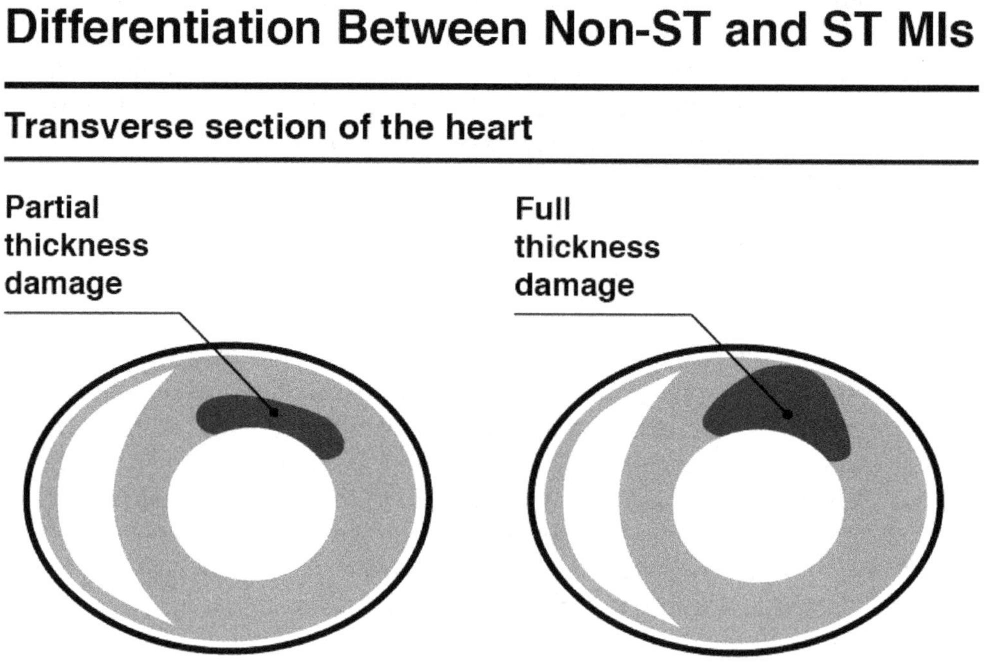

Treatment and Risk Scoring

Treatment for UA and NSTEMI is planned according to a risk score using the Thrombolysis in Myocardial Infarction (TIMI) tool. In the presence of UA or an NSTEMI, seven categories are scored: age, risk factors, a prior coronary artery stenosis, ST deviation on ECG, prior aspirin intake, presence and number of angina episodes, and elevated creatinine kinase (CK-MB) or troponins. In the presence of a STEMI, the TIMI tool scores eleven categories: age, angina history, hypertension, diabetes, systolic BP, heart rate,

Killip class, weight, anterior MI in an ECG, left bundle branch block (LBBB) in an ECG, and a treatment delay after an attack. The Global Registry of Acute Coronary Events (GRACE), or ACS risk calculator, is a common tool used to predict death during admission and six months, as well as three years after a diagnosis of Acute Coronary Syndrome (ACS).

ACS can be life threatening. Treatment and survival are time-dependent. Quick recognition by the nurse followed by a thorough focused assessment that includes evaluation of pain type, location, characteristic, and onset is essential. The MONA protocol is implemented immediately. The nurse should obtain a family, social, and lifestyle assessment to identify high-risk patients. An evaluation of recent medical history is imperative, since most ACS patients experience prodromal symptoms a month or more prior to the acute event. Establishing IV access is paramount for rapid administration of medications. Obtaining and reviewing an ECG and drawing and reviewing labs including troponins, CK-MB, complete blood count (CBC), C-reactive protein (CRP), electrolytes, and renal function will provide critical diagnostic data. A chest x-ray and echocardiogram will also add to the differential diagnosis. Immediate and long-term complications of ACS are cardiac dysrhythmia, heart failure (HF), and cardiogenic shock. Education should be provided to each patient about the diagnosis, risk factors, lifestyle modifications, and medications once the acute event has stabilized.

Aneurysm/Dissection

An **aneurysm** is an abnormal bulge or ballooning that can form within an artery, as seen in the image below. Depending on the location, the rupture of an aneurysm can result in hemorrhage, stroke, or death. The most common places for the formation of an aneurysm are the left ventricle (LV) of the heart, the aorta, the brain, and the spleen.

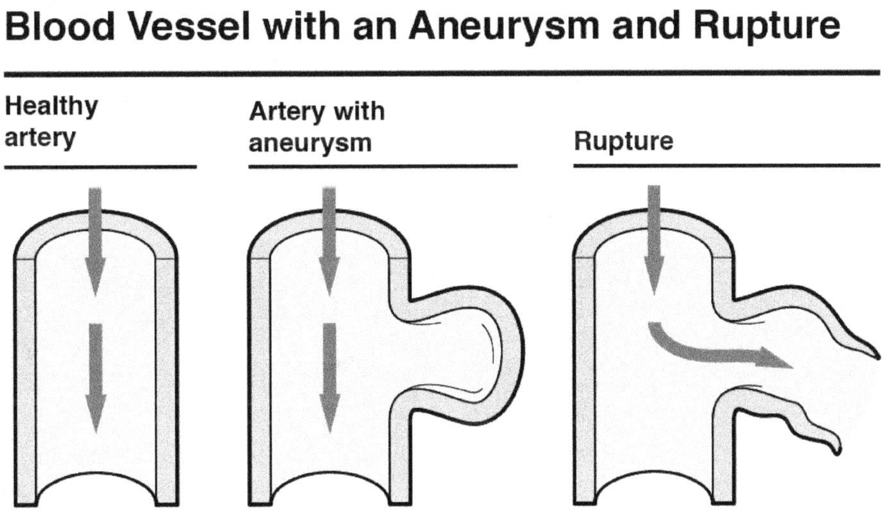

Anatomical Review

Generally, arteries carry oxygenated blood away from the heart to the organs and tissues of the body. The largest artery is the aorta, which receives blood directly from the LV of the heart. Oxygen-carrying blood continues to travel down the arterial system through successively smaller arteries that supply organs, ending with the arterioles that empty into the capillary bed.

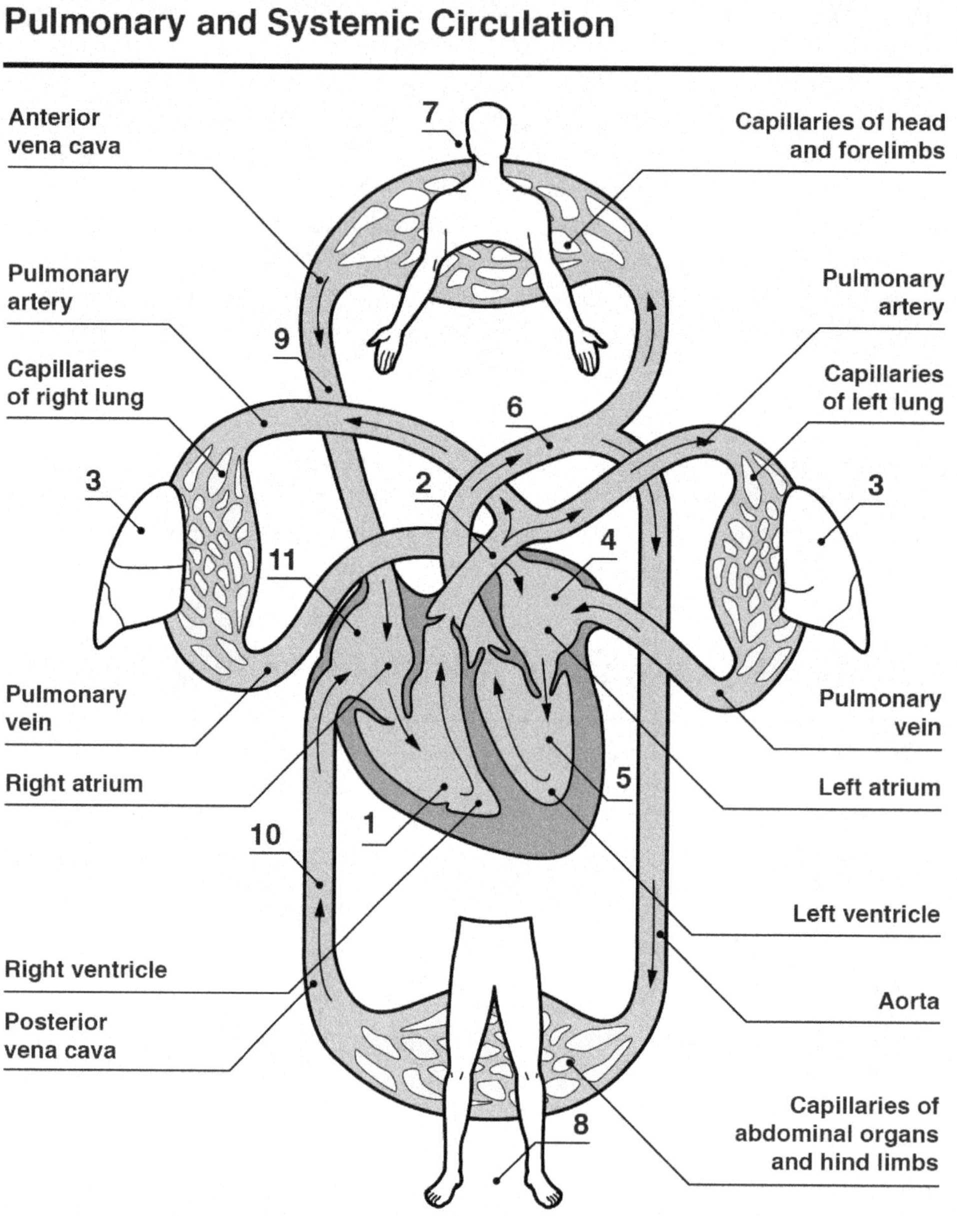

The capillary beds are drained on their opposite side by the venules, which return the now-deoxygenated blood back to the right atrium through progressively larger veins, ending in the great veins of the heart, known as the superior and inferior vena cava. The deoxygenated blood from the great veins moves into the right atrium, then the right ventricle, which pumps the blood to the lungs via the pulmonary artery to become oxygenated once again. The oxygenated blood flows from the pulmonary vein into the left atrium, then the LV, and into the aorta to repeat the cycle.

Arteries and Veins

There are three tissue layers in the structure of arteries and veins. The endothelium, or tunica intima, forms the inner layer. The middle layer, the tunica media, contains elastin and smooth muscle fibers, and connective tissue forms the outside coating called the tunica externa.

Arteries have a thicker elastin middle layer that enables them to withstand the fluctuations in pressure, which result from the high-pressure contractions of the LV. Arterioles regulate blood flow into the capillary bed through constriction and dilation, so they are the primary control structures for blood pressure regulation. Meanwhile, the venous side of circulation operates under very low pressures, so veins have no elastin in their structure; instead, they use valves to prevent backflow in those vessels working against gravity, as shown in the image below.

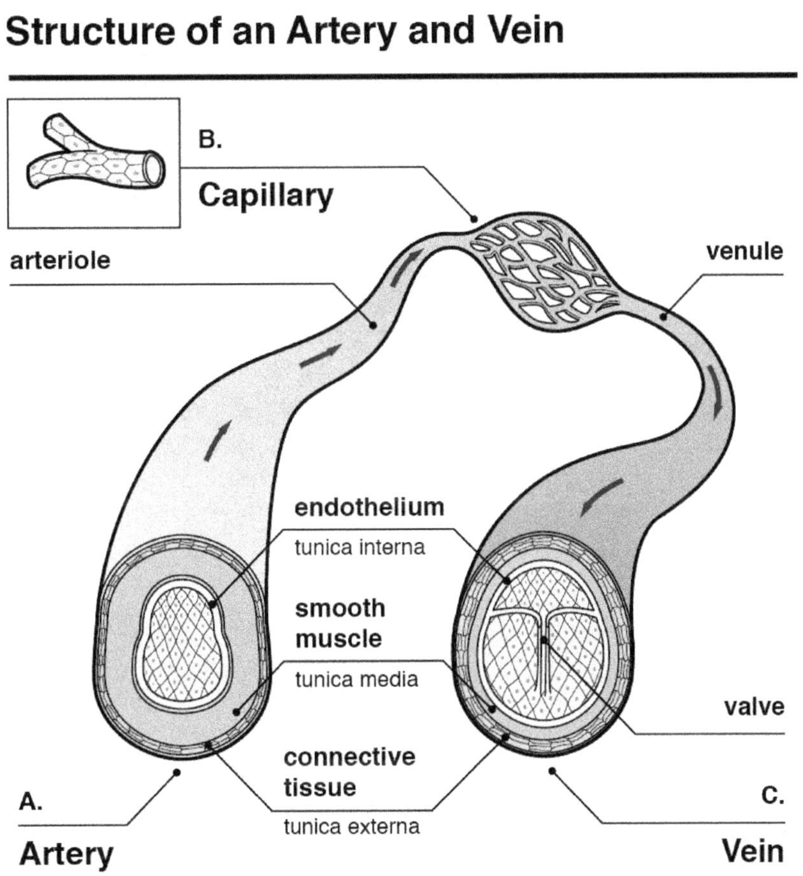

Left Ventricular Aneurysm

A left ventricular aneurysm (LVA) is a bulge or ballooning of a weakened area of the LV, generally caused by an MI. There are no symptoms of an LVA, which should be diagnosed with an echocardiogram and angiogram. Small LVAs usually do not require treatment. Clot formation is a common occurrence with LVAs. In the body's attempt to repair the aneurysm, the inflammatory process and the clotting cascade are initiated, both of which increase the propensity for clot formation. Patients are most likely prescribed anticoagulants. Rapid treatment for an MI reduces the incidence of LVA formation.

Aorta

The **aorta** stretches from the LV through the diaphragm into the abdomen and pelvis. In the groin, the aorta separates into two main arteries that supply blood to the lower trunk and the legs. An aneurysm can occur anywhere along the aorta; an abdominal aortic aneurysm (AAA) is the most common. Atherosclerosis, hypertension, diabetes, infection, inflammation, and injury such as from a fall or auto accident are frequent causes. The most common presenting symptoms with an AAA are chest pain and back pain. The clinician may be able to palpate a pulsating bulge in the abdomen. Nausea and vomiting may be present. Other symptoms include lightheadedness, confusion, dyspnea, rapid heartbeat, sweating, numbness, and tingling. When an AAA develops slowly over a period of years, it is less likely to rupture, in which case the patient should be regularly monitored with ultrasound imaging. Aneurysms greater than 2 inches (5.5 centimeters) will generally require surgical repair.

A thoracic aortic aneurysm occurs in the stretch of the aorta that lies within the chest cavity. The critical size for surgical intervention of a thoracic aortic aneurysm is 2.3 inches (6 centimeters). As with all surgeries in such close proximity to the heart, the risk-to-benefit ratio must be carefully weighed.

Treatment Options

If the AAA is small and slow-growing, a watch-and-wait approach is often taken. An abdominal ultrasound, computed tomography (CT), and MRI will aid in the determination of the most appropriate treatment. Surgical repair involves removing the damaged portion of the aorta and replacing it with a graft. Another minimally-invasive technique involves reinforcing the weakened area with metal mesh.

Brain

Bulging or ballooning in a blood vessel within the brain is the second most common site for an aneurysm. Another common site for aneurysms is where the internal carotid artery (ICA) enters the cranium; it branches into a system of arteries that provide blood flow to the brain, known as the *circle of Willis*. Most small brain aneurysms do not rupture and are found during various tests. An aneurysm may press on brain tissue and present with ocular pain or symptoms. However, a rupture is a medical emergency that can lead to stroke or hemorrhage. The most common symptom described by patients is "the *worst* headache of my life." A sudden, severe headache, stiff neck, blurred or double vision, photophobia, seizure, loss of consciousness, and confusion may also be reported.

Here's a graphic of the circle of Willis, which are interconnecting arteries at the base of the brain:

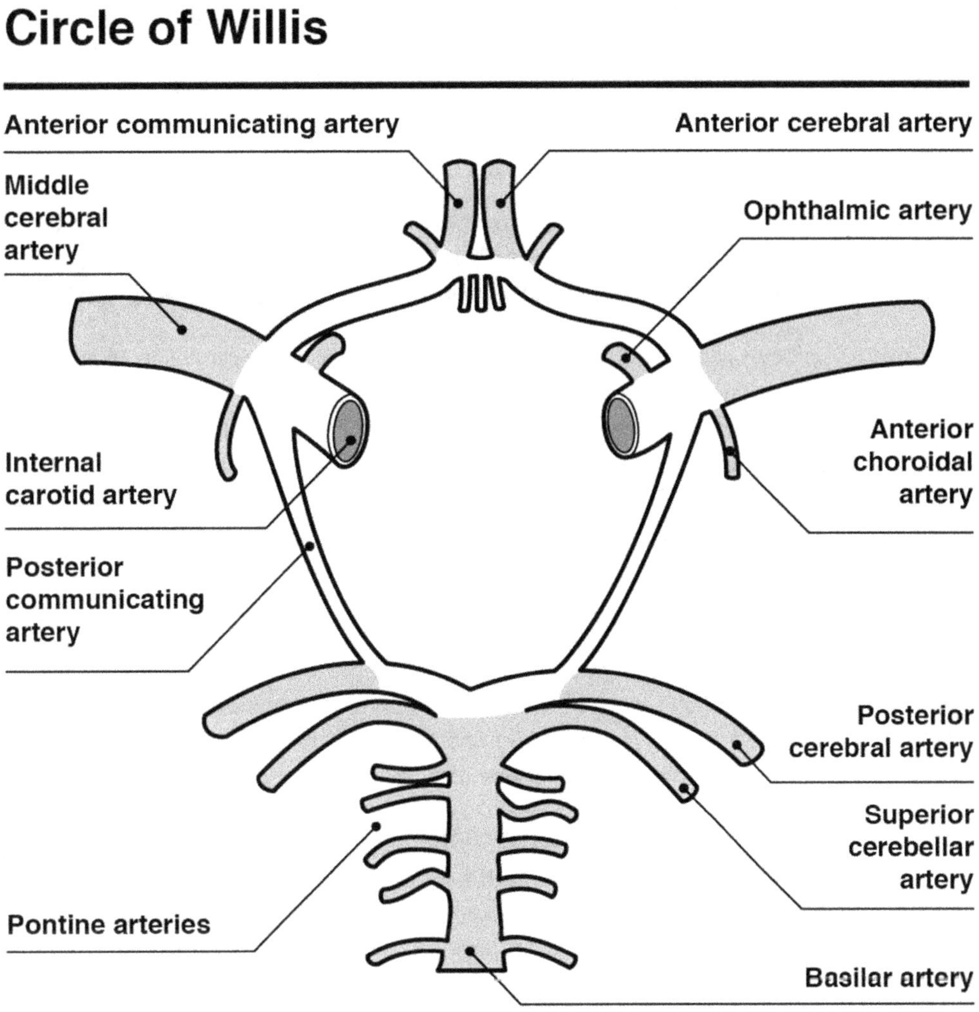

Risk Factors

A family history of aneurysm and certain other aneurysm risk factors are genetic. Other predisposing factors are an arteriovenous malformation (AVM) at the circle of Willis, polycystic kidney disease (PKD), and Marfan syndrome. Poor lifestyle choices, such as smoking and cocaine use, greatly increase the risk for aneurysm formation. There is a higher risk for individuals over the age of forty, women, patients who have experienced a traumatic head injury, and patients with hypertension.

Treatment Options

Depending on a brain aneurysm's cause, size, and symptoms, and the patient's general health, there are several treatment options. The most common surgical treatment is clipping. The bulge is clipped at the base to prevent blood from entering. The clip remains in place for life. Eventually, the bulge will shrink.

If the artery has been damaged by the aneurysm, an occlusion and bypass surgical procedure may be performed. The affected artery is closed off, and a new route that allows circulation to bypass the damage is created. The artificial development of an embolism, known as **endovascular embolization**, is another treatment option. A variety of substances such as plastic particles, glue, metal, foam, or balloons are coiled and inserted into the aneurysm to block blood flow.

A liquid embolic surgical glue is a new option to the standard coiling procedure: Onyx HD 500 is a vinyl alcohol copolymer that solidifies on contact with the blood in the aneurysm, sealing it. In the case of smaller aneurysms, a watch-and-wait approach may be taken. Bleeding, vasospasm, seizures, and hydrocephalus are the main complications related to a brain aneurysm.

Spleen

The **spleen** plays an important role in the regulation of red blood cells. The filtration action of the spleen removes worn-out or damaged red blood cells and microbes. It is also an important organ in the immune system, producing the white blood cells that fight infection and synthesize antibodies.

Although very rare, the spleen is the third most common site of an aneurysm. The exact cause of a splenic arterial aneurysm is unknown. However, the aneurysm represents a damaged splenic artery. Portal hypertension and multiple pregnancies produce an increase in intra-abdominal pressure that is thought to damage the splenic artery, leading to the formation of an aneurysm. Trauma and autoimmune disease are also known causes.

A splenic aneurysm is generally asymptomatic and found incidentally on diagnostic studies. An aneurysm of the splenic artery is treated by clipping.

Dissection

Dissection is a condition in which the layers of the arterial wall become separated and blood leaks in between the layers of the vessel. A dissection represents damage through more than one layer of an artery. It is a more serious form of aneurysm because all the layers are compromised.

A dissection is different from a rupture. With a dissection, blood leaks in and through the layers of an artery, but the artery remains structurally intact, albeit weakened. Blood is still contained within the vessel. When a rupture occurs, it is similar to the popping of a balloon. The integrity of the artery is disrupted, and blood leaks out of the artery. Dissections increase the risk of rupture. Medical management with beta-blockers is the treatment of choice for stable aortic dissections.

Summary

Symptoms of an aneurysm/dissection may be absent, vague, or difficult to identify. The consequences of a rupture are life-threatening. The expert clinician will ascertain a thorough patient and family history, including social factors and lifestyle choices. Autoimmune disorders, age, gender, a sedentary lifestyle, smoking, and drug or alcohol abuse are contributing factors to the development of an aneurysm. Rapid assessment, diagnosis, and treatment are essential. Vital signs, neurological status, and loss of consciousness should be closely monitored.

Cardiopulmonary Arrest

Cardiopulmonary arrest is a life-threatening emergency characterized by the sudden unexpected cessation of heart function, breathing, and consciousness caused by a disturbance in the electrical conduction of the heart. Immediate basic life support (BLS) followed by current advanced cardiac life support (ACLS) protocol is the treatment. Defibrillation is the treatment choice for cardiopulmonary arrest caused by ventricular tachycardia or fibrillation. The time between patient collapse and initiation of resuscitation efforts is the most important factor in patient survival.

The brain is the first organ impacted by loss of blood flow and oxygenation. Cardiac arrest lasting longer than 8 minutes has poor survival rates. A diagnostic work-up during and after stabilization will include an ECG, arterial blood gases (ABGs), troponins counts, CBC, electrolyte counts, and renal function labs.

Dysrhythmias

Dysrhythmia, also known as **arrhythmia**, is abnormal electrical activity of the heart. The heartbeat may be regular or irregular, too fast, or too slow.

Normally, the electrical conduction system of the heart begins with an impulse known as the **action potential** at the pacemaker sinoatrial (SA) node. The impulse travels across the right and left atria before activating the atrioventricular (AV) node.

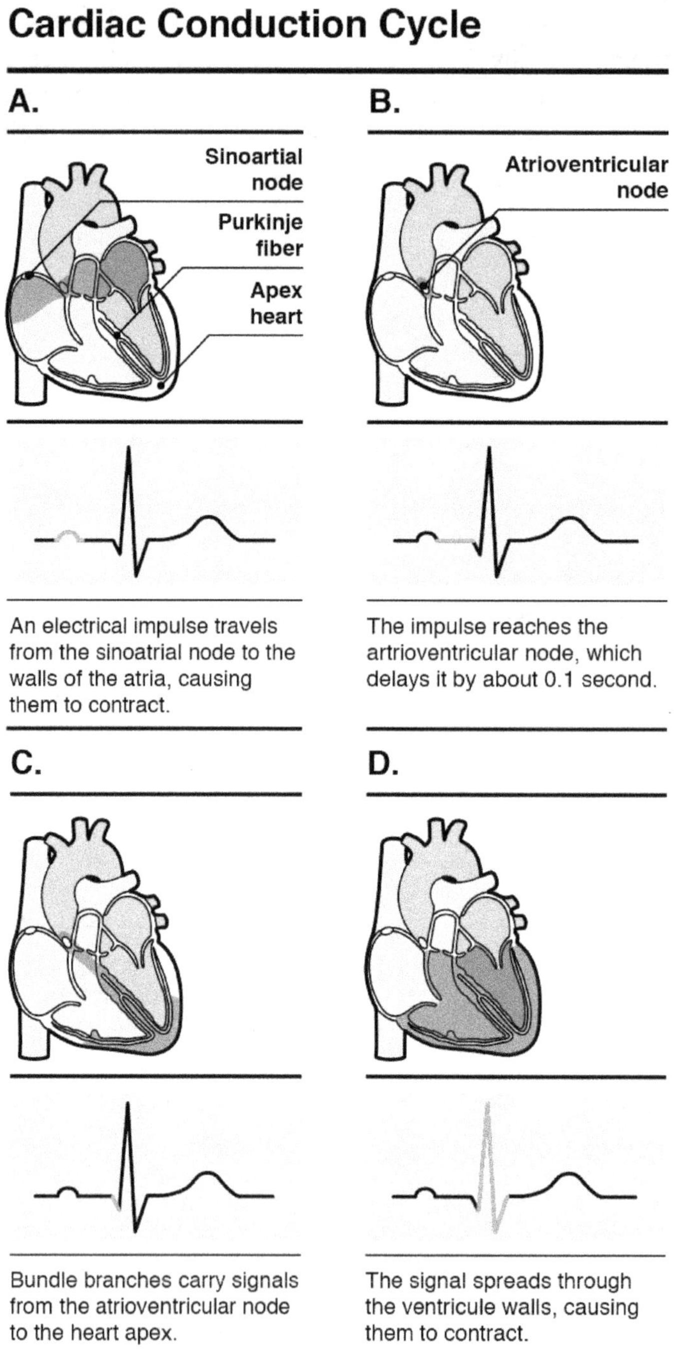

The pathway from the SA to the AV node is visualized on the ECG as the P wave. From the AV node, the impulse continues down the septum along cardiac fibers. These fibers are known as the **bundle of His**. The impulse then spreads out and across the ventricles via the Purkinje fibers. This is represented on the ECG as the QRS complex. The T wave represents the repolarization or recovery of the ventricles.

Electrical Events of the Cardiac Cycle

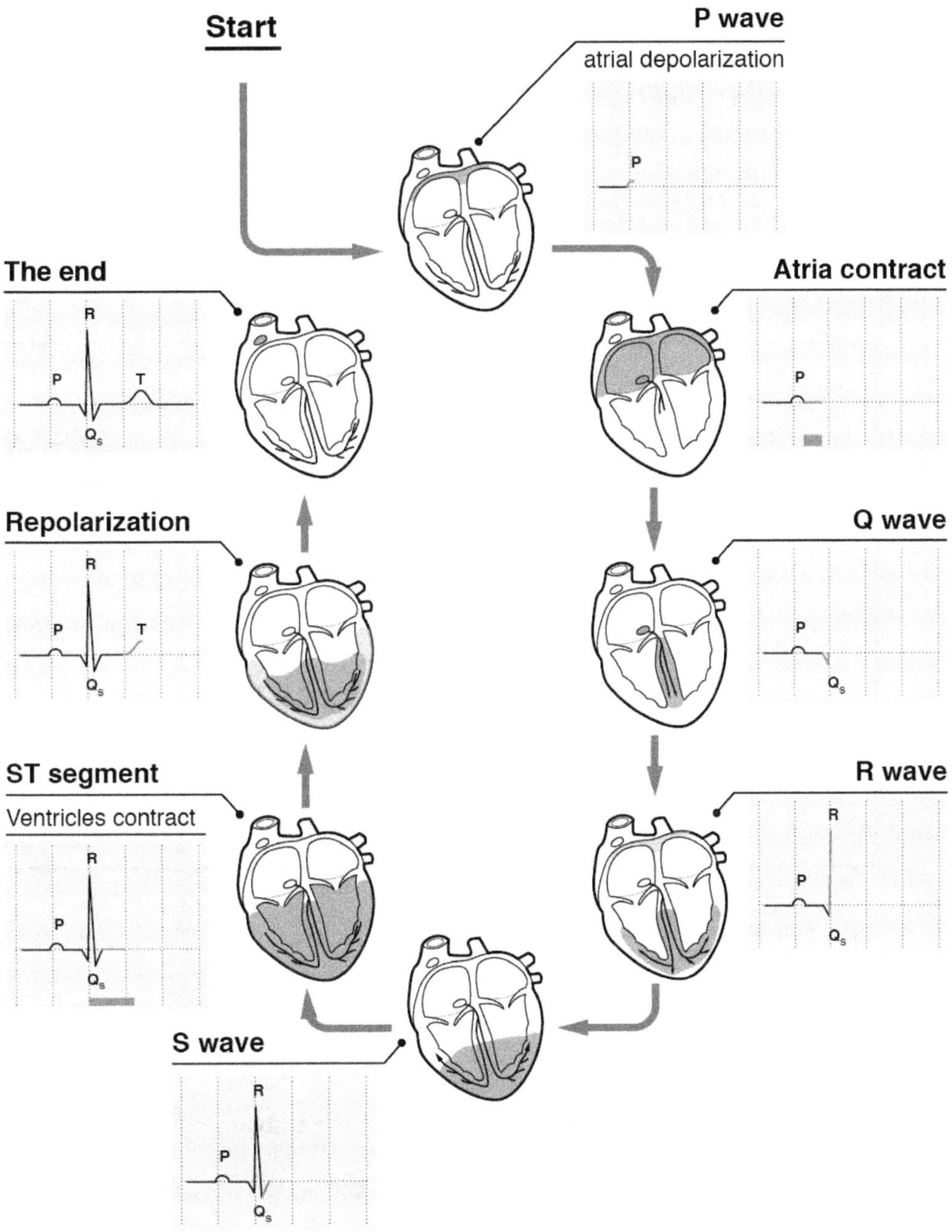

Properties of Cardiac Cells

Cardiac cells have four important properties: excitability, conductivity, contractility, and automaticity. **Excitability** allows the heart to respond to stimuli and maintain homeostasis. **Conductivity** is the ability to transfer the electrical impulse initiated at the SA node across cardiac cells. **Contractility** is the cardiac cells' ability to transform an action potential into the mechanical action of contraction and relaxation. **Automaticity** is the ability of cardiac cells to contract without direct nerve stimulation. In other words, the heart initiates its own impulse. If the SA node fails to initiate the impulse, the AV node will fire the impulse at a slower rate. If neither the SA nor the AV node fires the impulse, the cells within the bundle of His and the Purkinje fibers will fire to start the impulse at an even slower rate.

Action Potential

The **action potential** is a representation of the changes in voltage of a single cardiac cell. Action potentials are formed as a result of ion fluxes through cellular membrane channels, most importantly, the sodium (Na+), potassium (K+), and calcium (Ca+) channels. Electrical activity requires an action potential. Contraction of the cardiac muscle fibers immediately follows electrical activity.

Phases of an Action Potential

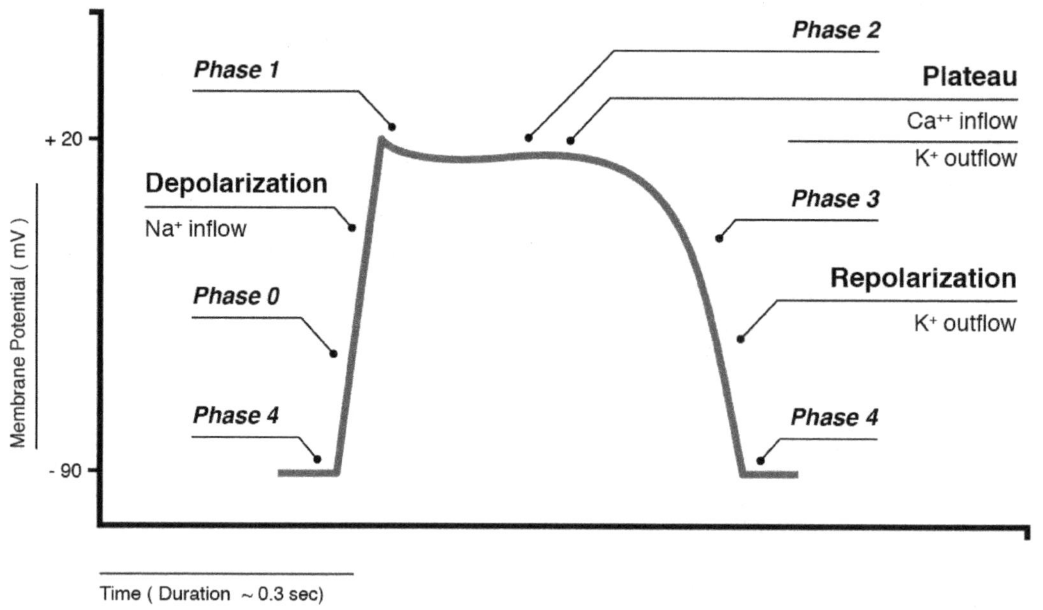

Phase 0: Depolarization

- Rapid Na+ channels are stimulated to open.
- The cardiac cell is flooded with Na+ ions, which change the transmembrane potential.
- The shift in potential is reflected by the initial spike of the action potential.
- Depolarization of one cell triggers the Na+ channels in surrounding cells to open, which causes the depolarization wave to propagate cell by cell throughout the heart.

Phases 1–3: Repolarization phases

- During these phases, represented as the plateau, Ca+ and some K+ channels open.
- Ca+ flows into the cells, and K+ flows out.
- The cell remains polarized, and the increased Ca+ within the cell trigger contraction of the cardiac muscle.

Phase 4: Completion of repolarization

- Ca+ channels close.
- K+ outflow continues.
- The cardiac cell returns to its normal state.

The cardiac cycle of **depolarization-polarization-depolarization** is represented on the ECG by the P wave, QRS complex, and T wave. A dysrhythmia can occur anywhere along the conduction system. It can be caused when an impulse from between the nodes or fibers is delayed or blocked. Arrhythmias also occur when an ectopic focus initiates an impulse, thereby disrupting the normal conduction cycle. Additional sources of damage to the conduction system include MIs, hypertension, coronary artery disease (CAD), and congenital heart defects.

Overview of Dysrhythmias

Abnormalities in the electrical conduction system of the heart may occur at the SA node, the AV node, or the His-Purkinje system of the ventricles. Careful evaluation of the ECG will aid in determining the location and subsequent cause of the dysrhythmia.

Dysrhythmias that occur above the ventricles in either the atria or the SA/AV nodes are known as **supraventricular dysrhythmias**. Common arrhythmias in this category are sinus bradycardia, sinus tachycardia, atrial fibrillation, atrial flutter, junctional rhythm, and sustained supraventricular tachycardia (SVT). **Atrioventricular** (AV) **blocks**, known as **heart blocks**, occur when the impulse is delayed or blocked at the AV node. The three types of heart block are first degree, second degree, and third degree, with first degree being the least severe and third degree being the most severe.

Ventricular dysrhythmias can be life-threatening because they severely impact the heart's ability to pump and maintain adequate cardiac output (CO). A bundle branch block (BBB), premature ventricular complexes (PVCs), sustained ventricular tachycardia (V-tach), ventricular fibrillation (V-fib), Torsades de pointes, and digoxin-induced ventricular dysrhythmias are the most common ventricular arrhythmias.

Supraventricular Dysrhythmias

Sinus Bradycardia

Sinus bradycardia occurs when the SA node creates an impulse at a slower-than-normal rate—less than 60 beats per minute (bpm). Causes include metabolic conditions, calcium channel blockers (CCB) and beta-blocker medications, MIs, and increased intracranial pressure. If symptomatic, treatment involves transcutaneous pacing and atropine.

Sinus Tachycardia

Sinus tachycardia occurs when the SA node creates an impulse at a faster-than-normal rate, also characterized as a rate greater than 100 bpm. Causes include physiological stress such as shock, volume loss, and heart failure, as well as medications and illicit drugs. Sinus tachycardia is typically treated by treating the underlying cause.

Atrial Fibrillation

Atrial fibrillation is the most common sustained dysrhythmia. It is caused when multiple foci in the atria fire randomly, thereby stimulating various parts of the atria simultaneously. The result is a highly irregular atrial rhythm. Ventricular rate may be rapid or normal. Fatigue, lightheadedness, chest pain, dyspnea, and hypotension may be present. Treatment goals are to improve ventricular pumping and prevent stroke. Beta-blockers and CCBs impede conduction through the AV node, thereby controlling ventricular rates, so they are the medications of choice. Cardioversion and ablation are also treatment options.

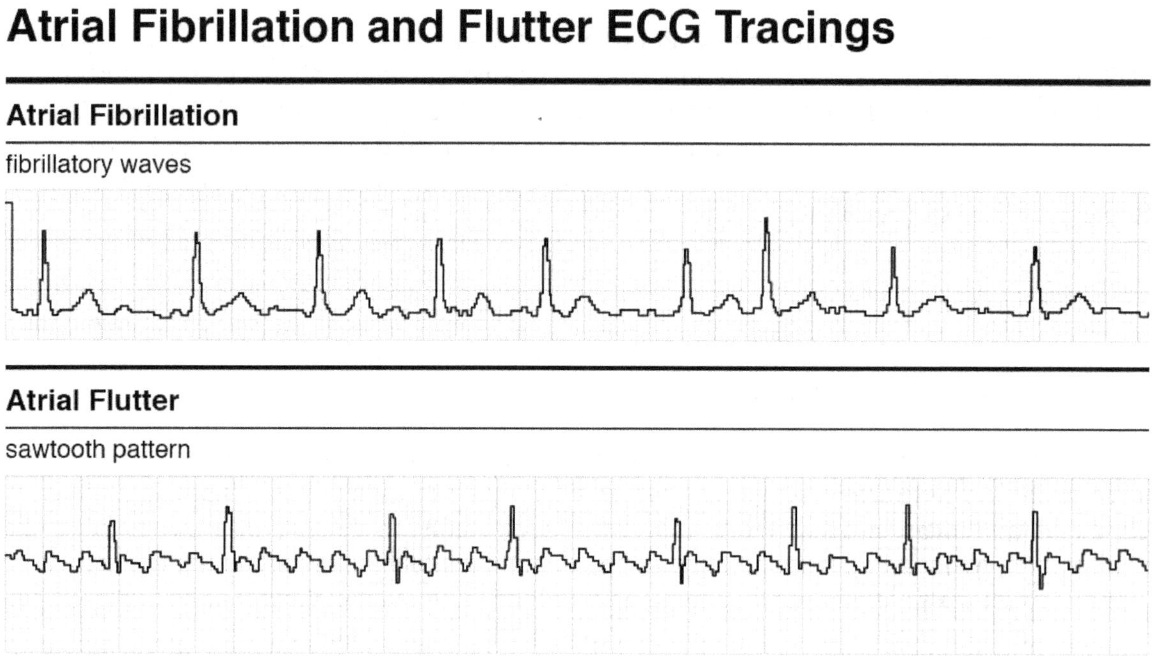

Atrial Flutter

Atrial flutter is caused by an ectopic atrial focus that fires between 250 and 350 times a minute. The AV node is unable to transmit impulses at that speed, so typically only one out of every two impulses reach the ventricles. Cardioversion is the treatment of choice to convert atrial flutter back to a sinus rhythm. CCBs and beta-blockers are used to manage ventricular rates.

Junctional Dysrhythmias

If either the SA node slows or its impulse is not properly conducted, the AV node will become the pacemaker. The heart rate for an impulse initiated at the AV junction will be between 40 and 60 bmp. The P wave will be absent on an EKG. Suggested treatment is similar to that of sinus bradycardia: transcutaneous pacing, atropine, and epinephrine.

Supraventricular Tachycardia

Sustained **supraventricular tachycardia** (SVT) is usually caused by an AV nodal reentry circuit. Heart rate can increase to 150 to 250 bpm. Interventions that increase vagal tone such as the Valsalva maneuver or carotid massage may slow the heart rate. Beta-blockers and CCBs may be given intravenously for immediate treatment or may be taken orally to prevent reoccurrence.

Heart Block

In **first-degree heart block**, the impulse from the SA node is slowed as it moves across the atria. On an ECG, the P and R waves will be longer and flatter. First-degree block is often asymptomatic.

Second-degree heart block is divided into two categories known as Mobitz type I and Mobitz type II. In Mobitz type I, the impulse from the SA node is increasingly delayed with each heartbeat until eventually a beat is skipped entirely. On an ECG, this is visible as a delay in the PR interval. The normal PR interval is 0.12–0.20. The PR interval will get longer until the QRS wave doesn't follow the P wave. Patients may experience mild symptoms with this dysrhythmia.

When some of the impulses from the SA node fail to reach the ventricles, the arrhythmia is a Mobitz type II heart block. Some impulses move across the atria and reach the ventricles normally, and others do not. On an ECG, the QRS follows the P wave at normal speed, but some QRS complexes are missing because the signal is blocked. Patients experiencing this dysrhythmia usually need a pacemaker.

A **third-degree heart block** is also known as complete heart block, or complete AV block. The SA node may continue to initiate the impulses between 80 and 100 bpm, but none of the impulses reach the ventricles. The automaticity of cardiac cells in the Purkinje fibers will prompt the ventricles to initiate an impulse; however, beats initiated in this area are between 20 and 40 bpm. The slower impulses initiated from the ventricles are not coordinated with the impulses from the SA node. Therefore, third-degree heart block is a medical emergency that requires a temporary to permanent pacemaker.

Bundle Branch Block

A **bundle branch block** (BBB) occurs when there is a delay or defect in the conduction system within the ventricles; a BBB may be designated as "left" or "right" to specify the ventricle at fault or as "complete" or "partial." The QRS complex will be widened or prolonged. Treating the underlying cause is the goal.

Premature Ventricular Complex

A **premature ventricular complex** (PVC) occurs when a ventricular impulse is conducted through the ventricle before the next sinus impulse. This may be caused by cardiac ischemia, heart failure, hypoxia, or hypokalemia. Treatment is to correct the cause, and long-term treatment is not indicated unless the patient is symptomatic.

Ventricular Tachycardia

Ventricular tachycardia (V-tach) occurs from a single, rapidly firing ectopic ventricular focus that is typically at the border of an old infarct (MI). This dysrhythmia is usually associated with CAD. Ventricular rates can be 150 to 250 bpm. However, the heart cannot pump effectively at those increased rates. Immediate cardioversion is the treatment of choice. Antidysrhythmic medications such as amiodarone, lidocaine, or procainamide may be given. An implantable cardioverter defibrillator (ICD) may be necessary.

Ventricular Tachycardia and Fibrillation ECG Tracings

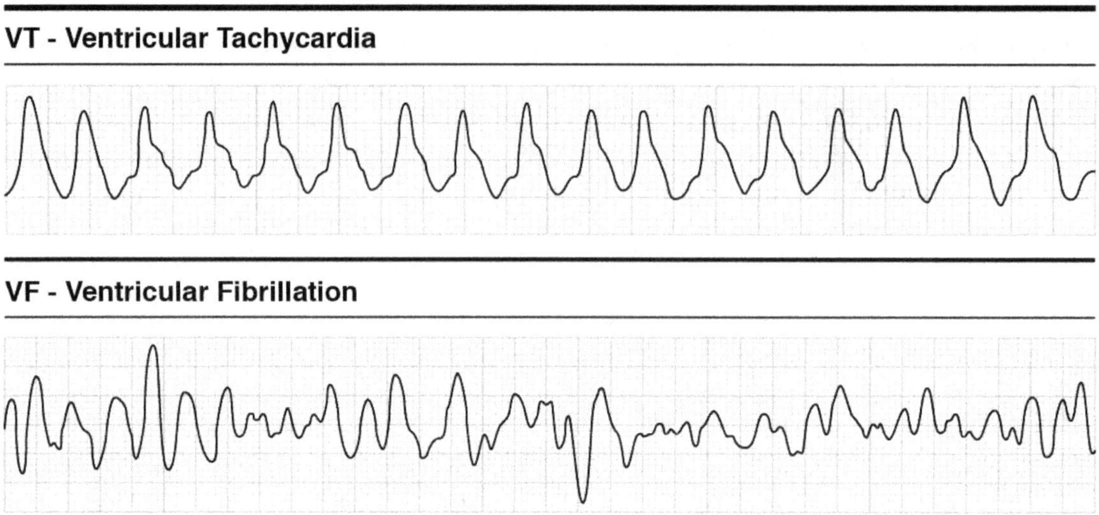

Ventricular Fibrillation

Ventricular fibrillation (V-fib) is a life-threatening emergency that requires immediate treatment. It is caused by multiple ventricular ectopic foci firing simultaneously, which forces the ventricles to contract asynchronously. Coordinated ventricular contraction is impossible in this scenario. The result is reduced cardiac output, and defibrillation is required. Lidocaine, amiodarone, and procainamide may be used.

Torsade de Pointes

Torsade de pointes is an atypical rapid undulating ventricular tachydysrhythmia. This rhythm has a prolonged QT interval. A variety of drugs cause QT-interval prolongation. The treatment is intravenous magnesium and cardioversion for sustained V-tach.

Torsade de Pointes ECG Tracing

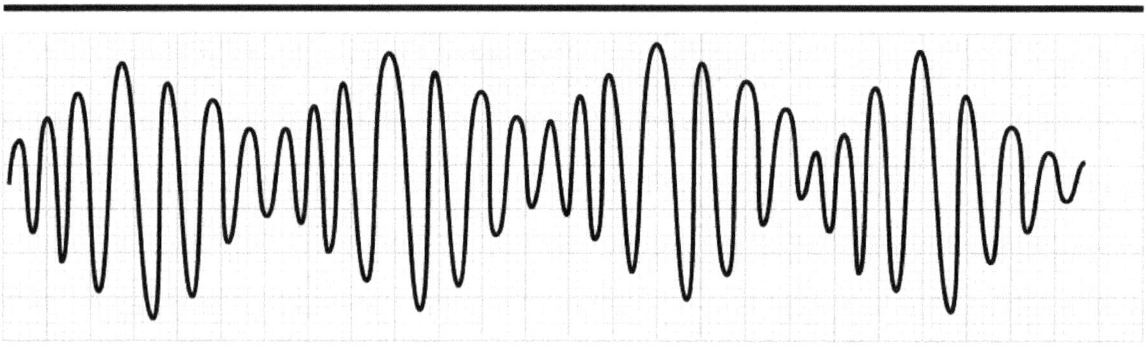

Digoxin-Induced Ventricular Dysrhythmias

Digoxin is a cardiac glycoside medication that increases the strength and regularity of the cardiac rhythm. It has a very narrow therapeutic range. Toxicity occurs when therapeutic levels are exceeded. Digoxin toxicity can mimic all types of dysrhythmias. Digoxin acts by increasing automaticity in the atria, ventricles, and the His-Purkinje system. It also decreases conduction through the AV node. Therefore, an AV block is the most common form of presenting dysrhythmia in the general population. Among the elderly, chronic toxicity is common as well, as it can be easily caused by drug-to-drug interactions and declining renal function.

Summary

Dysrhythmias range from asymptomatic to life-threatening. They can be divided into three major groups: supraventricular dysrhythmias, heart block, and ventricular dysrhythmias. Treatment is necessary when ventricular pumping and cardiac output are impacted. There are two phases of treatment. The first is to terminate the dysrhythmia using medications, defibrillation, or both. The second is long-term suppression with medications.

A complete medical history with an emphasis on current medications, comorbidities, and family history is paramount. Immediate nursing priorities include establishing IV access, monitoring vital signs, and administering oxygen as needed. Evaluation of the ECG, chest x-ray, and both laboratory and diagnostic values is required. Defibrillation, cardioversion, and transcutaneous pacing are other possibilities.

Endocarditis

By definition, endocarditis is the inflammation of the endocardium, or innermost lining of the heart chambers and valves. It is also called **infective endocarditis**, or **bacterial endocarditis**.

To review, there are three layers of tissue that comprise the heart. A double-layer serous membrane, known as the **pericardium**, is the outermost layer. The pericardium forms the pericardial sac that surrounds the heart. The middle and largest layer is the **myocardium**. Since an MI occurs when the heart muscle is deprived of oxygen, the myocardial layer of the heart is where the damage due to lack of oxygen occurs. The innermost layer that lines the heart chambers and also the heart valves is called the **endocardium**. Endocarditis occurs when the endocardial layer and heart valves become infected and inflamed.

The most common cause of endocarditis is a bloodstream invasion of bacteria. **Staphylococci** and **Streptococci** account for the majority of infective endocarditis occurrences. During medical or dental procedures—such as a colonoscopy, cystoscopy, or professional teeth cleaning—bacteria may enter the bloodstream and travel to the heart. Inflammatory bowel disease and sexually transmitted diseases also foster bacterial transmission to the bloodstream and, ultimately, the heart.

Risk factors for the development of endocarditis include valve and septal defects of the heart, an artificial heart valve, a history of endocarditis, an indwelling long-term dialysis catheter, parenteral nutrition or central lines in the right atrium, IV drug use, and body piercings. Patients taking steroids or immunosuppressive medications are susceptible to fungal endocarditis. Regardless of the source, the bacteria infect the inside of the heart chambers and valves. Clumps of infective bacteria, or vegetation, develop within the heart at the site of infection. The heart valves are a common infection site, which often results in incomplete closure of the valves.

The classic symptoms of endocarditis are fever, cardiac murmur, petechial lesions of the skin, conjunctiva, and oral mucosa. However, symptoms can range in severity. Flu-like symptoms, weight loss, and back pain may be present. Dyspnea and swelling of the feet and ankles may be evident. Endocarditis caused by Staphylococcus has a rapid onset, whereas Streptococcus occurs more slowly with a prolonged course.

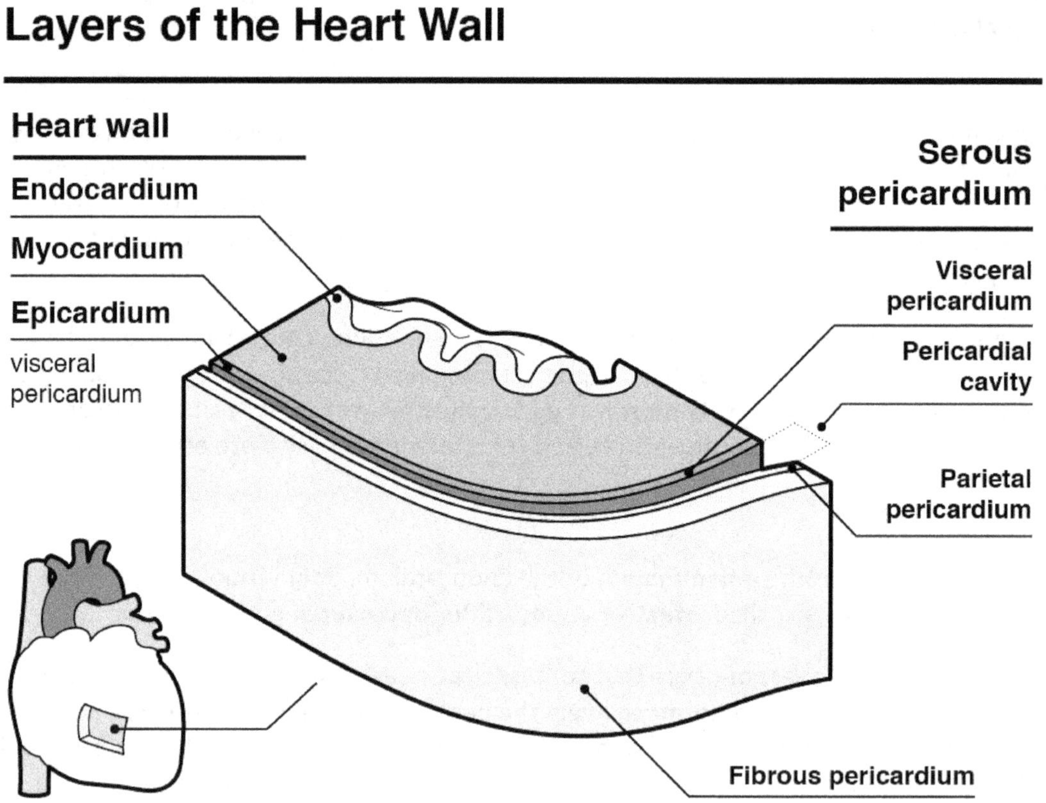

Antimicrobial treatment for four to six weeks is the standard of care. In some cases, two antimicrobials are used to treat the infection and prevent drug resistance. The objective of treatment is to eradicate the infection and treat complications. Surgery may be required for persistent recurring infections, one or more embolic occurrences, or if heart failure develops.

Left untreated, endocarditis can result in stroke or organ damage, as the vegetation breaks off and travels through the bloodstream and blocks circulation. The spread of infection and subsequent formation of abscesses throughout the body may also occur. Heart failure may develop when the infection hampers the heart's ability to pump effectively or with perforation of a valve.

A complete history and physical that includes inquiry about medications, recent surgeries, screening, and diagnostic testing may provide the crucial piece of information that identifies endocarditis in the face of otherwise vague symptom presentation. The nurse should anticipate the order for blood cultures, an erythrocyte sedimentation rate (ESR), a CBC, an ECG, a chest x-ray, and a transthoracic or transesophageal echocardiogram to identify the location of the infected area.

An in-depth patient interview and assessment by the nurse are essential. Diagnostic and laboratory results coupled with data from the patient interview will aid in early recognition and treatment of endocarditis. Because an incident of endocarditis places one at a higher risk for future infections, patient teaching should include informing all providers and dentists prior to treatment. Antibiotic prophylaxis may be indicated.

Heart Failure

Mechanism

Defined as the failure of the heart to meet the metabolic demands of the body, **heart failure** (HF) is a general term that refers to the failure of the heart as a pump. HF is a syndrome with diverse clinical features and various etiologies. The syndrome is progressive and often fatal. It may involve either or both sides of the heart. Based on ejection fraction (EF), it can be further categorized as diastolic or systolic HF.

Left-sided HF is also referred to as congestive heart failure (CHF) because the congestion occurs in the pulmonary capillary beds. As mentioned previously, oxygenated blood flows from the pulmonary artery into the left atrium, then the LV, and into the aorta for distribution through the systemic circulation.

Once the oxygenated blood has been delivered to end-point tissues and organs, it arrives at the capillary bed. The now-deoxygenated blood begins the return journey back to the heart by passing from the capillary beds into small veins that feed into progressively larger veins and, ultimately, into the superior and inferior vena cava. The vena cava empties into the right atrium. From the right atrium, blood flows into the right ventricle and then into the pulmonary system for oxygenation.

When the right ventricle is impaired, it cannot effectively pump blood forward into the pulmonary system. The ineffective forward movement of blood causes an increase of venous pressure. When venous pressure rises, the blood backs up and leaks into the tissues and the liver. The end result is edema in the extremities and congestion within the liver.

When the LV is impaired, it cannot effectively pump blood forward into the aorta for systemic circulation. The ineffective forward movement of blood causes an increase in the pulmonary venous blood volume, which forces fluids from the capillaries to back up and leak into the pulmonary tissues. This results in pulmonary edema and impaired oxygenation.

Ejection fraction (EF) is the percentage of blood volume pumped out by the ventricles with each contraction. The normal EF is 50 to 70 percent. An EF of 60 percent means that 60 percent of the available blood volume was pumped out of the LV during contraction. It is an important measurement for diagnosing and tracking the progression of HF. The EF also differentiates between diastolic and systolic HF.

Diastolic HF is currently referred to as HF with normal ejection fraction (HFNEF). The heart muscle contracts normally, but the ventricles do not adequately relax during ventricular filling. In systolic HF, or heart failure with reduced ejection fraction (HFrEF), the heart muscle does not contract effectively, so less blood is pumped out to the body.

Variables

There are several variables that both impact and are impacted by HF. A review of these variables will provide the backdrop for a closer look at the classification, sequelae, symptoms, and treatment of HF.

Cardiac output (CO, or Q) is the volume of blood being pumped by the heart in one minute. It is the product of heart rate multiplied by stroke volume. **Stroke volume** (SV) is the amount of blood pumped out of the ventricles per beat; *CO = HR × SV*. Normal CO is between four and eight liters per minute. Both CO and SV are reduced in HF.

Systemic vascular resistance (SVR) is related to the diameter and elasticity of blood vessels and the viscosity of blood. For example, narrow and stiff vessels and/or thicker blood will cause an increase in SVR. An increase in SVR causes the LV to work harder to overcome the pressure at the aortic valve. Conversely, larger and more elastic vessels and/or thin blood will decrease SVR and reduce cardiac workload.

Pulmonary vascular resistance (PVR) is the vascular resistance of the pulmonary circulation. It is the difference between the mean pulmonary arterial pressure and the left atrial filling pressure. Resistance and blood viscosity impact both SVR and PVR. However, pulmonary blood flow, lung volume, and hypoxic vasoconstriction are unique to the pulmonary vasculature.

Preload is defined as the amount of ventricular stretch at the end of diastole, or when the chambers are filling. In other words, preload is the amount of pressure from the blood that is being exerted against the inside of the LV. It is also known as left ventricular end-diastolic pressure (LVEDP) and reflects the amount of stretch of cardiac muscle sarcomeres. **Afterload** is the amount of resistance the heart must overcome to open the aortic valve and push the blood volume into the systemic circulation.

Classification

HF is closely associated with chronic hypertension, CAD, and diabetes mellitus. The New York Heart Association (NYHA) classification tool is most frequently used to categorize the stages and symptom progression of HF as it relates to heart disease.

- Stage I: Cardiac disease; no symptoms during physical activity
- Stage II: Cardiac disease; slight limitations on physical activity
- Stage III: Cardiac disease; marked limitations during physical activity
- Stage IV: Cardiac disease; unable to perform physical activity; symptoms at rest

Sequelae

HF may have an acute or chronic onset, but it is progressive. When CO is diminished, tissues are not adequately perfused, and organs ultimately fail. When the LV works harder because of increased preload or afterload, its muscular walls becomes thick and enlarged, resulting in ventricular hypertrophy. Ventricular hypertrophy causes ventricular remodeling (cardiac remodeling), which is a change to the heart's size, shape, structure, and physiological functioning.

The sympathetic nervous system responds to a diminished CO by increasing the heart rate, constricting arteries, and activating the renin-angiotensin-aldosterone system (RAAS). Elevated angiotensin levels raise BP and afterload, thereby prompting the heart to work harder. The reduced CO caused by HF can diminish blood flow to the kidneys. The kidneys respond to the decreased perfusion by secreting renin and activating the RAAS. As a result, the increase in aldosterone signals the body to retain Na^+ and water. Retained Na^+ and water leads to volume overload, pulmonary congestion, and hypertension. The body's response to reduced CO caused by HF can perpetuate a downward spiral. However, there are naturally-occurring natriuretic peptides that are secreted in response to elevated pressures within the heart. These peptides counteract fluid retention and vasoconstriction.

Atrial natriuretic peptide (ANP) is secreted by the atria. **B-type natriuretic peptide** (BNP) is secreted by the ventricles. Both ANP and BNP cause diuresis, vasodilation, and decreased aldosterone secretion, thereby balancing the effects of sympathetic nervous system response and RAAS activation. Elevated levels of BNP are a diagnostic indication of HF.

Symptoms of Heart Failure

Either an MI or a dysrhythmia can precipitate HF. The clinical presentation reflects congestion in the pulmonary and/or systemic vasculature. Treatment depends on the clinical stage of the disease. Common symptoms include:

- Dyspnea on exertion
- Fatigue
- Pulmonary congestion, which causes a cough and difficulty breathing when lying down
- Feelings of suffocation and anxiety that are worse at night
- Peripheral edema

The most common cause of HF exacerbation is fluid overload due to nonadherence to sodium and water restrictions. Patient education is extremely critical to avoiding and managing exacerbations. Congestive heart failure is a core measure, tied to patient satisfaction, patient education, subsequent readmissions in a defined period of time, and ultimately, to reimbursements.

Treatment

Therapy for HF focuses on three primary goals: reduction of preload, reduction of afterload (SVR), and inhibition of the RAAS and vasoconstrictive mechanisms of the sympathetic nervous system. Pharmacotherapy includes ACE inhibitors, angiotensin II receptor blockers (ARBs), diuretics, beta-blockers, vasodilators, and a cardiac glycoside.

The ACE inhibitors and ARBs interfere with the RAAS by preventing the body's normal mechanism to retain fluids and constrict blood vessels. Diuretics decrease fluid volume and relieve both pulmonary and systemic congestion. Beta-blockers and cardiac glycosides slow the HR and strengthen the myocardium to improve contractility. Vasodilators decrease SVR. In addition to a thorough physical exam and complete medical history, a clinical work-up will include a chest x-ray, a BNP and other laboratory values, an ECG, and perhaps an echocardiogram or MUGA scan to measure EF.

Summary

HF is a common debilitating syndrome characterized by high mortality, frequent hospitalizations, multiple comorbidities, and poor quality of life. A partnership between providers, nurses, and patients is paramount to managing and slowing disease progression. Patient education should include a discussion of the disease process, prescribed medications, diet restrictions, and weight management. Patients should know which symptoms require immediate medical care. Self-care can be the most important aspect of HF management. The nurse as educator performs an essential role in this and all disease management.

Hypertension

Hypertension (HTN) is an abnormally high BP (140/90 mmHg or higher). The diagnosis is based on two or more accurate readings that are elevated. HTN is known as "the silent killer" because it is asymptomatic. Several variables impact BP and understanding them is essential.

Variables

BP is the product of CO multiplied by SVR; *BP = CO × SVR*. CO is the volume of blood being pumped by the heart in one minute. It is the product of HR multiplied by SV; *HR × SV = CO*. SV is the amount of blood pumped out of the ventricles per beat.

SVR is related to the diameter of blood vessels and the viscosity of blood. The narrower the vessels or the thicker the blood, the higher the SVR. Conversely, larger-diameter vessels and thinner blood decrease SVR.

Mechanism

For HTN to develop, there must be a change in one or more factors affecting SVR or CO and a problem with the control system responsible for regulating BP. The body normally maintains and adjusts BP by either increasing the HR or the strength of myocardial contraction or by dilating or constricting the veins and arterioles.

When veins are dilated, less blood returns to the heart, and subsequently, less blood is pumped out of the heart. The result is a decrease in CO. Conversely, when veins are constricted, more blood is returned to the heart, and CO is increased. The arterioles also dilate or constrict. An expanded arteriole reduces resistance, and a constricted arteriole increases resistance. The veins and arterioles impact both CO and SVR. The kidneys contribute to the maintenance and adjustment of BP by controlling Na+, chloride, and water excretion and through the RAAS. Management of HTN will focus on one or more of the factors that regulate BP. Those regulatory factors are SVR, fluid volume, and the strength and rate of myocardial contraction.

Classification

HTN is classified as primary or secondary depending on the etiology. In **primary HTN**, the cause is unknown, but the primary factors include problems related to the natriuretic hormones or RAAS or electrolyte disturbances. Primary HTN is also known as essential or idiopathic HTN.

In **secondary HTN**, there is an identifiable cause. Associated disease states include kidney disease, adrenal gland tumors, thyroid disease, congenital blood vessel disorders, alcohol abuse, and obstructive sleep apnea. Products associated with secondary HTN are nonsteroidal anti-inflammatory drugs (NSAIDs), birth control pills, decongestants, cocaine, amphetamines, and corticosteroids.

HTN normally increases with age, and it is more prominent among African Americans. BP is classified according to treatment guidelines as normal, pre-HTN, Stage 1 HTN, and Stage 2 HTN. **Pre-HTN** is defined as systolic pressures ranging from 120 to 139 mmHg and diastolic pressures ranging from 80 to 89 mmHg. **Stage 1 HTN** ranges from 140 to 159 mmHg systolic and 90 to 99 mmHg diastolic pressures. In the more severe Stage 2 HTN, systolic pressures are 160 mmHg or higher, and diastolic pressures are 100 mmHg or higher.

Sequelae

Systolic pressure is the amount of pressure exerted on arterial walls immediately after ventricular contraction and emptying. This represents the highest level of pressure during the cardiac cycle. Diastolic pressure is the amount of pressure exerted on arterials walls when the heart is filling. This represents the lowest pressure during the cardiac cycle. In general, hypertension increases the risk of cardiovascular disease; diastolic HTN poses a greater risk.

Prolonged HTN damages the delicate endothelial layer of vessels. The damaged endothelium initiates the inflammatory response and clotting cascade. As mentioned, the diameter of veins, arterioles, and arteries changes SVR. When SVR is increased, the heart must work harder to pump against the increased pressure. In other words, the pressure in the LV must be higher than the pressure being exerted on the opposite side of the aortic valve by systemic vascular pressure. The ventricular pressure must overcome the aortic pressure for contraction and ventricular emptying to occur. When the myocardium works against an elevated systemic pressure for a prolonged period of time, the LV will enlarge, and HF may ensue.

Risk Factors

There are both modifiable and nonmodifiable risk factors associated with the development of HTN. Modifiable risk factors include obesity, a sedentary lifestyle, tobacco use, a diet high in sodium, dyslipidemia, excessive alcohol consumption, stress, sleep apnea, and diabetes. Age, race, and family history are nonmodifiable risk factors.

Treatment

First-line treatments include lifestyle changes and pharmacologic therapy.

Initial therapy includes diuretics, CCBs, ACE inhibitors, and ARBs. Diuretics decrease fluid volume. CCBs decrease myocardial contractility. Both ACE inhibitors and ARBs interfere with the RAAS by preventing the normal mechanism that retains fluids and narrows blood vessels. The result is decreased volume and SVR.

Hypertensive Crisis/Emergency

A **hypertensive crisis** is defined as a BP higher than 180/120 mmHg. BP must be lowered quickly to prevent end organ damage. Pregnancy, an acute MI, a dissecting aortic aneurysm, and an intracranial hemorrhage are associated with a hypertensive crisis. The therapeutic goal is to reduce the BP by 25 percent within the first hour of treatment with a continual reduction over the following 2 to 6 hours and an ongoing reduction to the target goal over a period of days. Short-acting antihypertensive medications administered intravenously is the primary treatment.

Summary

The astute nurse will conduct an in-depth patient interview to identify prescribed and illicit drug use, alcohol and tobacco use, family history, sleep patterns, and dietary habits. Patient education should include information about the Dietary Approach to Stop Hypertension (DASH) diet and alcohol in moderation with a limit of one to two drinks per day. Aerobic exercise and resistance training three to four times weekly for an average of 40 minutes is recommended. Information about prescribed hypertensive medications should also be reviewed with the patient.

Pericardial Tamponade

Cardiac tamponade, or **pericardial tamponade**, is a syndrome caused by the excessive accumulation of blood or fluid in the pericardial sac, resulting in the compression of the myocardium and reduced ventricular filling. It is a medical emergency with complications of pulmonary edema, shock, and death, if left untreated.

The pericardium, or outer layer of the heart wall, is a two-layer membrane that forms the pericardial sac, which envelops the heart. The parietal (outer) layer of the pericardium is made of tough, thickened fibrous tissue. This layer is attached to the mid-diaphragm and to the back of the sternum. These attachments keep the heart in place during acceleration or deceleration. The fibrous nature of the parietal layer prevents cardiac distention into the mediastinal region of the chest.

The visceral (inner) layer of the pericardium is a double-layered membrane. One layer is affixed to the heart. The second layer lines the inside of the parietal (outer) layer. The small space between the parietal and visceral layers is the pericardial space. The space normally contains between 15 and 50 milliliters of pericardial fluid. The pericardial fluid lubricates the membranes and allows the two layers to slide over one another as the heart beats.

A pericardial effusion develops when excess blood or fluid accumulates in the pericardial sac. If the effusion progresses, a pericardial tamponade will ensue. Because the fibrous parietal layer prevents cardiac distention, the pressure from the excessive blood or fluid is exerted inward, compressing the myocardium and reducing space for blood to fill the chambers. The normally low-pressure right ventricle and atrium are the first structures to be impacted by tamponade. Therefore, signs of right-sided HF such as jugular vein distention, edema, and hepatomegaly may be present.

Symptoms of a pericardial tamponade are dyspnea, chest tightness, dizziness, tachycardia, muffled heart sounds, and restlessness. Pulsus paradoxus is an important clinical finding in tamponade; it represents an abnormal BP variation during the respiration cycle and is evidenced by a decrease of 10 mmHg or more in systolic BP during inspiration. Pulsus paradoxus represents decreased diastolic ventricular filling and reduced volume in all four chambers of the heart. The clinical signs associated with tamponade are distended neck veins, muffled heart sounds, and hypotension. These clustered symptoms are known as **Beck's triad**.

Removal of the pericardial fluid via pericardiocentesis is the definitive therapy. A pericardiectomy or pericardial window may be performed to remove part of the pericardium. Fluid removed during the procedure is analyzed to determine the cause of the effusion. Malignancies, metastatic disease, and trauma are major causes of the development of pericardial effusions.

Identification and treatment of a tamponade requires emergent medical intervention. A rapid focused assessment of heart sounds and BP, including assessing for pulsus paradoxus, is a critical first step. An in-depth medical and surgical history can aid in identifying the etiology.

Pericarditis

Pericarditis is inflammation of the pericardium, which forms the pericardial sac that surrounds the heart.

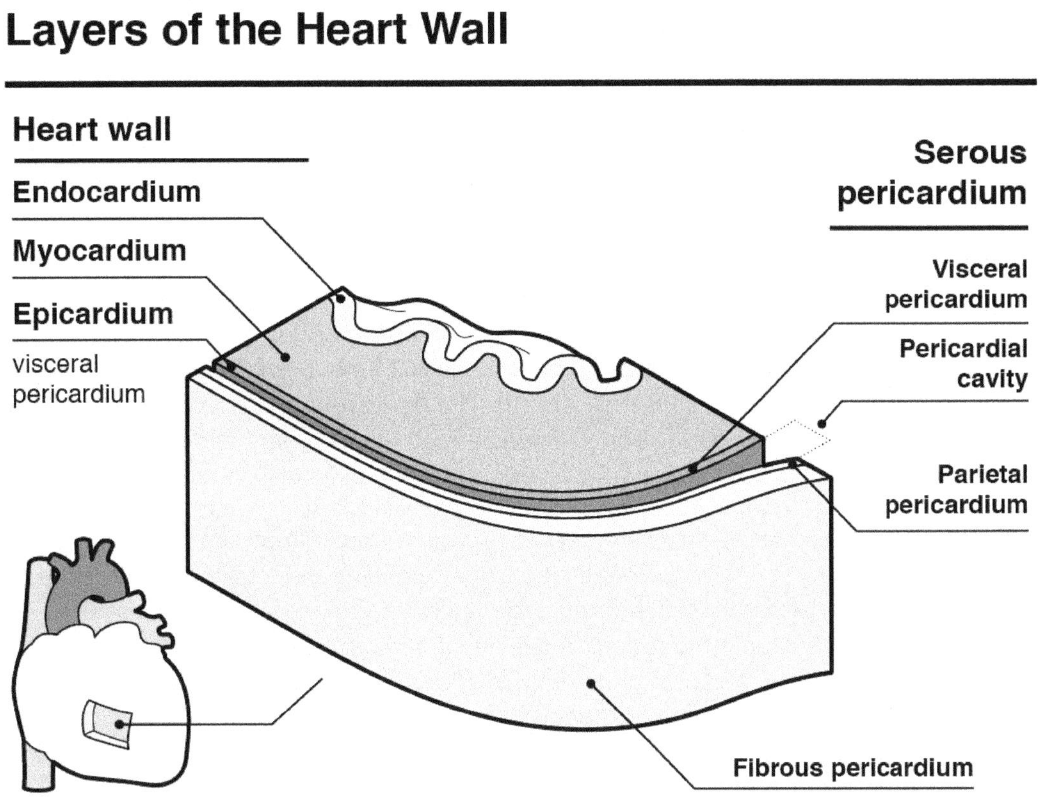

The pericardial sac consists of two layers. The pericardium, or outer layer of the heart wall, is a two-layer membrane that forms the pericardial sac, which envelops the heart.

The visceral (inner) layer of the pericardium is a double-layered membrane. One layer is affixed to the heart. The second layer lines the inside of the parietal layer (outer layer). The small space between the parietal and visceral layers is the pericardial space. The space normally contains between 15 and 50 milliliters of pericardial fluid. The pericardial fluid lubricates the membranes and allows the two layers to slide over one another as the heart beats.

The parietal (outer) layer of the pericardium is made of tough, thickened fibrous tissue. This layer is attached to the mid-diaphragm and to the back of the sternum.

These attachments keep the heart in place during acceleration or deceleration. The fibrous nature of the parietal layer prevents cardiac distention into the mediastinal region of the chest. It separates the heart from the surrounding structures, and it protects the heart against infection and inflammation from the lungs. The pericardium contains pain receptors and mechanoreceptors, both of which prompt reflex changes in the BP and HR.

Pericarditis can be either acute or chronic in presentation. Causes are varied and include an acute MI; bacterial, fungal, and viral infections; certain medications; chest trauma; connective tissue disorders such as lupus or rheumatic fever; metastatic lesions from lung or breast tumors; and a history of radiation therapy of the chest and upper torso. Frequent or prolonged episodes of pericarditis can lead to thickening and scarring of the pericardium and loss of elasticity. These conditions limit the heart's ability to fill with blood, and therefore limit the amount of blood being pumped out to the body. The result is a decrease in CO. Pericarditis can also cause fluid to accumulate in the pericardial cavity, known as **pericardial effusion**.

A characteristic symptom of pericarditis is chest pain. The pain is persistent, sharp, pleuritic, felt in the mid-chest, and aggravated by deep inhalation. Pericarditis may also cause ST elevation, thereby mimicking an acute MI, or it may be asymptomatic.

A pericardial friction rub is diagnostic of pericarditis. It is a creaky or scratchy sound heard at the end of exhalation. The rub is best heard when the patient is sitting and leaning forward. Stethoscope placement should be at the left lower sternal border in the fourth intercostal space. The rub is audible on auscultation and synchronous to the heartbeat. A pericardial friction rub is differentiated from a pleural friction rub by having patients hold their breath. The pericardial friction rub will remain constant with the heartbeat. Other presenting symptoms include a mild fever, cough, and dyspnea. Common laboratory findings are elevated white blood cell (WBC), ESR, or CRP levels.

The diagnosis of pericarditis is based on history, signs, and symptoms. Treatment goals are to determine the cause, administer therapy for treatment and symptom relief, and detect signs of complications. A thorough medical and surgical history will identify patients at risk for developing pericarditis. The physical assessment should evaluate the reported pain level during position changes, inspiration, expiration, coughing, swallowing, and breath holding. In addition, flexion, extension, and rotation of the neck and spine should be assessed for their influence on reported pain.

Peripheral Vascular Disease

Peripheral vascular disease (PVD) refers to diseases of the blood vessels that are outside the heart and brain. The term PVD is used interchangeably with **peripheral arterial disease** (PAD). It is the narrowing of peripheral vessels caused by atherosclerosis. The narrowing can be compounded by emboli or thrombi. Limb ischemia due to reduced blood flow can result in loss of limb or life. The primary factor for the development of PVD is atherosclerosis.

PVD encompasses several conditions: atherosclerosis, Buerger's disease, chronic venous insufficiency, deep vein thrombosis (DVT), Raynaud's phenomenon, thrombophlebitis, and varicose veins.

Risk Factors

CAD, atrial fibrillation, cerebrovascular disease (stroke), and renal disease are common comorbidities. Risk factors include smoking, phlebitis, injury, surgery, and hyperviscosity of the blood. Autoimmune disorders and hyperlipidemia are also common factors. The two major complications of PVD are limb complications or loss and the risk for stroke or heart attack.

Symptoms

Intermittent claudication (cramping pain in the leg during exercise) may be the sole manifestation of early symptomatic PVD. It occurs with exercise and stops with rest. Physical findings during examination may include the classic five Ps: pulselessness, paralysis, paresthesia, pain, and pallor of the extremity.

The most critical symptom of PVD is critical limb ischemia (CLI), which is pain that occurs in the affected limb during rest. Manifestations of PVD may include the following symptoms:

- Feet that are cool or cold to the touch
- Aching or burning in the legs that is relieved by sitting
- Pale color when legs are elevated
- Redness when legs are in a hanging-down (dependent) position
- Brittle, thin, or shiny skin on the legs and feet
- Loss of hair on feet
- Nonhealing wounds or ulcers over pressure points
- Loss of muscle or fatty tissue
- Numbness, weakness, or heaviness in muscles
- Reddish-blue discoloration of the extremities
- Restricted mobility
- Thickened, opaque toenails

Diagnostics

The ankle-brachial index (ABI) should be measured. The ABI is the systolic pressure at the ankle, divided by the systolic pressure at the arm. It is a specific and sensitive indicator of peripheral artery disease (PAD). The Allen test looks for an occlusion of either the radial or ulnar arteries. A Doppler ultrasonography flow study can determine the patency of peripheral arteries.

The patient should be assessed for heart murmurs, and all peripheral pulses should be evaluated for quality and bruit. An ECG may reveal an arrhythmia. Because the presence of atherosclerosis initiates an inflammatory response, inflammatory markers such as the D-dimer, CRP, interleukin 6, and homocysteine may be present. Blood urea nitrogen (BUN) and creatinine levels may provide indications of decreased organ perfusion. A lipid profile may reveal the risk for atherosclerosis. A stress test or angiogram may be necessary.

Treatment

The two main goals for treatment of PVD are to control the symptoms and halt the progression to lower the risk of heart attack and stroke. Specific treatment modalities depend on the extent and severity of the disease, the patient's age, overall medical history, clinical signs, and his or her preferences. Lifestyle modifications include smoking cessation, improved nutrition, and regular exercise. Aggressive treatment of comorbidities can also aid in stopping the progression. Pharmacotherapy may include anticoagulants and vasodilators.

Summary

The primary factor in PVD is atherosclerosis. Prevention should begin early and be centered on balanced nutrition and exercise, alcohol in moderation, and smoking cessation. Once diagnosed, management of PVD will include preventive measures and the incorporation of pharmacotherapeutics. Providing patient education about proper diet and exercise should occur during every patient encounter. The conscientious nurse will take advantage of an encounter to improve patient outcomes through education and referral.

Thromboembolic Disease

In simplest terms, a **thrombus** is a blood clot that forms in a vein. Clots can be caused by either a fat globule, gas bubble, amniotic fluid, or any foreign material that gets into the bloodstream. A DVT usually forms in the leg. A thrombus becomes an **embolus** when a fragment dislodges and travels through the circulatory system. The embolus will remain in the circulatory system until it reaches a vessel too narrow for its passage. An **embolism** occurs when the embolus lodges and prevents blood flow. In the cardiac cycle, veins begin at the capillary bed and get progressively larger as they return deoxygenated blood to the right side of the heart. From the right side of the heart, blood flows to the lungs.

A **pulmonary embolism** (PE) occurs when the embolus, or a fragment of the embolus, becomes lodged in the pulmonary circulation. A DVT frequently results in a PE. A **fat embolism** may form when fat globules pass into the small vessels and damage the endothelial lining. As the fat breaks down to free fatty acids, it causes toxic damage. When the damage occurs in the lungs, acute respiratory failure ensues.

Mechanism

A strong clinical link exists between clot formation and atherosclerosis, PAD, diabetes, and other factors contributing to heart disease. Anything that damages a vein's endothelial lining may cause a DVT to form. Damage to vessel lining can occur from smoking, cancer, chemotherapy, injury, or surgery. In addition to a damaged endothelial layer, increased age, dehydration, and viscous or slow-flowing blood increase the risk of DVT formation. Factors that slow blood flow are prolonged bed rest, sitting for extended periods, smoking, obesity, and HF. In the presence of atrial fibrillation, the atria do not empty adequately. Blood pools in the upper chambers, increasing the risk for clots to form.

Closed long-bone fractures carry a high risk for a fat embolism to develop because when the bone marrow is exposed as a result of a fracture, its particles can enter the bloodstream. Orthopedic procedures, a bone marrow biopsy, massive soft tissue injury, and severe burns are also associated with the development of an embolus. In addition, there are nontraumatic conditions associated with a fat embolism, such as prolonged corticosteroid therapy, pancreatitis, liposuction, fatty liver, and osteomyelitis.

Women who are pregnant or taking oral contraceptives are at risk for the development of an embolus. Estrogen increases plasma fibrinogen, some coagulation factors, and platelet formation, which lead to the hypercoagulability of the blood. During pregnancy, the expanding uterus can slow blood flow in the veins. The combined effects of hypercoagulability and slowed blood flow exacerbate the risk. During delivery, an embolus can form from the amniotic fluid and travel through maternal circulation. Therefore, during pregnancy and the subsequent postpartum period, women are at increased risk for DVT formation.

Symptoms

Swelling of the leg below the knee is a common symptom of a DVT. There may also be redness, tenderness, or pain over the area around the clot, but a DVT may be asymptomatic. When a DVT becomes a PE, the patient may experience difficulty breathing and a rapid HR. Reported symptoms may include chest pain, coughing up blood, fainting, and low BP. There is a 24- to 72-hour latent period from injury to onset in the development of a fat embolism.

Diagnosis and Treatment

The clinician will consider presenting signs and symptoms, the patient's and family's medical history, and an ultrasound to evaluate blood flow to identify a DVT. The differential diagnoses are pneumonia and a thrombus. A vena cava filter may be placed in the inferior vena cava to capture a clot or fragments. In life-threatening situations such as a PE, an IV thrombolytic may be used to break up the clot. Indications for thrombolytic therapy are chest pain lasting longer than 20 minutes, ST elevation in two leads, and less than 6 hours from the pain's onset. However, thrombolytic medications are absolutely contraindicated in a patient with active bleeding. Prior to the administration of a thrombolytic, the international normalized ration (INR) must be calculated to determine clotting time. In healthy people, an INR of 1.1 or below is considered normal. An INR range of 2.0 to 3.0 is an effective acceptable therapeutic range for people taking warfarin.

For long-term management, patient education should include anticoagulant medication therapy, the use of compression stockings, and avoidance of tight clothing. Patients should be instructed to regularly elevate their feet, avoid prolonged periods of sitting, and increase their exercise to counteract slowed blood flow.

Trauma

The causes of trauma can be categorized into three types, according to their potential degree of injury: penetrating injuries, blunt nonpenetrating injuries, and medical injuries that occur during an invasive procedure. **Penetrating injuries** are associated with knife and gunshot wounds. **Blunt nonpenetrating** injuries are most commonly due to automobile accidents. **Medical injuries** may occur during the implantation of a medical device, an endomyocardial biopsy, the placement of a Swan-Ganz catheter, and cardiopulmonary resuscitation (CPR).

Trauma is evaluated according to a prioritized systematic assessment approach that starts with the primary survey and proceeds to the secondary survey. The findings gathered during the surveys in conjunction with the type of injury identified will direct the treatment approach.

Types of Injuries

A penetrating injury is categorized by the mechanism of injury as low, medium, or high velocity. A knife wound is low velocity, disrupting just the surface penetrated. A handgun wound, or medium-velocity injury, damages more than the penetrated surface, but less than a high-velocity injury. A high-velocity injury is related to rifles and military weapons.

Penetrating chest trauma comprises a broad spectrum of injury and severity. Any structure within the thoracic cavity may be impacted, such as the heart and great vessels, the tracheobronchial tree, the esophagus, the diaphragm, and surrounding bony structures.

The following conditions may result from penetrating chest trauma: hemothorax, pneumothorax, or pneumomediastinum. These conditions compromise oxygenation and ventilation. A diaphragmatic rupture, pulmonary contusion, rib or sternal fractures, and esophageal or thoracic tears may be present.

A blunt nonpenetrating injury can also affect any of the components of the thoracic cavity. The major damage from both penetrating and nonpenetrating injuries involves derangement in the flow of air, blood, or both. If esophageal perforations are present, alimentary contents may leak into the bloodstream, causing sepsis. Blunt injuries can be further categorized according to the area of impact.

- Chest wall fractures, dislocations, or diaphragmatic injuries
- The pleural lining, the lungs, and upper digestive tract
- The heart, great arteries, veins, and lymphatics

Trauma Survey

The **primary survey** begins with the ABCDE resuscitation system: airway, breathing, circulation, disability or neurological status, and exposure. Adjuncts to the primary survey are x-rays, an EKG, laboratory testing, and the focused assessment with sonography in trauma (FAST) examinations.

Trauma patients may not be able to provide a historical account or verbalize symptoms. Injuries within the thoracic cavity can quickly become life-threatening. Hypoxia and hypoventilation are the major causes of death in chest trauma. Therefore, the FAST examinations can provide a timely diagnosis when compared to older methods of assessment. Blood and fluid tend to pool in dependent areas within the body. The primary FAST examination includes the hepatorenal recess (Morison pouch), the perisplencic view, the subxiphoid pericardial window, and the suprapubic window (Douglas pouch). The extended version (E-FAST) incorporates additional views of the thoracic cavity to assess for hemothorax and pneumothorax. These specific views can rapidly identify injuries and bleeding in the pericardial, pleural, and peritoneal areas. The ease and noninvasiveness of the FAST approach allows for serial examinations to observe changes and monitor progression.

The **secondary survey** incorporates the physical assessment beginning with the ample history acronym. Allergies, medication, past illnesses, last meal, and events, environment, or mechanism of injury are assessed. The head-to-toe physical assessment should be done using inspection, auscultation, percussion, and palpation, as appropriate.

The head, face, and neck are first assessed for injury. The presence of Battle's sign or raccoon's eyes may indicate intracranial bleeding. Central nervous system function is evaluated using the Glasgow Coma Scale (GCS). Motor, verbal, and eye responses are graded from total paralysis (3) to normal strength (15). Next, the chest, abdomen, pelvis, perineal, rectal, and genital areas are assessed for injury. Finally, the neurovascular status of the musculoskeletal system is evaluated.

In addition to sonographic and physical assessments, trauma scoring systems are used by clinicians to identify the severity of the trauma and to guide treatment, ensure continuous quality improvement, and direct future research.

Severity Scoring

Scoring the level of injury in a trauma patient has several applications, and there are a variety of tools available for use. **Field trauma** scoring can guide prehospital triage decisions, reduce time of transfer and treatment, and maximize resources. It also serves as a quality assurance measure between facilities and during transfer.

Trauma scoring tools are categorized according to the data points they evaluate as either physiologic, anatomical, or combined.

Physiologic Scoring Tools

The **Revised Trauma Score** (RTS) is the most common physiologic scoring tool in use. The RTS combines three parameters: the GCS, systolic blood pressure (SBP), and respiratory rate (RR). The best motor or eye-opening response can be substituted for the GCS in the presence of central nervous system influences such as drugs or alcohol.

Revised Trauma Score			
Coded Value	**GCS**	**Systolic Blood Pressure (mmHg)**	**Respiratory Rate (breaths per minute)**
0	3	0	0
1	4-5	< 50	< 5
2	6-8	50-75	5-9
3	9-12	76-90	> 30
4	13-15	> 90	10-30

The **Acute Physiology and Chronic Health Evaluation** (APACHE II) scoring tool incorporates the chronic health evaluation and comorbid conditions with the Acute Physiology Score (APS).

The **Emergency Trauma Score** (EMTRAS) uses patient data that is quickly available, and it does not require knowledge of anatomic injuries. EMTRAS comprises patient age, GCS, base excess, and prothrombin time (PT) to accurately predict mortality.

Anatomic and Combined Scoring Tools

The **Injury Severity Score** (ISS) tool is based on the Abbreviated Injury Scale (AIS). The ISS uses an anatomical scoring system to give an overall score for patients who have sustained multiple injuries, each of which is assigned an AIS score. Only the highest AIS score for each of six different body regions (head, face, chest, abdomen, extremities and pelvis, and external) is used. The ISS tool grades the severity of injury from minor injury (1) to lethal injury (6); the three most severely injured body regions have their score squared and added together to produce the ISS score. The Trauma and Injury Severity Scoring (TRISS) tool combines ISS, RTS, and the age of the patient to grade severity and predict mortality.

Summary

Regardless of the cause or degree of injury, the astute clinician begins the assessment with the primary survey. The secondary survey focusing on the head-to-toe physical assessment also includes evaluation of the FAST examination, x-rays, laboratory testing, and severity scoring tools. Although there is no universally accepted tool for scoring the severity of trauma, there are many valid tools. Coupled with clinician judgment, the assessment findings and severity scoring tools can improve and predict mortality.

Shock

Cardiogenic Shock

The clinical definition of **cardiogenic shock** is decreased CO and evidence of tissue hypoxia in the presence of adequate intravascular volume. It is a medical emergency and the most severe expression of LV failure. It is the leading cause of death following an MI with mortality rates between 70 and 90 percent without aggressive treatment. When a large area of the myocardium becomes ischemic, the heart cannot pump effectively. Therefore, SV, CO, and BP drastically decline. The result is end-point hypoperfusion and organ failure. Characteristics of cardiogenic shock include ashen, cyanotic, or mottled extremities; distant heart sounds; and rapid and faint peripheral pulses. Additional signs of hypoperfusion such as altered mental status and decreased urine output may be present.

Work-Up/Treatment

The key to survival in cardiogenic shock is rapid diagnosis, supportive therapy, and coronary artery revascularization. Diagnosis is based on clinical presentation, cardiac and metabolic laboratory studies, chest x-ray, ECG, echocardiogram, and invasive hemodynamic monitoring. Treatment is the restoration of coronary blood flow and correction of electrolyte and acid-base abnormalities.

Obstructive Shock

Obstructive shock occurs when the heart or the great vessels are mechanically obstructed. A cardiac tamponade or massive PE is a frequent cause of obstructive shock. Systemic circulatory collapse occurs because blood flow in or out of the heart is blocked. Generalized treatment goals for shock are to identify and correct the underlying cause. In the case of obstructive shock, the goal is to remove the obstruction.

Treatment begins simultaneously with evaluation. Stabilization of the airway, breathing, and circulation are primary, followed by fluid resuscitation to increase BP. Vital signs, urine flow, and mental status using the GCS should be monitored. Shock patients should be kept warm. Serial measurements of renal and hepatic function, electrolyte levels, and ABGs should be monitored.

Summary

Shock is characterized by organ blood flow that is inadequate to meet the oxygen demands of the tissue. The management goal for shock is to restore oxygen delivery to the tissues and reverse the perfusion deficit. This is accomplished through fluid resuscitation, increasing CO with inotropes, and raising the SVR with vasopressors.

Diabetes (Types 1 & 2)/Other Endocrine/Immunological

Diabetic Situations

Diabetes is a common diagnosis among patients in the United States. It is a disease in which the body's natural insulin response to blood glucose is compromised, causing hyperglycemia. **Hyperglycemia** is a dangerously high blood sugar that can damage the organs and tissues of the body.

The nursing assistant will become accustomed to taking care of patients with diabetes. These patients may have a special diabetic diet that restricts or counts carbohydrates; may need blood sugar levels taken before meals, upon rising, and before going to bed, depending on their specific orders; and will need special care in case their blood sugar becomes dangerously low or high.

Insulin is a hormone secreted by the pancreas in the body. No other organ secretes insulin. The **pancreas** is positioned behind the stomach in the body, making it conveniently situated to assist with the absorption and distribution of glucose that enters the body. Glucose enters through the food that one eats, is a type of sugar, and is necessary for metabolic functioning in the body. Insulin works in the blood stream to allow glucose to be absorbed into the cells of the body.

When the insulin response is compromised, as is the case in diabetes, it is no longer effective in moving glucose from the bloodstream into the cells of the body. The glucose then accumulates in the blood stream with nowhere to go, and the resulting state is called **hyperglycemia.** The cells of the body need glucose to survive and are unable to function if they are unable to obtain glucose from the bloodstream.

There are two main types of diabetic emergencies: **hypoglycemia**, in which the blood sugar is too low; and **hyperglycemia**, in which the blood sugar is too high.

Hypoglycemia is when the blood sugar of a patient drops below 70 milligrams per deciliter (mg/dL). Patients may develop this if they have had too much insulin or have not ingested enough dietary glucose. This can sometimes occur in a hospital or facility if a patient misses meals due to scheduled tests or procedures. The nursing assistant should be vigilant about the patient getting regular meals and if not, work with the nurse to keep them aware of the situation so that insulin dosages can be adjusted or meals can be obtained.

Symptoms of hypoglycemia include decreased level of consciousness, tremors, fatigue, excessive sweating, dizziness, and syncope (fainting). The patient may also become anxious, report blurred vision, headache, or have slurred speech.

If the nursing assistant sees signs of hypoglycemia, this should be reported immediately to the nurse. The nursing assistant should expect to collect a blood glucose reading and a set of vital signs. The nurse will likely administer prescribed oral glucose, IV dextrose, or perhaps parenteral glucagon to correct the blood sugar.

Hyperglycemia is a blood sugar level greater than 200 milligrams per deciliter. Normal blood sugar recommendations are usually between 70 and 130 milligrams per deciliter, but symptoms of hyperglycemia may not manifest until the blood sugar level is greater than 200 milligrams per deciliter. Hyperglycemia may go unnoticed since the patient may not have symptoms of high blood sugar. It is therefore important to obtain blood sugar levels as necessary, even if the patient is not showing symptoms.

Hyperglycemia can be caused by the patient not having adequate insulin and/or anti-diabetic medication management, ingesting more glucose than normal, illness that changes normal routine, or a personal crisis that has occurred causing emotional stress in the body.

The nursing assistant should recognize the most common symptoms of hyperglycemia: an increased need to urinate, called **polyuria**, and excessive thirst, called **polydipsia.** If hyperglycemia has caused complications such as **diabetic ketoacidosis** (an acidotic metabolic state in the body), a patient may display these two symptoms, as well as nausea, abdominal pain, fruity-scented breath, and/or confusion.

Diabetic ketoacidosis is a metabolic imbalance that can cause a condition called **diabetic coma**, when the blood sugar becomes so high that the patient loses consciousness. If diabetic coma is not treated, the patient may not survive.

If signs and symptoms of either hypoglycemia or hyperglycemia are present in the patient, the nursing assistant must report this immediately to the nurse in order to stabilize the patient's blood glucose.

Sudden Onset of Confusion or Agitation

Patients who have entered a facility or hospital may experience periods of confusion or agitation. This may be an acute situation for the individual or part of an ongoing diagnosis of dementia or Alzheimer's disease. A severe and acute situation that involves confusion and agitation is called **delirium**. The nursing assistant should be aware of these different situations, their causes, and what can be done to assist the patient back to normal functioning.

Confusion and agitation are symptoms of an underlying condition or disease. Patients who once were oriented to who they were, where they were, what circumstances brought them to the facility, and the time may become confused on one or all of these points. They will suddenly not understand and become uncertain about the facts of their situation.

A patient who is agitated may display an acute anxiety about seemingly small details of their stay at the hospital or facility, perhaps even becoming verbally or physically abusive toward staff. In either of these situations, if the confusion and agitation are new, they should be reported to the nurse immediately for further investigation. Usually if the cause can be found, the situation can be corrected.

Delirium is a mental disturbance involving confusion, decreased awareness of surroundings, and sometimes agitation that causes a patient to lose focus and attention. This condition is usually transient in nature, not lasting for long if appropriate interventions are applied. Delirium usually occurs in the presence of an illness, as a sign of drug toxicity, and in situations of dehydration, where the body's fluids and electrolytes are out of balance. A patient who is older, has Parkinson's disease, dementia, or a history of stroke may be at a greater risk to develop delirium.

Patients with dementia or Alzheimer's disease may be prone to periods of heightened agitation or confusion. A person with these conditions is also more prone to acute periods of delirium. **Dementia** is a chronic, long-term condition that involves decreased cognitive ability over time, while delirium happens quickly and usually does not last long.

The nursing assistant should work with the rest of the health care team to create an environment around the confused patient that is conducive to calm, collected behavior. This includes making the environment around the patient as stable as possible, without bright lights, loud and/or sudden noises, and unexpected interruptions to the patient's expected routine.

Including items in a patient's room such as family photographs and other familiar objects can be visual reminders to the patient about their circumstances.

If the patient has sensory deficits such as visual or hearing loss, the nursing assistant should ensure that these are addressed. The patient's hearing aid batteries should be kept refreshed, glasses and dentures in a place where they can be easily accessed, and assistive walking devices such as canes or walkers at hand if appropriate. Granting the patient as much freedom and familiarity as possible will assist the patient in functioning while in the facility.

The nursing assistant can help patients with confusion and agitation by listening to their needs, maintaining a calm, collected, and professional attitude, talking about what the daily tasks and expectations are, and reorienting the patient whenever necessary. The nursing assistant must work with patients based on their cognitive abilities to assure that they can work with the health care team effectively without becoming overwhelmed and confused.

Family members and/or friends of the patient are valuable resources when dealing with confusion, especially if it is a long-standing issue. The patient's loved ones may have developed some tips and tricks for helping the patient regain orientation that can be used by the health care team.

Endocrine Conditions

The endocrine system is responsible for hormone production and messaging. These hormones are produced by glands through the brain and body. They regulate a vast number of mental, emotional, and physiological functions, such as mood, growth, metabolism, sleep, sexual function, and reproduction. Consequently, some pathological conditions can have system-wide repercussions.

Adrenal Conditions

Located on top of each kidney, the adrenal glands are responsible for producing a number of hormones. These include sex hormones, such as DHEA and androstenedione; corticosteroids, such as cortisol; and mineralocorticoids, such as aldosterone. These hormones influence sexual function, metabolism, electrolyte balance, blood volume, blood pressure, immunity, and stress management. Dysfunctional conditions of the adrenal glands include the following:

Cushing's Syndrome

This disease results from an excess of glucocorticoid, which is responsible for producing steroids that manage inflammation and other stresses in the body. One example of a glucocorticoid is cortisol. Symptoms of Cushing's syndrome include excessive weight gain that cannot be managed, excessive growth of body hair, high blood pressure, and decreased elasticity in the skin. This disease is typically treated with medication that controls hormone production. In severe cases, adrenal surgery may be required.

Addison's Disease

This disease may be referred to as *adrenal insufficiency*. It results when the adrenal glands produce insufficient amounts of glucocorticoids and mineralocorticoids. Mineralocorticoids are another group of steroids influencing electrolyte and fluid balance. This can be the result of an underlying autoimmune disorder or systemic infection. Symptoms include fatigue and skin discoloration. Addison's disease is usually treated with steroid injections but may become a medical crisis if the patient goes into shock, a stupor, or a coma. This can occur if the patient does not realize he or she has the disease, as some of the primary symptoms can be quite generic.

Conn's Syndrome

This disease is characterized by excess aldosterone production. Symptoms include hypertension, muscle cramping, weakness, dehydration, and excessive thirst. It is usually treated by surgically removing any tumors on the adrenal glands, and the patient may be asked to minimize table salt consumption. If Conn's syndrome goes untreated, it can result in serious cardiovascular and kidney disease.

Adrenal Tumors

The presence of malignant or benign tumors on the adrenal glands may affect hormone production, which can cause one of the above disorders to develop.

Glucose-Related Conditions

The endocrine system handles processes related to the metabolism of glucose.

Disorders relating to glucose include the following:

Diabetes Mellitus

This is a condition that affects how the body responds to the presence of glucose. Glucose is needed for cell functioning, and all consumable calories eventually are converted to glucose in the body. A hormone produced by the pancreas, called **insulin**, is needed to break down food and drink into glucose molecules. In patients with type 1 diabetes, the pancreas fails to produce insulin, leading to high levels of glucose in the bloodstream. This can lead to organ damage, organ failure, or nerve damage. Patients with type 1 diabetes receive daily insulin injections or have a pump that continuously monitors their blood insulin levels and releases insulin as needed. These patients need to be careful to not administer excess insulin, as this will cause their blood sugar to become too low. Low blood sugar can lead to fainting and exhaustion and may require hospitalization.

In patients with type 2 diabetes, the pancreas produces insulin, but the body is unable to use it effectively. Patients with type 2 diabetes typically need to manage their condition through lifestyle changes, such as losing weight and eating fewer carbohydrate-rich and sugary foods. There are also some medications that help the body use the insulin that is present in the bloodstream. Gestational diabetes is a form of diabetes that some women develop during the second to third trimester of pregnancy, when their systems temporarily become resistant to insulin. High blood sugar in a pregnant woman can affect fetal growth and influence the baby's risk of becoming obese. Pregnant women with gestational diabetes are encouraged to exercise daily, avoid excessive weight gain, and carefully monitor their diet. Gestational diabetes is similar to type 2 diabetes in the way symptoms present and in treatment options.

Diabetic Ketoacidosis

This is an acute complication that primarily occurs in patients with type 1 diabetes who lack adequate insulin. When the body does not have enough insulin in the blood to break down macronutrients into glucose, it defaults to breaking down fatty acids into ketones for energy. This typically does not cause major issues in a person who does not have diabetes, as eventual insulin production and uptake will balance the level of ketones in the blood. In a patient with diabetes who cannot produce enough insulin, the body will continue to release fatty acids into the bloodstream. Eventually, this will result in too many ketones in the blood and will shift the body's pH level to an excessively acidic one. This is a crisis situation, and the patient may eventually go into a coma if left untreated. Symptoms include dehydration, nausea, sweet-smelling breath, confusion, and fatigue. Treatment includes oral or IV electrolyte and insulin administration. Diabetic ketoacidosis can occur with type 2 diabetes but occurs more frequently with type 1 diabetes. Often, a ketoacidosis event is the first indicator that a person may have diabetes.

Glycogenoses

Glycogenoses refer to a number of hereditary disorders in which the body is unable to convert stored glycogen to glucose when glucose is needed by the body. This inability is the result of the absence of an enzyme, although the specific enzyme that is missing can vary from patient to patient. Symptoms include failure to thrive (in infants), growth and development issues, kidney stones, confusion, and general weakness. More severe cases can result in chronic gout, seizures, coma, intestinal sores, and kidney failure. These disorders are usually treated by timing carbohydrate consumption so that blood sugar levels remain stable throughout the day.

Metabolic Syndrome/Syndrome X

Metabolic syndrome, or **Syndrome X**, refers to the presence of comorbid cardiovascular and insulin-related conditions. Patients diagnosed with metabolic syndrome must have three or more of the following conditions: hypertension, elevated fasting blood glucose levels, low HDL cholesterol, high triglycerides, and excess belly fat. This syndrome is believed to result from insulin resistance, causing high blood glucose, insulin, and lipid levels. Patients with metabolic syndrome tend to be overweight or obese and at an increased risk of organ failure, heart attacks, and strokes. They often suffer from another underlying condition, such as diabetes or polycystic ovary syndrome, that leads to metabolic syndrome. Metabolic syndrome is often treated with prescription medications that lower cholesterol and blood pressure, but diet and exercise changes are strongly recommended. Weight loss is a key component in managing metabolic syndrome.

Thyroid Conditions

Located at the front of the throat, the thyroid is one of the most influential glands in the endocrine system. The hormones it produces are involved in a multitude of functions throughout the body, including an assortment of metabolic, muscle, and digestive functions. Thyroid hormones also play a key role in neurological processes. When thyroid conditions develop, they can cause systemic effects. Testing for thyroid conditions goes beyond simply testing thyroid hormone levels. It can also include a physical exam, blood tests to determine how much thyroid-stimulating hormone (TSH) is being produced by the pituitary gland, tests to determine blood antibody levels, ultrasounds to check for tumors, and uptake tests to determine the rate at which the thyroid uses iodine.

Hyperthyroidism

When patients are diagnosed with **hyperthyroidism**, they may also be referred to as having an **overactive thyroid**, which results in the overproduction of T4 and/or T3 hormones. Symptoms include feelings of anxiety, trouble focusing, feeling overheated, gastrointestinal problems such as diarrhea, insomnia, elevated heart rate, and unexplained weight loss. Hyperthyroidism is commonly caused by Grave's disease, an autoimmune disorder. The extent to which symptoms of Grave's disease manifest can be broad, depending on the severity of the disease. Family history, stress, smoking, and pregnancy can increase the risk of developing Grave's disease. Women under the age of forty are most likely to be diagnosed. Medical treatment options can include methimazole and propylthiouracil, two common antithyroid medications. Prescription corticosteroids may also be used. In nonpregnant patients, radioactive iodine may be used. This is a long-term, repeat-dose solution that can sometimes result in hypothyroidism, which can be easier to treat. In serious cases, some or all of the thyroid may be removed, although this also usually results in hypothyroidism. It is also recommended that most patients with Grave's disease modify their lifestyle to limit stress, eat a healthy diet, and exercise regularly.

Hypothyroidism

When patients are diagnosed with **hypothyroidism**, they may also be referred to as having an underactive thyroid, which results in the underproduction of T4 and/or T3 hormones. Symptoms include depression, excessive fatigue, chills, dry skin, lowered heart rate, gastrointestinal problems such as constipation, and unexplained weight gain. Hypothyroidism is commonly caused by Hashimoto's disease, another autoimmune disease that affects thyroid functioning. This disease is usually treated with synthetic thyroid hormone replacement therapy, which involves taking a daily dose of the T4 hormone. T3 supplementation is rare, as it is derived from T4. Hypothyroidism can also be caused by the presence of too much iodine. The thyroid uses iodine to make T4 and T3 hormones. If there is too much iodine in the blood, the pituitary gland releases less TSH. The low levels of TSH can later result in the thyroid not producing enough T4 and/or T3 hormones. In some cases of hypothyroidism, surgery is required.

Goiter

A **goiter** refers to any enlargement in the thyroid gland. Goiters can occur in healthy thyroids or in thyroids producing abnormal levels of hormones. Their presence can indicate a lack of iodine, an autoimmune disease, an injury, or cancer.

Thyroid Cancer

Thyroid cancer is rare but can result in goiters and thyroid dysfunction. Thyroid cancer is more common in people who have nodes or goiters already present on the thyroid, which later turn malignant. The disease is also more prevalent in people who have been exposed to radiation. Thyroid cancer is usually treated through surgery, and thyroid hormone replacement therapy is a part of follow-up treatment.

Immunocompromised Patients

An **immunocompromised** person refers to any individual who has a less than optimally functioning immune system. This could be the result of a genetic disorder, a viral or cancerous disease, medication, injury, surgery, age, or nutrition. An immunocompromised person is more susceptible to infection and illness than someone whose immune system is functioning optimally.

HIV/AIDS

The human immunodeficiency virus (HIV) is a sphere-shaped virus that is a fraction of the size of a red blood cell. There are primarily two types of HIV: HIV-1 and HIV-2. HIV-2 is not highly transmissible and is poorly understood. It has mainly affected people in West Africa. HIV-1 is more severe and more highly transmissible. It is the dominant strain among global HIV cases, and when literature and media refer to HIV, this is usually the type that is being referred to.

HIV is highly contagious. It is found in human bodily fluids and can be transmitted through infected breast milk, blood, mucus, and sexual fluids. The most common forms of transmission are through anal or vaginal sex, but transmission can also occur through contaminated syringe use, blood transfusions, or any other method where membranes are compromised. Once in the body, HIV attacks and destroys

CD4/T cells. These cells are responsible for attacking foreign bodies (e.g., bacteria, infections, other viruses). As the body's CD4/T-cell count diminishes, the patient is left immunocompromised.

The HIV-1 type can be broken further into four groups: M, N, O, and P. M is the most commonly seen group globally. Within group M, there are nine different subtypes of HIV. These are noted as A, B, C, D, E, F, G, H, J, and K. Subtype B is prevalent in the Western world, and most research has been conducted on this subtype. This research has led to the manufacturing of antiretroviral (ARV) drugs. Antiretroviral therapy (ART) has been a major breakthrough in the management of HIV and in the quality of life for patients with HIV. In conjunction with medical care, many patients with HIV are able to have completely normal, healthy, active lives. It is important to treat HIV as early as possible. The better a patient's HIV is managed, the lower his or her viral load. Viral load refers to how much HIV is present in a patient's blood; when a viral load is low, transmission of the disease is far less likely to occur. With ART, many patients with HIV are viral-suppressed, and some even have an undetectable viral load. Viral load in other transmitting fluids, such as semen, cannot be detected but the virus is still present. Therefore, transmission is still possible, and all precautions should be taken.

Globally, most HIV patients have subtype C, but subtypes are mixing as travel and migration become more widespread. Most subtypes can be treated with ART, though these drugs were researched and manufactured to treat subtype B. However, ART is not always physically available or financially accessible in countries that need it most.

Without early intervention or adequate managed care of HIV, the virus can deteriorate the host body's immune system to a point where it cannot be rehabilitated. This stage is marked by extremely low levels of CD4/T cells (less than two hundred cells per cubic millimeter of blood) and is referred to as **acquired immunodeficiency syndrome** (AIDS). When a patient's HIV diagnosis progresses to AIDS, he or she often succumbs to serious chronic diseases, such as cancer. Mild illnesses, such as a cold or flu, can also be fatal to someone with AIDS. Not everyone who is diagnosed with HIV will also be diagnosed with AIDS. Once diagnosed with AIDS, the patient has approximately one to three years to live unless he or she receives adequate treatment.

Patients Receiving Chemotherapy

Chemotherapy is a broad term referring to the use of drugs in cancer treatment. This type of therapy is intended to target and treat the entire body, especially in advanced stages of cancer where malignant cells may be widespread. However, it may also be used in earlier stages of cancer to eliminate many of the cancerous cells. This is done with the intention that the patient will go into remission and potentially not experience cancer again in the future. If this does not seem like a viable prognosis, chemotherapy can be used to control early stages of cancer from advancing. In advanced stages of cancer, chemotherapy can be used to manage pain and suffering from cancerous tumors, even if the patient's prognosis is poor.

The aggressiveness of chemotherapy (such as which drugs are used, dosing amount, and frequency) is contingent on many factors, such as the type and stage of cancer. Chemotherapy treatment plans also consider the patient's personal and medical history. Since this form of treatment is so aggressive, it is often effective in reducing or eliminating cancer cells. However, chemotherapy can also kill healthy cells in the process. The intensity of this side effect varies by person, but almost all patients experience some degree of immunocompromise. This is because chemotherapy almost always inadvertently targets bone marrow, where white blood cells are made.

White blood cells, especially neutrophils, play an important role in fighting infection. When there are not enough white blood cells present in the patient's blood, he or she can become seriously ill from sickness or infection that would be mild in a healthy person. Medical personnel usually monitor neutrophil counts during and between chemotherapy cycles to make sure these levels do not fall too low. Chemotherapy cycles can last up to six months, and patients are considered to have a compromised immune system for the entire time they are undergoing chemotherapy. Once a full cycle of chemotherapy ends, it takes approximately one month for the immune system to return to its normal state.

Patients undergoing chemotherapy should be especially mindful of personal hygiene habits such as handwashing and showering, as well as avoiding cuts, scrapes, insect bites, or other instances where the skin may break. They may also need help taking care of a pet and handling pet waste or other trash. Additionally, it is important to practice extra caution when handling foods, such as cooking meats well, avoiding unpasteurized foods, washing produce with produce cleaner, cooking many foods that typically could be eaten raw, and avoiding certain moldy cheeses. They also need to be more careful of their surroundings in public places; since these areas tend to be dirtier and more populated, there is an increased risk of contracting infections. Medical personnel and those visiting the patient should be aware of these practices as well.

Urological/Renal

Genitourinary

Foreign Bodies

The emergency care of the male patient who presents with purulent or mucopurulent penile discharge, dysuria, hematuria, or painful intercourse is focused on identifying the cause. Prompt treatment is necessary to prevent renal damage and systemic complications. In addition to obtaining routine lab studies and cultures, the provider will inquire if the patient has a recent history of catheterization of the urethra due to medical intervention or self-induced. Anecdotal reports indicate that insertion of foreign bodies into the urethra for autoerotic purposes is a rare occurrence, and in most cases, is associated with preexisting psychiatric disease.

Depending on the dimensions of the object, a local reaction may not be apparent immediately, which means that any infection may be advanced by the time the patient seeks treatment. The diagnosis is most often identified by the physical examination and patient report. Diagnostic imaging studies and laboratory data are collected to assess the extent of infection and inflammation and to determine the optimal method for retrieval of the foreign body. Common methods of retrieval include endoscopy, surgical removal by suprapubic cystotomy, and urethrotomy. Treatment for localized effects of the existence of the foreign body will include antimicrobial therapy appropriate to results of the cultures and referral for psychiatric care. If the condition has progressed beyond the urethra and bladder, aggressive management is necessary to prevent sepsis.

Infection

Infections of the male genitourinary (GU) tract are considered to be complicated infections because the infective process has overcome the naturally robust defenses of the male urinary tract. Common conditions resulting in infection include the inflammation of the prostate gland, the epididymis, testes, kidney, bladder, urethra; unprotected sexual intercourse; and the use of urinary catheters. Additional contributing factors to the incidence of infection include a history of previous urinary tract infections (UTIs), enlargement of the prostate gland, changes in voiding habits such as the onset of nocturia, comorbid diabetes or HIV infection, immunosuppressive therapy, and previous surgical intervention of the urinary tract. Painful urination, defined as *dysuri*a, is the most common presenting manifestation, and complaints of coexisting dysuria, urinary frequency, and urgency are considered to be 75 percent predictive for UTI. Additional manifestations are dependent on the cause but may include fever, tachycardia, flank pain, suprapubic pain, penile discharge, scrotal masses and tenderness, and enlargement of the inguinal lymph nodes.

The diagnosis depends on the patient's history; presenting manifestations and physical examination; cultures of the urine, penile discharge, and blood; and assessment of kidney function. If obstruction of any portion of the urinary tract is suspected, additional diagnostic studies may include ultrasound, CT scans, and IV pyelogram (IVP). The infection will be treated with third-generation antimicrobial therapy, fluid resuscitation, antipyretics, analgesics, and urinary analgesics. The successful treatment of sexually transmitted infections requires adherence to the agent-specific medication regimen and the protocol for the treatment of all sexual partners and follow-up care. Emergency care of the patient with a UTI is focused on prompt identification of any obstructive pathology, treatment of infection and pain, preservation of kidney function, and prevention of systemic disease.

Priapism

Priapism is a urological emergency manifested by the enlargement of the penis that is unrelated to sexual stimulation and is unrelieved by ejaculation. Low-flow priapism is the most common form and is not associated with evidence of trauma but is due to dysfunction of the detumescence mechanism that is responsible for the relaxation of the erect penis. High-flow priapism results from abnormal arterial blood to the penis as a result of trauma to the GU system. The cause of low-flow priapism is most often idiopathic; however, the most common cause of the condition in children is sickle cell disease. Additional conditions that may cause this form of priapism include dialysis, vasculitis, spinal cord stenosis, bladder and renal cancer, and some medications, including heparin, cocaine, and omeprazole. High-flow priapism is due to straddle injuries or, most commonly, injury to the arteries of the penis by the injection of medications into the vasculature of the penis.

Prompt treatment of low-flow priapism within 12 hours of the onset of symptoms is necessary to prevent long-term alterations in erectile function. The primary cause is identified and treated if possible, followed by aspiration of fluid from the corpora cavernosa at the base of the penis, with or without saline irrigation, which is an effective treatment in 30 percent of cases. If aspiration and irrigation are unsuccessful, a vasoconstrictive agent such as phenylephrine can be instilled at 5-minute intervals until the erection is entirely resolved. If these interventions fail to eradicate the priapism, temporary or permanent surgical placement of a shunt between the corpus cavernosum and the glans penis or corpus spongiosum is necessary to restore venous drainage. Treatment of high-flow priapism involves cauterization and/or evacuation of areas of bleeding. Emergency treatment is focused on identification of the specific condition and prompt resolution of the erection.

Renal Calculi

Nephrolithiasis is defined as the process of stone or calculi formation in the pelvis of the kidney. The pain associated with this condition is referred to as **renal colic** and most often reflects the stretching and distention of the ureter when the stone leaves the kidney. The most common cause is insufficient fluid intake that concentrates stone-forming substances in the kidney. In order of occurrence, calculi are composed of calcium (75 percent) due to increased absorption of calcium by the GI tract, struvite (15 percent) as a result of repeated UTIs, uric acid (6 percent) due to increased purine intact, and cysteine (1 percent) due to an intrinsic metabolic defect in susceptible individuals. In addition, AIDS medications, some antacids, and sulfa drugs are also associated with stone formation. Renal calculi are more common in men than women, are associated with obesity and insulin resistance, and have a familial tendency.

Diagnosis is based on the patient's history and physical examination. Common lab studies include CBC, coagulation studies, kidney function tests, and C-reactive protein. Imaging studies may include ultrasonography, KUB films, and CT scans. Treatment options are based on the likelihood that the stone will be expelled spontaneously from the urinary system, given the size and location of the stone. Common interventions include aggressive fluid management, antimicrobial therapy, and pain management. If necessary, to prevent mechanical damage to the organs or the progression of the condition to urosepsis, the stone may be surgically removed, or the patient may undergo extracorporeal shock wave lithotripsy. The emergency care is focused on preventing damage to the urinary tract, restoring fluid volume, managing pain, and preventing progression of the illness to systemic urosepsis. Patient education regarding the essential follow-up care is critical to the prevention of recurrent calculi formation.

Torsion

Torsion refers to the abnormal twisting of the structures of the spermatic cord, which results in ischemia in the ipsilateral testicle that causes irreversible damage to fertility if not relieved within 6 hours. The condition is most common in infants, due to the mobility of the undescended testicles, and in adolescents, due to the abnormal attachment of fascia and muscles to the spermatic cord. The Testicular Workup for Ischemia and Suspected Torsion (TWIST) is the scoring system used to quantify the risk associated with the condition. The TWIST is used by emergency providers and then validated by the physician, most commonly a urologist, and the score is based on swelling of the testicle, hardened texture of the testicle, absence of the cremasteric reflex, nausea and vomiting, and placement of the testicles at a higher than normal position in the scrotum. The resulting risk factor may be low, intermediate, or high. A low TWIST score may indicate an alternative cause for the patient's manifestations. An intermediate risk requires the use of ultrasound to confirm the diagnosis, while the patient with a high-risk TWIST score requires immediate surgical intervention to prevent long-term dysfunction.

Nonoperative treatments include manual manipulation of the testicle guided by Doppler imaging. If the procedure is successful, surgical stabilization of the spermatic cord structures is required. Immediate surgical repair is required if the procedure is unsuccessful. If the affected testicle is nonviable and is removed, a testicular prosthesis will be inserted after wound healing is complete. Analgesics and antianxiety medications will be included in the treatment plan. Caregivers must be aware that the condition can reoccur. Emergency care of the patient requires immediate intervention based on the calculation of the TWIST score to prevent necrosis of the affected testicle.

Trauma

Organs of the GU tract include the bladder, urethra, and external genitalia, all of which are subject to varied sources of trauma. The bladder is commonly injured by blunt trauma that results from pelvic fractures and is also affected less commonly by penetrating trauma. The different segments of the male urethra can be injured as a result of pelvic fractures, straddle-type injuries, or from penetrating injuries that may be self-inflicted. The penis and scrotum are subject to blunt trauma, often due to sports injuries and other varied injuries that may be self-inflicted.

The diagnosis depends on the history of the precipitating event and the physical examination. Trauma to the GU tract may not be life-threatening; however, the GU injuries are often secondary to other injuries affecting the pelvis, spine, kidney, and abdomen, which warrant immediate attention. Common lab studies include CBC, prothrombin time, type and cross match, and urinalysis. Ultrasonography and CT scans are used in addition to studies specific to the bladder and testes, which include retrograde urethrogram, retrograde cystogram, and nuclear med studies. Established prehospital trauma care is required. Emergency treatment is aimed at identifying and correcting the underlying injury and preserving the function of the GU tract and includes fluid replacement, antimicrobial therapy, and pain management. Referrals to urologists, orthopedists, and other specialists must be made as necessary. In the event of self-inflicted injuries, psychiatric referrals are also appropriate.

Urinary Retention

Urinary retention may be acute or chronic and is defined as cessation of urination or incomplete emptying of the bladder. It occurs more often in older men, and common causes include prostate gland enlargement, neurogenic bladder due to diabetes or other chronic diseases, urethral strictures and other anatomic abnormalities, and the use of anticholinergic medications. Urinary retention in younger men is most commonly due to pelvic or spinal cord trauma. Unrelieved urinary retention can result in urinary tract infections due to stasis of the urine or renal failure due to the retrograde pressure of the accumulated urine. Common manifestations include suprapubic distension, pain, a history of contributing neurological diseases, and possible systemic signs such as fever and tachycardia. The condition also may be asymptomatic or characterized by urinary frequency or overflow incontinence, with loss of small amounts of urine accompanied by sensations of bladder fullness.

Diagnosis depends on the patient's history, including the presence of causative conditions and physical examination. Common lab studies include CBC, BUN, creatinine, electrolytes, urinalysis, ultrasound, urodynamic testing, and cystoscopy. The emergency treatment of acute urinary retention is aimed at draining the accumulated urine, protecting kidney function, addressing the underlying issue, and preventing systemic effects and recurrence. Urethral or suprapubic catheterization or a percutaneous nephrostomy may be done to drain the urine from the bladder, while urethral catheterization can also be used to obtain urodynamic measurements and to evaluate postvoid volumes after treatment. Clean technique self-catheterization is done by patients with chronic urinary retention due to neurogenic causes. If surgical removal of a portion or all of the bladder is required to repair traumatic damage or to remove malignant tumors, a urinary diversion will be created to maintain kidney function.

Gynecology

Abnormal Bleeding Dysfunction (Vaginal)

Abnormal or irregular uterine bleeding is defined as episodes of bleeding that are not caused by any specific pathology, systemic illness, or normal pregnancy. It is most often due to alterations in the hormonal stimulation of the endometrium by some source. The bleeding episodes vary widely as to the amount of blood loss and the duration and frequency of the episodes in the same individual. The most common cause of this anovulatory cycle is the presence of an abnormal pregnancy, which may be a threatened or incomplete abortion or an ectopic pregnancy. There are several additional conditions associated with abnormal uterine bleeding, including polycystic ovarian syndrome, thyroid dysfunction, and liver dysfunction that affects estrogen metabolism. Endometrial fibroids, polyps, hyperplasia, or cancer can also cause abnormal uterine bleeding. The condition is more common in adolescent women and women over the age of forty.

Once an abnormal pregnancy has been excluded, common diagnostic studies include CBC, Pap smear, thyroid and liver function tests, coagulation studies, and hormonal assays. Routine imaging studies are recommended only if the pelvic examination is unacceptable, as might occur in a patient with morbid obesity. However, pelvic ultrasonography is recommended in all patients who present with abnormal bleeding and are at high risk for cancer. Any identified pathology will be treated first; however, there are general guidelines for idiopathic ovulatory dysfunction, which include age-specific treatment protocols for the use of oral contraceptives as the initial treatment. Oral contraceptives suppress the thickening of the endometrial lining, regulate the menstrual cycle, and decrease menstrual flow, which reduces the risk of iron-deficiency anemia. In the event of the failure of medical treatment, hysterectomy may be recommended. The emergency care of the patient with abnormal bleeding is focused on hemostasis, aggressive fluid replacement, and treatment of the cause, which may require surgical intervention.

Foreign Bodies

Foreign bodies that exceed the dimensions of the female vagina may precipitate an emergency. While this condition is more common in children than adult females, adolescents and adults can present with tampons, condom portions, or other foreign objects that were inserted intentionally or as a form of abuse. Common presenting manifestations include vaginal bleeding and malodorous vaginal discharge and vulvar irritation. In most instances, the effects of the foreign body are limited to the vagina unless the wall of the vagina is penetrated, which can result in abdominal manifestations. Additionally, if the patient is immunocompromised, severe infection may result. Untreated or repeated episodes can result in the formation of fistulae between the vagina and the rectum, bladder, or abdominal cavity; pain with intercourse; and persistent bleeding.

The diagnosis depends on the patient's presenting history and physical examination; however, if the patient is a child or an adolescent, special care is required for both questioning the patient about the precipitating events and in the conduct of the physical examination. Depending on the size and location of the foreign body, sedation and/or anesthesia may be necessary to examine the patient, regardless of age, and to remove the foreign body. CT scans and ultrasonography may be necessary to identify the extent of any injury caused by the object. In most cases, removal of the object is the treatment of choice; however, perforation of the vagina, fistula formation, or infection require additional treatment and a surgical referral. In addition to the removal of the foreign body, emergency care also requires a thorough investigation of any evidence of abuse, consistent with agency policy. Referral to a mental health professional may also be indicated in the event of self-inflicted injury.

Hemorrhage

Hemorrhage in women can be due to abnormal uterine bleeding, hemorrhagic cystitis, trauma to the GU system or the bony pelvic structure, kidney injury or dysfunction, self-inflicted trauma, abuse, complications of pregnancy and childbirth, rupture of an ovarian cyst, or tumor. Manifestations relate to the specific cause but commonly include some degree of vaginal bleeding, flank or suprapubic pain, vital signs indicative of hypovolemia, hematuria, and neurological deficits or crepitus resulting from pelvic trauma. The emergency assessment of the patient with hemorrhage of the gynecologic (GYN) system will be consistent with the Advanced Trauma Life Support protocol. While the diagnosis depends on the history of the precipitating event and the physical examination, prompt use of ultrasonography, CT scanning, pelvic angiography, cystography, and/or retrograde urethrography are required to identify the source of the hemorrhage and to guide treatment. In addition, common lab studies include CBC, coagulation studies, type and screen, electrolytes, ABGs, and urinalysis.

There are several protocols for injury pattern recognition in the patient with pelvic trauma that include treatment recommendations for each category. The emergency treatment of postpartum hemorrhage is discussed in a subsequent section. The initial intervention for these events is the treatment of the underlying condition, in addition to the restoration of hemostasis with aggressive replacement of crystalloid and colloid solutions and appropriate referrals for all instances of suspected abuse, either self-inflicted or from another source.

Infection

The most common sexually transmitted infective agent in the United States is chlamydia, which is spread by unprotected vaginal, oral, or anal sexual activity. The organism can also be transmitted to an infant delivered vaginally by an infected mother. Risk factors common to all sexually transmitted diseases (STDs) include a history of multiple sexual partners, unprotected sexual intercourse, coinfection with other infective agents, and young age, with most infections occurring in women from fifteen to twenty-four years old.

Chlamydial infections may be asymptomatic, which has prompted the U.S. Preventive Services Task Force to recommend routine screening of all females fifteen to twenty-four years of age and all females older than twenty-four who have identifiable risk factors for chlamydia. Manifestations are specific to the involved organs, as either contained to the vagina and cervix or affecting the uterus and fallopian tubes, and include abnormal vaginal bleeding, rectal and vaginal discharge, and possible infection of the conjunctiva if the patient is pregnant. Diagnostic tests for lower tract infections include Pap smear, pregnancy tests, cultures, and HIV tests, while the diagnosis of infection of the upper GYN tract includes ultrasonography and CT scanning. Untreated infections often result in pelvic inflammatory disease (PID), infertility, and chronic pelvic pain. The treatment of lower tract infection is the administration of a single dose of azithromycin that is witnessed and confirmed by a health care provider to decrease costs of noncompliance. More complicated infections require extended antibiotic therapy to avoid long-term complications.

Gonorrheal infections are associated with risk factors, manifestations, complications, and diagnostic studies, similar to chlamydial infections. Newborns are treated prophylactically for gonorrhea infections; however, emergency care of a child with a gonorrheal infection involves collection of appropriate samples for possible forensic investigation. Untreated gonorrhea can progress to PID, and rarely, to gonococcemia or fatal systemic shock. Typical treatment includes ceftriaxone and azithromycin. Syphilis can progress through four stages if left untreated, with manifestations ranging from the initial chancre at the point of contact to systemic neurological effects, including dementia. Penicillin is the treatment of choice, and the dosage protocol is specific to the stage of the infection when diagnosed.

PID is a potential complication of untreated or recurrent infection by any of the organisms that are sexually transmitted; however, PID most commonly results from chlamydial infection. The infection and inflammation proceed from the vagina through the cervix to the uterus and fallopian tube, with eventual progression to the abdominal cavity. The most common presenting manifestations include lower abdominal pain and possible abnormal vaginal discharge. Untreated, the condition leads to systemic manifestations that include fever and elevated sedimentation rate. Complaints of upper right quadrant pain may be associated with Fitz-Hugh–Curtis perihepatitis, which may present with jaundice and altered liver function studies. Diagnosis is made by the patient's history and physical and the exclusion of pregnancy or other pelvic pathology as the cause of the patient's pain. Treatment is focused on the relief of pain, resolution of the infection, decreasing the risk of long-term effects including sterility and the risk for obstetrical failure, and preventing further transmission of the infective agent. Antibiotic therapy is the treatment of choice and is generally effective in up to 75 percent of cases of PID, with surgery indicated for patients who do not respond to antibiotics.

Ovarian Cysts

An **ovarian cyst** is defined as a discrete accumulation of fluid in an ovary resulting from an alteration in hormonal function. It can form at any point in a female's lifetime. Risk factors for benign ovarian cysts include a history of breast cancer, infertility treatment, smoking, hypothyroidism, and tubal ligation, while malignant cysts are associated with a positive family history, advancing age, Caucasian ethnicity, infertility, nulliparity, early menarche, delayed menopause, and a history of breast cancer. Most cysts are asymptomatic but may be associated with abdominal bloating, early satiety, change in bowel habits, and weight loss and severe abdominal pain if the cysts rupture. Diagnosis is made by the patient's history and physical examination in addition to pelvic ultrasonography, CA-125 measurement, and pregnancy testing. Initial treatment of simple cysts is observation and/or the use of oral contraceptive medications. If cysts grow in size or are associated with increasingly severe manifestations, laparoscopic removal of the cyst and/or the ovary is indicated.

Sexual Assault/Battery

Sexual assaults are the result of violent, nonconsensual sexual actions against the victim. Common manifestations include the presence of sperm or blood, contusions, local evidence of forceful vaginal penetration, orthopedic injuries, abdominal trauma, and lacerations. The emergency care of the victim of sexual assault is focused on identifying and treating all injuries; appropriate testing and preventive treatment for all possible STDs, HIV, and hepatitis; prescribing preventive antibiotic therapy; and administering interventions aimed at preventing posttraumatic stress disorder (PTSD). Although assault victims are often reluctant to provide a detailed account of the assault, emergency providers are responsible for meticulous and comprehensive documentation to protect the patient's rights. In addition, referrals to appropriate community resources for post-emergency care should be made prior to the patient's discharge from the acute care facility. The patient should also be referred to a GYN for follow-up evaluation for potential infections or complications.

Trauma

The pelvic organs may be affected by blunt trauma, penetrating trauma, and injury due to trauma of adjacent structures such as pelvic fractures. Wounds may be due to automobile accidents, sports injuries, attacks by another person, gunshot wounds, or self-inflicted trauma. Penetrating wounds of the urethra can interrupt urine flow, while penetrating wounds of the vagina and uterus can compromise the abdominal cavity, leading to systemic effects. Blunt trauma to the lower abdomen can cause intrauterine bleeding and kidney contusions, which can compromise fluid volume status. In addition, all patients presenting with a history of trauma and complaints of groin pain should be assessed for the presence of pelvic fractures.

Common diagnostic studies include CBC, electrolytes, coagulation studies, type and screen, radiography, ultrasonography, CT scanning, urinalysis, and possible paracentesis to assess for penetration of the abdomen. Treatment is specific to the specific injuries and commonly includes fluid resuscitation, possible transfusion, Foley catheter insertion, and orthopedic, surgical, and GYN referrals as necessary. Possible surgical interventions include stabilization of pelvic fractures, possible hysterectomy due to severe blunt or penetrating trauma, or removal of ischemic ovaries.

Depending on the extent of the injuries, the patient may be assessed by the Revised Trauma Score, which is a risk prediction assessment tool used to assess the probability of survival in trauma patients. The patient's initial data set obtained upon arrival in the ER is used to calculate the risk. Parameters include the Glasgow Coma Scale score, the systolic BP, and the respiratory rate. Possible scores range from 0 to 7.8, and a score greater than 5.0 is associated with 80 percent or greater chance of survival. Emergency care of the patient with GYN trauma is based on the ABCDE protocol with attention to the possibility of "hidden" injuries that are not readily apparent.

Obstetrical

Abruptio Placenta

Abruptio placenta refers to the premature separation of the placenta from the uterine wall and is the most significant cause of hemorrhage in the third trimester. Descriptive terms for the condition include the identification of the degree of separation (either partial or complete), or the location of the separation (either marginal or central). Clinically, Class 0 indicates only the identification of a blood clot in the expelled placenta, while the manifestations in Classes 1, 2, and 3 progress from mild vaginal bleeding to hemorrhage, from mild uterine pain to tetanic or continuous contractions, from normal vital signs to maternal shock, from absent fetal distress to fetal demise, and from normal clotting to fibrinogen deficiency and hemorrhage. The exact cause is not known. However, there are several common risk factors, including maternal hypertension, which occurs in 40 percent of the cases of abruptio placenta; smoking; trauma in the form of car accidents, falls, or assaults; cocaine or alcohol abuse; maternal age greater than thirty-five or less than twenty years old; and previous history of abruptio placenta.

Depending on the patient's presenting manifestations, diagnostic studies include CBC, coagulation tests, type and screen, Kleihauer-Betke test in Rh-negative mothers to identify fetal-to-maternal transfer of blood, a nonstress test, fetal monitoring, and the possible use of ultrasonography; however, ultrasounds have a low sensitivity for identifying the separation of the placenta. The emergency care of the patient starts with fetal monitoring, initiation of IV access for fluid resuscitation with crystalloids and colloids, assessment and correction of any coagulopathy, administration of RhoGAM as needed, consideration of steroids for fetal lung maturity in preterm newborns, and preparation for delivery of the newborn.

Ectopic Pregnancy

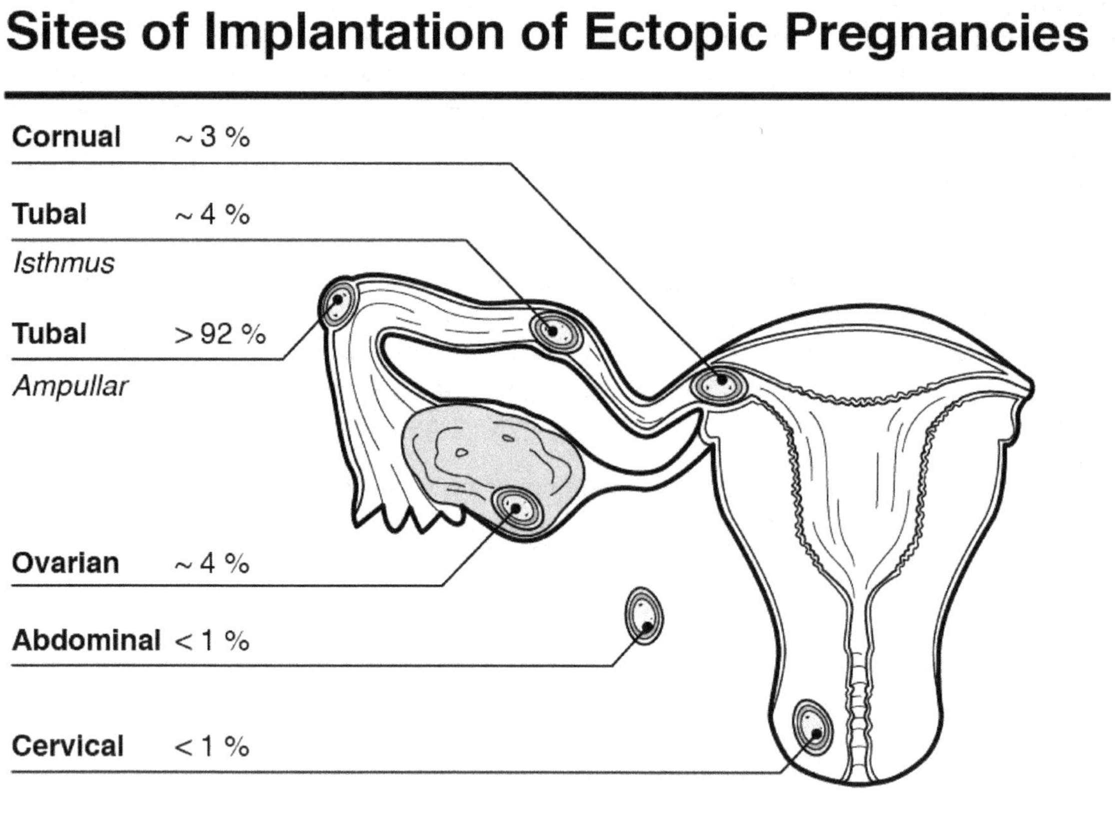

An ectopic pregnancy results from the abnormal implantation of the fertilized ovum at an alternative anatomical site—most commonly the fallopian tube—that is physiologically incapable of sustaining the pregnancy. An undetected or untreated ectopic pregnancy is a life-threatening emergency. The majority of patients do not have any identifiable risk factors; however, the most common defect is an alteration in the structure of the fallopian tubes that impedes the movement of the fertilized ovum to the appropriate site in the uterus. Common causes of damage to the fallopian tubes include PID, a history of previous ectopic pregnancies, smoking (because it decreases the motility of the fallopian tube), the use of intrauterine devices (IUDs), and assisted reproduction, which doubles the risk for this disorder. Although the three classic symptoms are pain, amenorrhea, and vaginal bleeding, only 40 to 50 percent of patients with an ectopic pregnancy present with all three manifestations. Additional manifestations will be dependent on the implantation site, most commonly the fallopian tube, or rarely, the abdomen, and the "age" of the pregnancy, and may include signs of early pregnancy or abnormal signs such as dizziness, weakness, flu symptoms, and in the extreme, cardiac arrest.

To decrease the morbidity associated with undiagnosed ectopic pregnancies, all women of childbearing age who present with pain, vaginal bleeding, and amenorrhea must be screened for pregnancy. Testing of the urine and serum for beta human chorionic gonadotropin (βHCG) will be positive before the first missed menstrual period, and transvaginal ultrasonography is the recommended imaging modality. Laparoscopy is the treatment of choice for patients who are experiencing pain or hemodynamic instability. Intramuscular methotrexate, which impedes DNA synthesis and prevents cellular replication, is the recommended expectant treatment for ectopic pregnancy. The protocol requires an initial assessment of βHCG, liver and kidney function, blood type, Rh status, and bone marrow function. Methotrexate is administered in a single dose, and its effectiveness is measured by evidence of decreasing βHCG levels. Emergency treatment of an ectopic pregnancy is focused on identification of the location and characteristics of the abnormal pregnancy and the patient's systemic manifestations, which may include hemorrhage and cardiac arrest.

Emergent Delivery

An emergent delivery occurs when a pregnant patient presents with signs of imminent delivery as manifested by complete effacement and dilation of the cervix; strong, effective uterine contractions; and possible visualization of the presenting part at the vaginal orifice. The Emergency Medical Treatment and Labor Act (EMTALA) dictates that all patients who present to the ER must be treated; however, in the case of an imminent delivery, the provider must decide whether delivery in the ER or transfer to the obstetrical department is the most appropriate course for the individual patient. An emergent delivery will trigger the department protocol that includes notification of all personnel required to care for the mother and newborn after the delivery.

Maternal and fetal vital signs, fetal monitoring, IV access, and baseline lab studies will be initiated. Trained personnel will facilitate the delivery, resuscitate and warm the newborn, assess the newborn's Apgar score at 1 and 5 minutes after delivery, monitor the delivery of the placenta, and maintain surveillance of uterine involution. Prompt transfer of the mother and baby to the postpartum unit and newborn nursery, respectively, is required. In addition to common obstetrical and fetal complications, an emergent delivery due to the rapid descent of the fetus may also include vaginal and/or perineal lacerations. Emergency care of this patient is based on the presenting manifestations and the agency-specific protocol for emergent deliveries.

Newborn Apgar Assessment			
	Score of 0	Score of 1	Score of 2
Appearance (skin color)	Blue or pale	Pink body but blue extremities	Pink; no cyanosis
Pulse	Absent	< 100 bpm	> 100 bpm
Grimace (irritability reflex)	No response	Feebly cries or grimaces when stimulated	Cries or pulls away when stimulated
Activity (muscle tone)	None	Some flexion in the limbs	Flexed limbs that resist extension
Respiration	Absent	Gasping, weak, or irregular	Strong cry

Hemorrhage

Postpartum hemorrhage is commonly defined as the loss of more than 500 milliliters following a vaginal delivery or 1000 milliliters after a Caesarean section (C-section) in a pregnancy that has progressed for at least twenty weeks. Less substantial losses can result in alterations in fluid volume status in patients with comorbidities such as anemia, cardiac disease, dehydration, or preeclampsia, which means that postpartum hemorrhage is the loss of any amount of blood that results in altered hemodynamic status. There are multiple contributing factors; however, the most common precipitating pathophysiology for hemorrhage is uterine atony. These factors are related to tone, tissue, trauma, or thrombosis. Alterations in tone may be due to uterine atony resulting from distention of the uterine muscles in prolonged labor or with a large-for-gestational-age (LGA) newborn. Tissue alterations include retained placental tissue or placenta accreta. Trauma may result from manipulation of the fetus during delivery, history of previous C-section, prolonged labor, and internal version and extraction of a second twin. Alterations in coagulation may be due to preexisting coagulopathies.

The diagnosis depends on the presenting manifestations of postpartum vaginal bleeding and deteriorating hemodynamic status. Commonly, the emergency care of postpartum hemorrhage includes notification of obstetrical, anesthesia, and surgical suite providers; type and cross match for six units of packed red blood cells (PRBCs); assignment of data recording to one provider; aggressive fluid management, including appropriate blood products; assessment of the placenta for missing fragments of tissue; baseline lab studies, including CBC, coagulation studies, renal function tests, and electrolytes; and oxygen by mask. The goal of treatment is to reverse the coagulopathy, resolve the underlying defect, and maintain close surveillance of the contractility of the uterus, or surgical intervention in the event of massive hemorrhage.

Hyperemesis Gravidarum

Hyperemesis gravidarum is an acute form of nausea and vomiting that is associated with fluid volume depletion, resulting in ketosis and up to a 5 percent weight loss. This extreme form of "morning sickness" may also be manifested by fatigue, weakness, dizziness, sleep disturbance, and mood changes. Diagnostic studies include urinalysis to assess acid-base balance and to rule out UTI, liver function studies to rule out hepatitis, CBC, and thyroid function studies. Obstetrical ultrasonography is done to assess the condition of the pregnancy and to confirm the number of fetuses.

The condition typically begins before eight weeks of gestation and rarely persists beyond twenty to twenty-two weeks of gestation. The symptomatic treatment includes close assessment of the fluid volume status and vital signs, antiemetics, and IV fluid replacement. In the event of severe nutritional deficits, acid-base dysfunction, or electrolyte imbalance, hospitalization may be required. The emergency care of the patient with hyperemesis gravidarum is focused on correction of fluid volume deficit, resolution of ketosis and electrolyte imbalances, and relief from nausea and vomiting.

Neonatal Resuscitation

In the United States, 50 percent of all newborn deaths occur in the first 24 hours after delivery. The two most common causes of newborn distress are perinatal asphyxia and extreme prematurity. Neither of these conditions is 100 percent predictable; therefore, all emergency departments must have skilled personnel and all appropriate resources to care for these patients. Additional complications that must be recognized include the presence of pneumothorax, esophageal atresia, multiple gestation, and/or congenital anomalies.

Emergency providers must be knowledgeable about the events of the newborn's transition from intrauterine to extrauterine life with respect to respiratory and cardiovascular adaptation. Respiratory adaptation requires the absorption or removal of the amniotic fluid from the airways and alveoli. In the full-term newborn, there are physiological fetal and maternal resorption mechanisms, which together with the stresses of delivery, decrease the amount of fluid that remains at birth; however, these mechanisms are less effective in preterm newborns. Cardiovascular adaptation involves the redirection of blood flow through the heart and the pulmonary vasculature with normal closure of the ductus arteriosus and the foramen ovale in the heart as a result of changes in the systemic and pulmonary vascular resistance.

The emergency resuscitation of the newborn begins with thermoregulation, which focuses initially on prevention of heat loss, prior to the application of additional heat. The goal is to achieve an initial axillary temperature of 36.5°C (97.7°F). Airway management initially involves clearance of amniotic fluid from the airway. It is recommended that only bulb syringes are used because catheters may stimulate a vagal response, resulting in apnea, bradycardia, and hypotension. Drying and clearing of secretions often provide sufficient stimulation to induce spontaneous respirations; however, rubbing the back or tapping the feet may be necessary. Supplemental oxygen therapy will be initiated depending on heart rate, color, and oxygen saturation. The pulse oximetry goal for full-term newborns is 92 to 96 percent and 88 to 92 percent for premature newborns. If there is sustained bradycardia (less than sixty beats per minute) and cyanosis, mechanical ventilation is required. Additional emergency measures will be ineffective unless a patent airway and an effective ventilatory pattern are present. IV or ET tube administration of epinephrine to stimulate cardiac function, intravenous infusion of 0.9 percent normal sodium chloride for volume expansion and reversal of metabolic acidosis, and cardiac compresses consistent with the PALS protocol will be instituted as necessary.

Placenta Previa

Placenta previa is defined as the abnormal placement of the placenta with either complete coverage of the internal cervical os (complete) by the placenta, or location of the placenta within two centimeters of the internal cervical os (marginal). The condition generally presents with painless vaginal bleeding during the third trimester of pregnancy and is associated with the possibility of hemorrhage at the onset of labor, due to cervical dilation and the relative inability of the lower uterine segment to effectively contract the vessels of the exposed maternal implantation site. Risk factors for this condition include maternal age greater than thirty-five years, infertility treatments, increased number of previous pregnancies, multiple births, previous C-sections, previous abortions, previous placenta previa, and smoking or cocaine use.

Once the condition is identified, the patient can be safely observed as long as the maternal and fetal monitoring parameters remain stable. Betamethasone therapy is indicated for the maturation of the fetal lungs if the pregnancy duration is less than thirty-four weeks. At the first sign of bleeding, immediate surgery is necessary. The care of the patient who presents with hemorrhage without prior identification of the placenta previa will trigger the agency protocol for obstetrical emergencies, which will include the transvaginal ultrasound confirmation of the condition and preparations for emergency surgery, including coagulation studies and type and cross match for six units of blood. Depending on the cause of the placenta previa, surgical removal of the uterus may be the only alternative surgical approach.

Postpartum Infection

There are several infectious conditions that may occur after a vaginal or Caesarean birth or during breastfeeding. There is rarely sufficient postpartum observation of the new mother to identify the onset of infection, usually from the second to the tenth postpartum day, which is manifested by a temperature greater than 38°C (100.4°F). Common infectious conditions include endometritis, postsurgical wound infections, perineal cellulitis, urinary tract infections, mastitis, and inflammation of the pelvic veins. The manifestations are specific to the anatomical site of the infection, while the causative agents are most often commonly occurring pathogens in the vagina and abdomen. Research indicates that the occurrence of severe sepsis is associated with preexisting conditions, including chronic liver disease, chronic kidney disease, congestive heart failure, and lupus.

Routine diagnostic studies include CBC; electrolytes; coagulation studies; blood, cervical, and wound cultures; and urinalysis. Ultrasonography is used to identify abscess formation, while CT and MRI scans are used to identify septic pelvic thrombosis or other systemic infection such as appendicitis. Antimicrobial treatment is specific to site of the infection. Emergency care of the patient with a postpartum infection is focused on aggressive fluid replacement to support hydration and hemodynamic status, identification of the source of the infection, and administration of the appropriate antimicrobial agent. Patients who present with thrombosed pelvic veins may also require anticoagulant therapy that will necessitate in-hospital care. All patients with systemic manifestations will be considered for admission, and all patients who present with infection will require follow-up care with an obstetrician.

Preeclampsia, Eclampsia, HELLP Syndrome

Preeclampsia is characterized by the onset of hypertension and proteinuria after twenty weeks of gestation and may persist for four to six weeks postpartum. The cause is unknown; however, there is evidence of alterations in the endothelium of the vasculature accompanied by vasospasm. Risk factors include nulliparity, maternal age over forty years old, family history, chronic renal disease, obesity, hypertension, and diabetes. Early manifestations include visual disturbances, altered mental state, dyspnea, facial edema, and possible upper right quadrant pain. Severe manifestations include hypertension on bedrest, increasing liver enzymes with increased pain, progressive renal dysfunction, pulmonary edema, and thrombocytopenia. Routine labs, fetal nonstress testing, and corticosteroids for lung maturation are done prior to delivery, which is the only known cure.

Eclampsia is the life-threatening complication of severe preeclampsia that is manifested by the onset of seizure activity and/or the development of coma and is associated with hypertension, proteinuria, intrauterine fetal growth delay, and diminished amniotic fluid. There are no specific diagnostic tests, and while the specific etiology is unknown, there are indications that the condition results from the interchange of maternal and fetal tissue or allografts. Magnesium sulfate is recommended for short-term use for 24 to 48 hours to stabilize the patient for delivery, which is the only curative measure.

HELLP syndrome is also associated with significant maternal and fetal mortality, resulting from liver rupture and strokes due to cerebral edema or hemorrhage. The syndrome is characterized by hemolysis of RBCs, elevated liver enzymes, and low platelet levels (HELLP). Some authorities consider HELLP syndrome to be a severe form of preeclampsia, while others view it as a separate entity. The coagulation defects and liver dysfunction are the result of microvascular changes in the endothelium in the presence of hypertension; however, the cause is unknown. Risk factors are similar to risk factors for preeclampsia. Manifestations include elevated liver enzymes, coagulation defects including thrombocytopenia and hemolytic anemia, and right upper quadrant pain, and there are classification systems that assess the condition according to the extent of hepatic dysfunction. The treatment involves stabilization of the patient and prompt delivery with attention to correction of the coagulation defects and liver dysfunction. The emergency care of all of these life-threatening conditions is focused on treating hypertension, safe delivery of the fetus, and prevention of associated complications.

Preterm Labor

Most neonatal deaths in the United States are due to preterm labor, which is defined as the onset of uterine contractions that are of adequate strength and frequency to result in effacement and dilation of the cervix between twenty- and thirty-seven-weeks' gestation. Although the exact etiology is unclear, the most significant predictor for preterm labor is a positive history for preterm labor. Additional risk factors include abruptio placenta, cervical incompetence due to prior surgery, uterine fibroids, cervical infections, fetal distress, and placental defects due to systemic conditions that include diabetes, hypertension, smoking, and alcohol and drug abuse.

The routine testing for a patient with a history of second-trimester pregnancy loss includes coagulation studies, cultures for chlamydia and gonorrhea, glucose tolerance assessment, and immune antibody studies. Two additional parameters—the cervical length as measured by transvaginal ultrasonography and the fetal fibronectin level (fFN)—are used to assess the risk for preterm labor in a patient with inconclusive manifestations. Preterm labor is treated with tocolytic agents and progesterone. The primary purpose of tocolytic therapy is to delay delivery for up to 48 hours to optimize the effect of betamethasone therapy on fetal lung maturation, thereby decreasing the incidence of respiratory distress syndrome in the newborn. Tocolytic therapy with magnesium sulfate is recommended for preterm labor from twenty-four to thirty-three weeks of gestation. Common side effects of magnesium sulfate are headache, lethargy, blurred vision, and facial flushing. Toxic manifestations include respiratory depression and cardiac arrest. Progesterone is believed to prevent preterm labor by direct effect on the uterus after the placenta is fully formed, and it may also be used to delay delivery. The emergency care of the patient with preterm labor is focused on confirming the presence of true labor, assessing fetal health, and administering tocolytic agents and progesterone, which help inhibit the labor process.

Threatened Spontaneous Abortion

Abortion is defined as any form of early pregnancy loss; however, the term **miscarriage** appears more commonly in lay literature. Up to 80 percent of spontaneous abortions occur in the first trimester and may be categorized as threatened, inevitable, incomplete, complete, or missed. In addition, abortions are labeled as sporadic or recurrent. Chromosomal anomalies of the fetus are generally accepted as the most common cause of early abortions. In addition, several maternal risk factors have been identified that may be associated with first- or second-trimester pregnancy losses. Advanced maternal age and a history of type 1 diabetes, renal disease, severe hypertension, thyroid dysfunction, anatomical defects of the uterus, illicit drug use, smoking, alcohol abuse, and non-ASA NSAID use have all been associated with an increased risk of an initial or recurrent early pregnancy loss.

The diagnosis of a threatened spontaneous abortion will be based on the patient's history and physical, lab studies, and ultrasonography. The first priority is to confirm the presence of the pregnancy; therefore, lab studies will include the assessment of βhCG (human gonadotropin hormone) in addition to CBC with differential, blood and Rh typing, hemoglobin and hematocrit, and coagulation studies. Transabdominal and transvaginal ultrasonography are the recommended imaging modalities. Treatment is dependent on the stage of the pregnancy, the presenting manifestations, and in some cases, the patient's preference for the treatment approach. A threatened abortion of a first-trimester pregnancy will be treated with expectant management, which includes close observation of maternal hemodynamic status and blood loss. If the abortion continues to an incomplete abortion, surgical or pharmacologically-induced evacuation of the products of conception will be considered. Emergency treatment is focused on the prevention and/or treatment of hemorrhage and the prevention of infection.

Trauma

Trauma care of pregnant women requires attention to the needs of two patients—mother and fetus—and the injury and complication risks are dependent on the gestational age of the fetus. Motor vehicle accidents, which include seat belt injuries in addition to blunt trauma, and domestic partner violence are the most common causes of trauma in pregnant women, and it is also noted that substance abuse is commonly related to these injuries. Research suggests that, collectively, accidental and violent trauma are responsible for more maternal injuries and death than all other complications of pregnancy. Patient complaints of pain must be differentiated as to an obstetrical or non-obstetrical etiology. There is an inherent risk of the onset of preterm labor and abruptio placenta with all maternal trauma.

The emergency care of the pregnant patient is focused on the assessment of maternal hemodynamic status and fetal wellbeing. Lab studies aimed at the identification and assessment of traumatic injuries may include CBC, electrolytes, glucose, blood typing and cross match, Rh typing, pregnancy testing, coagulation studies, urinalysis for presence of infection and/or RBCs, Kleihauer-Betke testing, toxicology screening, D-dimer testing for identification of placental abruption, and testing for a base deficit that may indicate intra-abdominal injury. In addition to the attention to special concerns related to the pregnancy, the trauma protocol will be initiated according to agency protocol. The emergency care of a pregnant trauma victim is focused on assessment of both patients, identification and emergency treatment of all injuries, preparations for emergency delivery of the fetus as necessary, prevention and/or treatment of hemorrhage, and appropriate fluid volume support. Emergency providers will also report the occurrence of domestic or criminal violence as mandated by applicable HIPAA and state laws.

Musculoskeletal/Neurological/Integumentary

Dementia/Alzheimer's Disease

Dementia

Dementia is a general term used to describe a state of general cognitive decline. Although Alzheimer's disease accounts for up to 80 percent of all cases of dementia in the United States, the remaining two million cases may result from any one of several additional causes. The destruction of cortical tissue resulting from a stroke, or more commonly from multiple small strokes, often results in altered cognitive and physical function, while repetitive head injuries over an extended period also potentially result in permanent damage, limiting normal brain activity. Less common causes of dementia include infection of the brain by prions (abnormal protein fragments), as in Creutzfeldt-Jakob disease or the human immunodeficiency virus (HIV); deposition of Lewy bodies in the cerebral cortex as in Parkinson's disease; and reversible conditions such as vitamin B-12 deficiency and altered function of the thyroid gland. The onset and progression of the disease relate to the underlying cause and associated patient comorbidities.

Alzheimer's Disease

Alzheimer's disease is a chronic progressive form of dementia with an insidious onset that is caused by the abnormal accumulation of amyloid-β plaque in the brain. The accumulation of this plaque eventually interferes with neural functioning, which is responsible for the progressive manifestations of the disease. Although the exact etiology is unknown, environmental toxins, vascular alterations due to hemorrhagic or embolic events, infections, and genetic factors have all been proposed as the triggering mechanism for the plaque formation. The progression of the disease and the associated manifestations are specific to the individual; however, in all individuals, there is measurable decline over time in cognitive functioning, including short-term and long-term memory, behavior and mood, and the ability to perform activities of daily living (ADLs).

The diagnosis is based on the patient's presenting history and manifestations, imaging studies of the brain, protein analysis of the cerebrospinal fluid (CSF), and cognitive assessment with measures such as the Mini-Mental State Exam. Current treatments are only supportive, although cholinesterase inhibitors and N Methyl D aspartate receptor antagonists may slow the progression of the manifestations for a limited period if administered early in the course of the disease. All patients will suffer an eventual decline in all aspects of cognitive functioning, with the average survival rate dependent on the presence of comorbidities and the level of care and support available to the patient.

Experiencing a fall with or without a resulting fracture, somatic illnesses, and caregiver strain are the most common reasons for emergency department visits in this population. The nursing care of the patient with Alzheimer's disease in the emergency department must focus on patient safety because the usual chaotic environment of the department is disorienting to the confused patient. Safeguards against increased confusion and wandering, which is a common behavior in this patient population, should be implemented. In addition, the entire family unit should be assessed by the interdisciplinary health team to identify any alterations of family process or additional resources that are required for adequate patient care after discharge from the emergency department or the acute care facility.

Chronic Neurological Disorders

Multiple Sclerosis

Multiple sclerosis (MS) is a chronic disease manifested by progressive destruction of the myelin sheath and resulting plaque formation in the central nervous system (CNS). The precipitating event of this autoimmune disease is the migration of activated T cells to the CNS, which disrupts the blood-brain barrier. Exposure to environmental toxins is considered to be the likely trigger for this immune response. These alterations facilitate the antigen-antibody reactions that result in the demyelination of the axons. The onset of this disease is insidious, with symptoms occurring intermittently over a period of months or years. Sensory manifestations may include numbness and tingling of the extremities, blurred vision, vertigo, tinnitus, impaired hearing, and chronic neuropathic pain. Motor manifestations may include weakness or paralysis of limbs, trunk, and head; diplopia; scanning speech; and muscle spasticity. Cerebellar manifestations include nystagmus, ataxia, dysarthria, dysphagia, and fatigue.

The progress of the disease and presenting clinical manifestations vary greatly from one individual to another; however, there are common forms of the disease that relate to the expression of the clinical manifestations or disability and the disease activity over time. An initial episode of neurological manifestations due to demyelination that lasts for at least 24 hours is identified as a clinically isolated episode of MS. The potential for progression of the disease to the relapsing-remitting form of MS is predicted by magnetic resonance imaging (MRI) studies indicating the presence or absence of plaque formation. The remaining forms of MS are all associated with increasing disability related to the disease over time. The relapsing-remitting form is common to 85 percent of all patients diagnosed with MS and presents a variable pattern of active and inactive disease. The manifestations may resolve, decrease in severity, or become permanent after a relapse. In the primary-progressive form of MS that affects 10 percent of patients diagnosed with MS, the disease is constantly active without periods of remission. The secondary-progressive form of MS is identified as the progression of the relapsing-remitting form to a state of permanently active disease without remission.

Acute exacerbations of MS are treated with interferon or another of the seven disease-modifying drugs (DMDs), which are used to decrease the frequency of relapses and slow the progression of the disease. Research indicates that the medications are most effective when therapy is begun as soon as the diagnosis is confirmed. Other treatments are symptomatic and may treat conditions such as bladder infections, gastrointestinal (GI) disorders, and muscle spasticity. Patients with MS most commonly access care in the emergency department for non-neurological conditions, including GI disorders, falls, and bladder infections, and management of the manifestations associated with acute relapses.

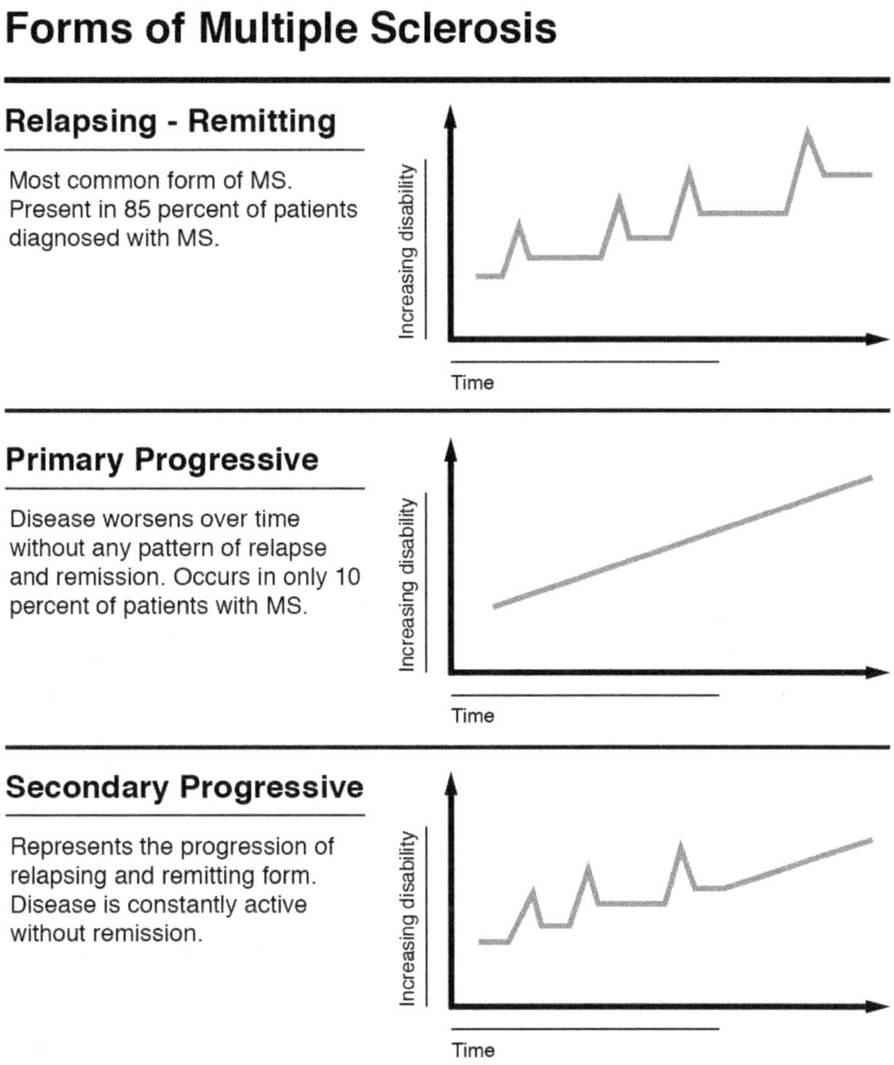

Myasthenia Gravis

Myasthenia gravis is also an autoimmune disease of the CNS that is manifested by severe muscle weakness resulting from altered transmission of acetylcholine at the neuromuscular junction due to antibody formation. Relapses and remissions are common, and these relapses may be triggered by infection, increases in body temperature due to immersion in hot water, stress, and pregnancy. Subjective manifestations include weakness, diplopia, dysphagia, fatigue on exertion, and bowel and bladder dysfunction. Objective manifestations include unilateral or bilateral ptosis of the eye, impaired respiratory function, impaired swallowing, and decreased muscle strength. Tensilon testing and electromyography, which measures muscle activity over time, are used to diagnose this disorder, while anticholinesterase agents and immunosuppressant agents are the mainstays of treatment. Additional treatments include plasmapheresis to decrease circulating antibodies and removal of the thymus gland to slow T-cell production.

Patients in myasthenic crisis due to a lack of cholinesterase may present in the emergency department with hypertension and severe muscle weakness that requires mechanical ventilation. Tensilon therapy may temporarily reduce the symptoms. Patients in cholinergic crisis due to an excess of cholinesterase exhibit hypotension, hypersecretion, and severe muscle twitching, which eventually results in respiratory muscle fatigue requiring ventilatory support. Atropine is used to control manifestations of this complication.

Guillain-Barré Syndrome

The most common form of **Guillain-Barré syndrome** (GBS) is acute immune-mediated demyelinating polyneuropathy. This rare syndrome may develop two to four weeks after a bacterial or viral infection of the respiratory or GI systems or following surgery. The most common causative organisms are *C. jejuni* and cytomegalovirus that may produce a subclinical infection that occurs unnoticed by the patient prior to the development of the acute onset of GBS. Other causative agents that are associated with GBS include the Epstein-Barr virus, *Mycoplasma pneumoniae*, and varicella-zoster virus. There is also an association between GBS and HIV. Current research is focused on investigating any association between the Zika virus and GBS; however, to date, there is little evidence of that relationship because there are few laboratories in the United States with the technology needed to identify the virus. The incidence of GBS has also been associated with vaccine administration; however, accumulated data does not support these claims.

The manifestations present as an acute onset of progressive, bilateral muscle weakness of the limbs that begins distally and continues proximally. The syndrome is the result of segmental demyelination of the nerves with edema, resulting from the inflammatory process. Additional presenting manifestations include pain, paresthesia, and abnormal sensations in the fingers. The progressive muscle weakness peaks at four weeks and potentially involves the arms, the muscles of the core, the cranial nerves, and the respiratory muscles. Involvement of the cranial nerves may result in facial drooping, diplopia, dysphagia, weakness or paralysis of the eye muscles, and pupillary alterations. Alterations in the autonomic nervous system also may result in orthostatic hypotension, paroxysmal hypertension, heart block, bradycardia, tachycardia, and asystole. Respiratory manifestations include dyspnea, shortness of breath, and dysphagia. In addition, as many as 30 percent of patients will progress to respiratory failure requiring ventilatory support due to the demyelination of the nerves that innervate the respiratory muscles.

The syndrome is diagnosed by the patient's history and laboratory studies to include electrolytes, liver function analysis, erythrocyte sedimentation rate (ESR), pulmonary function studies, and the assessment of CSF for the presence of excess protein content. In addition, electromyography and nerve conduction studies are used to identify the signs of demyelination, which confirms the diagnosis.

The emergency care of the patient with Guillain-Barré syndrome follows the Airway, Breathing, Circulation (ABC) protocol. Intubation with assisted ventilation is indicated in the event of hypoxia or decreasing respiratory muscle function as evidenced by an ineffective cough or aspiration. Cardiac manifestations vary according to the progression of the disease and are treated symptomatically. Placement of a temporary cardiac pacemaker may be necessary to treat second- or third-degree heart block. Treatment with plasmapheresis to remove the antibodies and intravenous (IV) immunoglobulin (Ig) to interfere with the antigen expression must be initiated within two to four weeks of the onset of symptoms to induce progression to the recovery phase of the syndrome. Care of the patient in the recovery phase must also address the common complications of immobility. Emergency care providers often make the initial diagnosis of this rare disease and therefore must be alert for the presenting manifestations that can progress rapidly to respiratory failure.

Headaches and Head Conditions

Temporal Arteritis

Temporal arteritis, also known as **giant cell arteritis**, is an inflammatory disorder of unknown origin that manifests as inflammatory changes in the intima, media, and adventitia layers of the artery as well as scattered accumulations of lymphocytes and macrophages that result in ischemic changes distal to the damaged areas. The condition is more common in women over fifty years of age, and current research indicates that infection and genetics also may be related to the development of the disease. The onset may be acute or insidious, and common signs and symptoms include head pain, neck pain, jaw claudication (jaw pain caused by ischemia of the maxillary artery), visual disturbances, shoulder and pelvic girdle pain, and general malaise and fever. The condition is diagnosed by a patient history of the onset of the headaches or the change in the characteristics of the headache in patients with chronic headaches, elevated ESR, and temporal artery biopsy that confirms the diagnosis. The condition is immediately treated with steroids if possible, or alternatively with cyclosporine, azathioprine, or methotrexate.

The onset of ophthalmic alterations requires emergency care because any loss of vision before treatment is initiated will be irreversible. In addition, if treatment is delayed beyond two weeks after the onset of the initial vision loss, vision in the unaffected eye will be lost as well. Additional complications are related to steroid therapy and include stroke, myocardial infarction, small-bowel infarction, vertebral body fractures, and steroid psychoses. Even with successful treatment that prevents irreversible vision alterations, the patient with temporal arteritis has a lifelong risk of inflammatory disease of the large vessels.

Migraine

Migraine headaches are often preceded by an aura, which may be visual or sensory. The pulsatile pain associated with migraine headaches is described as throbbing and constant and most often localizes to one side of the head. Other manifestations include photophobia, sound sensitivity, nausea and vomiting, and anorexia. The pain increases over a period of one to two hours and then may last from 4 to 72 hours. The exact cause of the migraine headache syndrome is not well understood; however, there is strong evidence of a genetic link and some support for the role of alterations in neurovascular function and neurotransmitter regulation. Risk factors include elevated C-reactive protein and homocysteine levels, increased levels of TNF-alpha and adhesion molecules (systemic inflammation markers), increased body weight, hypertension, impaired insulin sensitivity, and coronary artery disease. The diagnosis is determined by the patient's history, laboratory testing for inflammatory markers, and imaging studies and lumbar puncture, as indicated by the severity of the patient's condition.

The treatment for migraine headaches may be preventive, therapeutic, and/or symptomatic. Medications used to prevent migraine headaches are used for those patients with chronic disease who have fourteen or more headaches per month. Antiemetics are used to lessen nausea and vomiting, while opioids may be prescribed even though their use in migraine management is not recommended. The emergency care of the patient with a migraine headache is focused on establishing the differential diagnosis and correcting fluid volume alterations that may result from vomiting. Although most patients who seek emergency care are diagnosed with migraine headaches, the importance of early intervention for temporal arteritis, stroke, or brain tumor requires a prompt diagnosis.

Increased Intracranial Pressure

Under normal circumstances, there is a dynamic equilibrium among the bony structure of the cranium, brain tissue, and extracellular fluid that comprise approximately 85 percent of the intracranial volume; the blood volume that comprises 10 percent of the volume; and the CSF that occupies the remaining 5 percent of the volume of the cranium. If any one of these volumes increases, there must be a compensatory decrease in one or more of the remaining volumes to maintain normal intracranial pressure (ICP) and optimal cerebral perfusion pressure (CPP).

The CPP represents the pressure gradient for cerebral perfusion and is equal to the difference between the mean arterial pressure (MAP) and the ICP ($MAP - ICP = CPP$). The process of autoregulation maintains optimal CPP by dilation and constriction of the cerebral arterioles; however, if the MAP falls below 65 millimeters of mercury or rises above 150 millimeters of mercury, autoregulation is ineffective, and cerebral blood flow is dependent on blood pressure (BP). Once this mechanism fails, any increase in volume potentially will cause an increase in the ICP. For instance, normal ICP may be maintained in the presence of a slow-growing tumor; however, a sudden small accumulation of blood will cause a sharp increase in the ICP. Eventually, all autoregulatory mechanisms will be exhausted in either circumstance, and the ICP will be increased. In an adult in the supine position, the normal ICP is 7 to 15 millimeters of mercury, while an ICP greater than 15 millimeters of mercury is considered abnormal, and pressures greater than 20 millimeters of mercury require intervention.

Conditions associated with increased ICP include space-occupying lesions such as tumors and hematomas; obstruction of CSF or hydrocephalus; increased production of CSF due to tumor formation; cerebral edema resulting from head injuries, strokes, infection, or surgery; hyponatremia; hepatic encephalopathy; and idiopathic intracranial hypertension. Early manifestations of increased ICP include blurred vision with gradual dilation of the pupil and slowed pupillary response, restlessness, and confusion with progressive disorientation as to time, then to place, and finally to person.

Later signs include initially ipsilateral pupillary dilation and fixation, which progresses to bilateral dilation and fixation; decorticate or decerebrate posturing; and Cushing's triad of manifestations that include bradycardia, widening pulse pressure, and Cheyne-Stokes respirations. ICP monitoring will be used to assess all patients requiring emergency care for any condition that is potentially associated with increased ICP. Depending on the underlying pathology, common interventions for increased ICP include sedation and paralysis, intubation and hyperventilation to decrease the $PaCO_2$, infusion of mannitol, an osmotic diuretic, and hypertonic saline IV solutions. Emergency providers understand that sustained elevations of ICP are associated with a poor prognosis, and therefore, the underlying cause and manifestations must be treated aggressively.

Meningitis

Meningitis is defined as the infection and resulting inflammation of the three layers of the meninges, the membranous covering of the brain and spinal cord. The causative agent may be bacterial, viral, parasitic, or fungal, which commonly occurs in patients who are HIV positive. The most common bacterial agent is *S. pneumoniae*, while meningococcal meningitis is common in crowded living spaces. However, the development and use of the meningococcal vaccine (MCV 4) has reduced the incidence in college students and military personnel. The *Haemophilus influenzae* type B (Hib) vaccine has decreased the incidence and morbidity of the HI meningitis in infants, and the pneumococcal polysaccharide vaccine (PPSV) is being used to prevent meningitis in at-risk populations, such as immunocompromised adults, smokers, residents in long-term care facilities, and adults with chronic disease.

General risk factors for bacterial infection of the meninges include loss of, or decreased function of, the spleen; hypoglobinemia; chronic glucocorticoid use; deficiency of the complement system; diabetes; renal insufficiency; alcoholism; chronic liver disease; otitis media; and trauma associated with leakage of the CSF. Bacterial meningitis is infectious, and early diagnosis and treatment are essential for survival and recovery. Emergency providers understand that even with adequate treatment, 50 percent of patients with bacterial meningitis will develop complications within two to three weeks of the acute infection, and long-term deficits are common in 30 percent of the surviving patients. The complications are specific to the causative organism, but may include hearing loss, blindness, paralysis, seizure disorder, muscular deficiencies, ataxia, hydrocephalus, and subdural effusions. In contrast, the incidence of viral meningitis is often associated with other viral conditions such as mumps, measles, herpes, and infections due to arboviruses such as the West Nile virus. The treatment is supportive, and the majority of patients recover without long-term complications; however, the outcome is less certain for patients who are immunocompromised, less than two years old, or more than sixty years old.

The classic manifestations of bacterial meningitis include fever, nuchal rigidity, and headache. Additional findings may include nausea and vomiting, photophobia, confusion, and a decreased level of consciousness. Patients with viral meningitis may report the incidence of fatigue, muscle aches, and decreased appetite prior to the illness. Infants may exhibit a high-pitched cry, muscle flaccidity, irritability, and bulging fontanels.

The diagnosis of meningitis is determined by lumbar puncture; CSF analysis; cultures of the blood, nose, and respiratory secretions and any skin lesions that are present; complete blood count (CBC); electrolytes; coagulation studies; serum glucose to compare with CSF glucose; and procalcitonin to differentiate bacterial meningitis from aseptic meningitis in children. There is a small risk of herniation of the brain when the CSF is removed during the lumbar puncture, and while a computerized tomography (CT) scan may be done to assess the risk, emergency providers understand that effective antibiotic treatment must be initiated as quickly as possible to prevent the morbidity associated with bacterial meningitis. The results of the Gram stain of the CSF and blood will dictate the initial antibiotic therapy, which will be modified when the specific agent is identified. Additional interventions include seizure precautions, cardiac monitoring, and ongoing assessment of respiratory and neurological function. Patients with bacterial meningitis may require long-term rehabilitation.

Seizure Disorders

A **seizure** is defined as a chaotic period of uncoordinated electrical activity in the brain, which results in one of several characteristic behaviors. Although the exact cause is unknown, several possible triggers have been proposed as noted below. The recently revised classification system categorizes seizure activity according to the area of the brain where the seizure initiates, the patient's level of awareness during the seizure, and other descriptive features such as the presence of an aura. The unclassified category includes seizure patterns that do not conform to the primary categories. Seizures that originate in a single area of the brain are designated as **focal seizures**, while seizures that originate in two or more different networks are designated as **generalized seizures**. The remaining seizures in the onset category include seizures without an identified point of onset and seizures that progress from focal seizures to generalized seizures.

Risk factors associated with seizures include genetic predisposition, illnesses with severe temperature elevation, head trauma, cerebral edema, inappropriate use or discontinuance of antiepileptic drugs (AEDs), intracerebral infection, excess or deficiency of sodium and glucose, toxin exposure, hypoxia, and acute drug or alcohol withdrawal. Patients are encouraged to identify any conditions that may be triggers for their seizure activity. Although the triggers vary greatly from one patient to another, commonly identified events include increased physical activity, excessive stress, hyperventilation, fatigue, acute ETOH (ethyl alcohol) ingestion, exposure to flashing lights, and inhaled chemicals, including cocaine.

The tonic phase presents as stiffening of the limbs for a brief period, while the clonic phase is evidenced by jerking motions of the limbs. These manifestations may be accompanied by a decreased level of consciousness, respiratory alterations and cyanosis, incontinence, and biting of the tongue. Absence seizures are manifested by a decreased level of awareness without abnormal muscular activity. The manifestations of the postictal phase include alterations in consciousness and awareness and increased oral secretions. Seizure disorders are diagnosed by serum lab studies to assess AED levels and to identify excess alcohol and recreational drugs, metabolic alterations, and kidney and liver function. Electroencephalography (EEG) and the enhanced magnetoencephalography are used to identify the origin of the altered electrical activity in the brain, and MRI, skull films, and CSF analysis are used to rule out possible sources of the seizure disorder such as tumor formation.

Seizure disorders are treated with AEDs that stabilize the neuron cell membrane by facilitating the inhibitory mechanisms or opposing the excitatory mechanisms. Patients with a chronic seizure disorder, or epilepsy, usually require a combination of medications to minimize seizure activity. Elderly patients respond differently to the AEDs and may require frequent assessment and revision of the care plan. The emergency care of the patient with seizures is focused on patient safety during and after the seizure and the cessation and prevention of the seizure activity. Prolonged seizure activity is defined as *status epilepticus*, which is the occurrence of multiple seizures, each lasting more than 5 minutes over a 30-minute period. This life-threatening condition is commonly the result of incorrect usage of AEDs or the use of recreational drugs. Emergency care of this condition includes the immediate administration of phenytoin and benzodiazepines, in addition to possible general anesthesia if the medication therapy is not effective.

Shunt Dysfunctions

Increased production or decreased absorption and drainage of CSF results in hydrocephalus. This condition develops in infants, due to premature birth, intracranial hemorrhage, and genetic defects such as spina bifida, while in older children and adults, CSF accumulations due to hemorrhagic disease and tumor formation result in a significant increase in ICP due to the presence of a rigid cranium. In any event, emergency care of hydrocephalus is necessary to prevent physical and intellectual deficits.

If tumor formation is responsible for the development of hydrocephalus, removal of the tumor commonly results in an 88 percent reduction in the ICP. Research indicates that medical interventions are only minimally effective, and while surgical interventions have greater efficacy in select patients, 75 percent of patients with hydrocephalus will require the placement of a shunt for long-term drainage of the CSF. A CSF shunt facilitates the flow excess CSF from the ventricle to a distant anatomical site such as the peritoneum (the most common site), the atria, and the pleural space. The catheter has a one-way flow pressure valve that limits the rate of flow of the CSF from the cerebral ventricle to the distant absorption site and a reservoir that provides percutaneous access to the shunt. The catheter is positioned in the ventricle and then tunneled subcutaneously to the collection site, allowing the excess CSF to flow from the ventricle to be reabsorbed, thereby decreasing the ICP.

Infections of the shunt manifest with similar signs of increased ICP in addition to possible purulent drainage, skin erosion and erythema, abdominal pain, and signs of peritonitis. Fever may or may not be present and is not necessary to confirm the diagnosis. Noninfectious complications related to the catheter include mechanical failure, migration of the distal catheter due to the patient's growth, and initial mispositioning of the catheter. Obstruction of the catheter accounts for 50 to 80 percent of all shunt failures, with the proximal catheter and shunt valve identified as the most common sites of obstruction due to choroid ingrowth or deposition of blood and cellular debris. Obstruction of the distal catheter, which occurs most often at the abdominal entry site, is less common and may be due to twisting of the catheter or from obstruction by inflammatory cellular debris or pseudocyst formation.

Emergency providers understand that the manifestations of each of these complications are age-dependent, with infants experiencing bulging of the fontanels and increasing head circumference in addition to other expected signs of increased ICP, such as headache, vomiting without nausea, changes in the level of consciousness, irritability, bradycardia, seizures, and visual alterations. Patients and care providers must be alert for these changes to access appropriate emergency care. Previous shunt revision or infection are associated with an increased risk of shunt failure, which typically occurs two to four months after insertion of the catheter. MRI scans, shunt series radiographs and nuclear medicine studies, and ultrasounds are used to assess the integrity and position of the catheter. Emergency management includes initiating a neurosurgical consultation, close observation of all vital signs for the advancement of the increased ICP, identification of the cause of the malfunction, treatment of any infection, and drainage of the excess CSF through the reservoir.

Spinal Cord Injuries

Injuries to the spinal cord are associated with severe and often irreversible neurological deficits and disabilities. **Spinal cord injuries** (SCIs) may be due to one or a combination of the following types of injury: direct traumatic injuries of the spinal cord, compression of the spinal cord by bone fragments or hematoma formation, or ischemia resulting from damage to the spinal arteries. The anatomical location of the SCI predicts the degree of sensory and motor function that will be lost. In addition, the injury will be labeled as **paraplegia** if the lesion is at the T1 to the T5 level, affecting only the lower extremities, or **tetraplegia** if the lesion is at the C1 to the C7 level, affecting both the upper and lower extremities in addition to respiratory function. SCIs may be categorized as complete or incomplete depending on the degree of impairment.

While complete SCIs are associated with complete loss of sensory-motor function, incomplete lesions are determined by the actual portion of the spinal cord that is affected. Central spinal cord syndrome is an incomplete SCI that involves upper extremity weakness or paralysis with little or no deficit noted in the lower extremities. Anterior spinal cord syndrome is also an incomplete SCI that is associated with loss of motor function, pain, and sensation below the injury; however, the sensations of light touch, proprioception, and vibration remain intact. In addition, Brown-Sequard syndrome is an incomplete lesion of one-half of the spinal cord, which results in paralysis on the side of the injury and loss of pain and temperature sensation on the opposite side of the injury.

Emergency providers understand that the injury to the spinal cord is an evolving process, which means that the level of the injury can rise one to two spinal levels within 48 to 72 hours after the initial insult. An incomplete injury may progress to a complete injury during this time due to the effects of altered blood flow and resulting edema and the presence of abnormal free radicals. Essential interventions aimed at minimizing or preventing this progression include establishing and maintaining normal oxygenation, arterial blood gas (ABG) values, and perfusion of the spinal cord.

SCIs are also associated with three shock syndromes, including hemorrhagic shock, spinal shock, and neurogenic shock. Hemorrhagic shock from an acute or occult source must be suspected in all SCIs below the T6 level that present with hypotension. Spinal shock refers to the loss of sensory-motor function that may be temporary or permanent depending on the specific injury. At the same time, the patient must be monitored for signs of neurogenic shock, which presents with a triad of symptoms that include hypotension, bradycardia, and peripheral vasodilation. This complication is due to alterations in autonomic nervous system function, which causes loss of vagal tone. Most often, it occurs with an injury above the T6 level, resulting in decreased vascular resistance and vasodilation. Neurogenic shock may also be associated with hypothermia due to vasodilation; rapid, shallow respirations; difficulty breathing; cold, clammy, pale skin; nausea; vomiting; and dizziness. Emergency treatment of neurogenic shock includes IV fluids and inotropic medications to support the BP and IV atropine and/or pacemaker insertion, as needed, to treat the bradycardia. If a patient presents with neurological deficits eight or more hours after sustaining an SCI, high-dose prednisone may be administered to reverse the manifestations of neurogenic shock.

Emergency management of SCIs is focused on preventing extension of the injury and long-term deficits with immobilization and interventions based on the Airway, Breathing, and Circulation protocol. Cervical SCIs result in an 80 to 95 percent decrease in vital capacity, and mechanical ventilation is often required for lesions at this level. Support of the circulation is addressed in the treatment of neurogenic shock. Other supportive treatment interventions are aimed at minimizing the effects of immobility. Emergency providers are aware that patients with complete SCIs have less than a 5 percent chance of recovery; however, more than 90 percent of all patients with SCIs eventually return home and regain some measure of independence.

Stroke

A **stroke** is defined as the death of brain tissue due to ischemic or hemorrhagic injury. Ischemic strokes are more common than hemorrhagic strokes; however, the differential diagnosis of these conditions requires careful attention to the patient's history and physical examination. In general, an acute onset of neurological symptoms and seizures is more common with hemorrhagic stroke, while ischemic stroke is more frequently associated with a history of some form of trauma. The National Institutes of Health (NIH) Stroke Scale represents an international effort to standardize the assessment and treatment protocols for stroke. The scale includes detailed criteria and the protocol for assessment of the neurological system. The stroke scale items are to be administered in the official order listed and there are directions that denote how to score each item.

Ischemic Stroke

Ischemic strokes result from occlusion of the cerebral vasculature as a result of a thrombotic or embolic event. At the cellular level, the ischemia leads to hypoxia that rapidly depletes the ATP stores. As a result, the cellular membrane pressure gradient is lost, and there is an influx of sodium, calcium, and water into the cell, which leads to cytotoxic edema. This process creates scattered regions of ischemia in the affected area, containing cells that are dead within minutes of the precipitating event. This core of ischemic tissue is surrounded by an area with minimally-adequate perfusion that may remain viable for several hours after the event. These necrotic areas are eventually liquefied and acted upon by macrophages, resulting in the loss of brain parenchyma. These affected sites, if sufficiently large, may be prone to hemorrhage, due to the formation of collateral vascular supply with or without the use of medications such as recombinant tissue plasminogen activator (rtPA). The ischemic process also compromises the blood-brain barrier, which leads to the movement of water and protein into the extracellular space within 4 to 6 hours after the onset of the stroke, resulting in vasogenic edema.

Nonmodifiable risk factors for ischemic stroke include age, gender, ethnicity, history of migraine headaches with aura, and a family history of stroke or transient ischemic attacks (TIAs). Modifiable risk factors include hypertension, diabetes, hypercholesterolemia, cardiac disease including atrial fibrillation, valvular disease and heart failure, elevated homocysteine levels, obesity, illicit drug use, alcohol abuse, smoking, and sedentary lifestyle. The research related to the occurrence of stroke in women indicates the need to treat hypertension aggressively prior to and during pregnancy and prior to the use of contraceptives to prevent irreversible damage to the microvasculature. In addition, it is recommended that to reduce their risk of stroke, women with a history of migraine headaches preceded by an aura should ameliorate all modifiable risk factors, and all women over seventy-five years old should be routinely assessed for the onset of atrial fibrillation.

Heredity is associated with identified gene mutations and the process of atherosclerosis and cholesterol metabolism. Hypercholesterolemia and the progression of atherosclerosis in genetically-susceptible individuals are now regarded as active inflammatory processes that contribute to endothelial damage of the cerebral vasculature, thereby increasing the risk for strokes. There are also early indications that infection also contributes to the development and advancement of atherosclerosis.

The presenting manifestations of ischemic stroke must be differentiated from other common diseases, including brain tumor formation, hyponatremia, hypoglycemia, seizure disorders, and systemic infection. The sudden onset of hemisensory losses, visual alterations, hemiparesis, ataxia, nystagmus, and aphasia are commonly, although not exclusively, associated with ischemic strokes. The availability of reperfusion therapies dictates the emergent use of diagnostic imaging studies, including CT and MRI scans, carotid duplex scans, and digital subtraction angiography to confirm the data obtained from the patient's history and physical examination. Laboratory studies include CBC, coagulation studies, chemistry panels, cardiac biomarkers, toxicology assays, and pregnancy testing as appropriate.

The emergency care of the patient who presents with an ischemic stroke is focused on the stabilization of the patient's ABCs, completion of the physical examination and appropriate diagnostic studies, and initiation of reperfusion therapy as appropriate, within 60 minutes of arrival in the emergency department. Reperfusion therapies include the use of alteplase (the only fibrinolytic agent that is approved for the treatment of ischemic stroke), antiplatelet agents, and mechanical thrombectomy. Emergency providers must also be alert for hyperthermia, hypoxia, hypertension or hypotension, and signs of cardiac ischemia or cardiac arrhythmias.

Hemorrhagic Stroke

Hemorrhagic strokes are less common than ischemic strokes; however, a hemorrhagic stroke is more likely to be fatal than an ischemic stroke. A hemorrhagic stroke is the result of bleeding into the parenchymal tissue of the brain due to leakage of blood from damaged intracerebral arteries. These hemorrhagic events occur more often in specific areas of the brain, including the thalamus, cerebellum, and brain stem. The tissue surrounding the hemorrhagic area is also subject to injury due to the mass effect of the accumulated blood volume. In the event of subarachnoid hemorrhage, ICP becomes elevated with resulting dysfunction of the autoregulation response, which leads to abnormal vasoconstriction, platelet aggregation, and decreased perfusion and blood flow, resulting in cerebral ischemia.

Risk factors for hemorrhagic stroke include older age; a history of hypertension, which is present in 60 percent of patients; personal history of stroke; alcohol abuse; and illicit drug use. Common conditions associated with hemorrhagic stroke include hypertension, cerebral amyloidosis, coagulopathies, vascular alterations including arteriovenous malformation, vasculitis, intracranial neoplasm, and a history of anticoagulant or antithrombotic therapy.

Although the presenting manifestations for hemorrhagic stroke differ in some respect from the those associated with ischemic stroke, none of these such manifestations is an absolute predictor of one or the other. In general, patients with hemorrhagic stroke present with a headache that may be severe, significant alterations in the level of consciousness and neurological function, hypertension, seizures, and nausea and vomiting. The specific neurological defects depend on the anatomical site of the hemorrhage and may include hemisensory loss, hemiparesis, aphasia, and visual alterations.

Diagnostic studies include CBC, chemistry panel, coagulation studies, and blood glucose. Non-contrast CT scan or MRI are the preferred imaging studies. CT or magnetic resonance angiography may also be used to obtain images of the cerebral vasculature. Close observation of the patient's vital signs, neurological vital signs, and ICP is necessary.

The emergency management of the patient with hemorrhagic stroke is focused on the ABC protocol, in addition to the control of bleeding, seizure activity, and increased ICP. There is no single medication used to treat hemorrhagic stroke; however, recent data suggests that aggressive emergency management of hypertension initiated early and aimed at reducing the systolic BP to less than 140 millimeters of mercury may be effective in reducing the growth of the hematoma at the site, which decreases the mass effect. Beta-blockers and ACE inhibitors are recommended to facilitate this reduction. Endotracheal intubation for ventilatory support may be necessary; however, hyperventilation is not recommended due to the resulting suppression of cerebral blood flow. While seizure activity will be treated with AEDs, there is controversy related to the prophylactic use of these medicines. Increased ICP requires osmotic diuretic therapy, elevation of the head of the bed to 30 degrees, sedation and analgesics as appropriate, and antacids. Steroid therapy is not effective and is not recommended.

Patients who present with manifestations of hemorrhagic stroke with a history of anticoagulation therapy present a special therapeutic challenge due to the extension of the hematoma formation. More than 50 percent of patients taking warfarin who suffer a hemorrhagic stroke will die within thirty days. This statistic is consistent in patients with international normalized ratio (INR) levels within the therapeutic range, with increased mortality noted in patients with INRs that exceed the therapeutic level. Emergency treatment includes fresh frozen plasma, IV vitamin K, prothrombin complex concentrates, and recombinant factor VIIa (rFVIIa). There are administration concerns with each of these therapies that must be addressed to prevent any delays in the reversal of the effects of the warfarin.

Transient Ischemic Attack

A **transient ischemic attack** (TIA) is defined as a short-term episode of altered neurological function that lasts for less than one hour; it may be imperceptible to the patient. The deficit may be related to speech, movement, behavior, or memory and may be caused by an ischemic event in the brain, spinal cord, or retina. The patient's history and neurological assessment according to the NIH Stroke Scale establish the diagnosis. Additional diagnostic studies include CBC, glucose, sedimentation rate, electrolytes, lipid profile, toxicology screen, 12-lead ECG, and CSF analysis. Imaging studies include non-contrast MRI or CT, carotid Doppler exam, and angiography.

Emergency care of the patient with a TIA is focused on the assessment of any neurological deficits and the identification of comorbid conditions that may be related to the attack. Hospital admission is required in the event of an attack that lasts more than one hour, if the patient has experienced more than a single attack in a one-week period, or if the attack is related to a cardiac source such as atrial fibrillation or a myocardial infarction. The $ABCD^2$ stroke risk score calculates the patient's risk for experiencing a true stroke within two days after the TIA based on five factors (see the table below). Interventions aimed at stroke prevention in relation to the risk stratification as calculated by the $ABCD^2$

score are specific to underlying comorbidities; however, treatment with ASA and clopidogrel is commonly prescribed.

ABCD² Stroke Risk Score		
	1 Point	2 Points
***A*ge**	≥ 60 years	
***B*lood Pressure**	SBP ≥ 140 mmHg DBP ≥ 90 mmHg	
***C*linical Features**	Speech impairment but no focal weakness	Focal weakness
***D*uration of Symptoms**	≤ 59 minutes	≥ 60 minutes
***D*iabetes**	Diagnosed	
Total Score (denotes risk for stroke (CVA) within 2 days after TIA)	0-3 points = 1% risk 4-5 points = 4.1% risk 6-7 points = 8.1% risk	

Trauma

The Advanced Trauma Life Support protocol is a standardized procedure for the assessment and treatment of trauma patients. Injuries that are immediately fatal or occur minutes to hours after the initial injury are most often due to hemorrhage, cardiovascular collapse, and failed oxygenation, while deaths that occur days to weeks after an injury are commonly due to sepsis and multisystem organ failure. The primary survey or assessment of a trauma victim follows an ABCDE protocol: *A* refers to airway management; *B* refers to respiratory effort; *C* refers to circulation, including hemorrhage; *D* refers to gross mental status and mobility; and *E* addresses exposure such as hypothermia and environmental conditions. The results of the assessment dictate the interventions, while at the same time, monitoring devices are employed, a nasogastric tube and an indwelling urinary catheter are inserted, and lab samples for type/cross match, glucose, and ABGs are obtained. The CT scan is the most useful imaging study; however, ultrasound, angiography, and A&P chest and pelvic films are also used. Fluid resuscitation is calculated according to estimated blood loss consistent with a standardized trauma protocol. Once the interventions have been initiated, a second assessment is performed that includes examination of every orifice and body system to identify additional or worsening injuries. Emergency providers understand that the source of any deterioration in a patient's condition after stabilization is most often associated with changes in the airway, breathing, or circulation.

Trauma related to burns, hypothermia, and high-voltage electrical burns require additional consideration. Burn injuries may require chemical neutralization, excision of eschar formation to prevent compartment syndrome, aggressive fluid replacement, and ventilatory support. Resuscitative efforts for patients with hypothermia should not be discontinued until the patient's core temperature has been brought to normal with warm IV solution. Myonecrotic damage due to high-voltage electrical burns may not be visible but can result in direct myocardial injury and life-threatening hyperkalemia due to muscle damage.

Acute care institutions are obligated to provide adequate skilled personnel, equipment, and resources to address the emergency needs of the trauma patient according to the agency's designated trauma care level.

Med Surg Practice Test #1

1. The nurse is assessing the abdomen of a thirty-year-old female patient with appendicitis. Which finding is the nurse most likely to assess?
   a. Soft abdomen
   b. Periumbilical pain
   c. Absent bowel sounds
   d. Abdominal pulsations

2. Which assessment data is of greatest concern when present in a patient with pneumonia?
   a. Capillary refill greater than 3 seconds
   b. 9,000 white blood cells per microliter
   c. Respiratory rate of 20 breaths per minute
   d. Productive cough

3. Which intervention should the nurse NOT include while maintaining seizure precautions for a patient with epilepsy?
   a. Padded side-rails
   b. Suction by the bedside
   c. Side-rails down
   d. Ambu-bag in room

4. The nurse in the emergency department is assessing a nineteen-year-old college student who presents with sudden onset of headache that is associated with neck stiffness and fever. In caring for the patient with meningitis, the nurse understands that which of the following observations is correct?
   a. The presence of a skin rash eliminates the diagnosis of viral meningitis.
   b. Brain herniation after lumbar puncture is more common in immunosuppressed patients.
   c. The CSF protein level is decreased in bacterial meningitis.
   d. The MCV4 vaccine has dramatically decreased the incidence of meningitis in patients in long-term care facilities.

5. While working with a withdrawn patient, how should the medical-surgical nurse respond?
   a. Enable the patient to establish the pace
   b. Remain the lead of the conversation
   c. Include short, quick movements
   d. Discourage verbal expression of anxiety triggers

6. While completing morning rounds, the medical-surgical nurse is introduced to a new patient; a 23-year-old female dressed like popular singer Diana Ross and mimicking her behavior. How should the medical-surgical nurse chart this defense mechanism finding?
   a. Projection
   b. Introjection
   c. Rationalization
   d. Identification

7. The medical-surgical nurse provides patient education before administering a new treatment for a patient with myasthenia gravis. Which description provided by the nurse accurately describes the reason for administering immunosuppressive therapy for this patient?
   a. Decrease autoantibody production
   b. Promote excretion of autoantibodies
   c. Increase autoantibody production
   d. Block autoantibody receptors

8. The nurse is caring for a patient in the emergency department who has manifestations of diverticulitis. The patient asks the nurse to explain the difference between diverticulosis and diverticulitis. Which of the following statements is correct?
   a. Diverticulosis rarely occurs in adults.
   b. Diverticulitis is associated with chronic NSAID use.
   c. The initial treatment for diverticulitis is surgery to remove the affected bowel segment.
   d. The patient's age at onset of diverticulosis is associated with the risk of diverticulitis.

9. When taking a history from a pregnant woman with placenta previa, the nurse would expect the patient to report which of the following?
   a. Maternal age of twenty-eight years
   b. First pregnancy
   c. Previous C-section
   d. One previous vaginal delivery

10. Which condition does the medical-surgical nurse attribute the patient's painful reddish-purple blistering rash to?
   a. Lupus erythematosus
   b. Vitiligo
   c. Stevens-Johnson syndrome
   d. Lyme disease

11. Which statement is typical of data the nurse collects on a woman hospitalized with abruptio placenta?
   a. "I am a smoker."
   b. "I am twenty-five years old."
   c. "I do not drink alcohol."
   d. "I have no history of placental abruption."

12. Which treatment intervention should be implemented in the plan of care for a patient with acute renal failure?
   a. Sulfonylureas
   b. Intravenous contrast studies
   c. Bed rest
   d. High-protein diet

13. Which analgesic, a dye known to numb pain within the urinary tract, should the medical-surgical nurse administer while caring for the patient with a urinary tract infection?
   a. Meperidine
   b. Phenazopyridine
   c. Naprosyn
   d. Ceftriaxone

14. How long should the medical-surgical nurse auscultate the apical heart rate while completing a focused assessment?
   a. 15 seconds
   b. 30 seconds
   c. 60 seconds
   d. 120 seconds

15. A patient overdosed on acetaminophen after retrieving it from their visitor's purse during visiting hours. While providing emergent care with the code response team, which medication should the nurse administer to counteract the effects of this poisoning?
   a. Atropine
   b. Acetylcysteine
   c. Naloxone
   d. Flumazenil

16. The nurse is caring for a patient in the emergency department with a non-ST elevation myocardial infarction (NSTEMI). Using the Thrombolysis in Myocardial Infarction (TIMI) tool, which of the following categories would the nurse NOT assess?
   a. Age
   b. ST deviation on ECG
   c. Left bundle branch block
   d. Prior aspirin intake

17. The nurse is administering an intravenous infusion of magnesium sulfate to a pregnant woman at thirty-two weeks' gestation who is experiencing preterm labor. When the patient reports facial flushing to the nurse, which action should the nurse take FIRST?
   a. Stop the infusion
   b. Notify the physician
   c. Reduce the rate of the infusion
   d. Continue to monitor the patient

18. While caring for a 54-year-old patient with rheumatoid arthritis and long-term corticosteroid use, which side effect does the medical-surgical nurse consider?
   a. Hypotension
   b. Weight Loss
   c. Hyperglycemia
   d. Thickening Skin

19. The nurse in the emergency department is admitting a patient who has sustained electrical burns 3 hours ago. The patient is awake, alert, and oriented, and vital signs are BP 136/70, HR 86, normal sinus rhythm, T 97.6 °F, pulse oximetry 97 percent, respiratory rate 18. The patient's skin is intact with one area of redness over the anterior chest wall. Two hours after admission, the patient is in cardiac arrest. What is the most likely cause of this complication?
   a. Hypovolemic shock
   b. Pulmonary edema
   c. Myocardial perforation
   d. Myonecrosis of skeletal muscle

20. Which of the following test results is consistent with pulmonary edema of a non-cardiogenic origin?
   a. Chest x-ray with bilateral pulmonary infiltrates
   b. Elevated blood levels of *B*-type natriuretic peptide (BNP)
   c. ABG analysis revealing hypoxemia
   d. A pulmonary artery wedge pressure of 12 mmHg

21. The nurse is teaching the family of a patient with early Alzheimer's disease about medication options to treat the disease. Which statement by the patient's daughter indicates an understanding of the effects of these medications?
   a. "Early treatment may cure my mom's Alzheimer's disease."
   b. "Hopefully, medication can place my mom in remission."
   c. "We may be able to slow the disease progression with early treatment."
   d. "Early treatment has not been shown to have an effect on this disease."

22. The medical-surgical nurse notes jugular vein distention during a head-to-toe physical assessment of a 63-year-old patient. Which cause does the nurse consider may be responsible for this finding?
   a. Right-sided heart failure
   b. Decreased pressure in circulation in lungs
   c. Fluid volume deficit
   d. Hypotension

23. The nurse is caring for a patient with congestive heart failure and is reviewing their medications with them during medication teaching. The patient expresses concern about their potassium level after recalling an issue with low potassium when prescribed a diuretic in the past. Which medication does the nurse explain is a potassium-sparing diuretic during this teaching?
   a. Lasix® (furosemide)
   b. Demadex® (torsemide)
   c. Aldactone® (spironolactone)
   d. Microzide® (hydrochlorothiazide)

24. The nurse administers intramuscular methotrexate to a woman with an ectopic pregnancy. Which parameter should the nurse evaluate to determine the effectiveness of this medication?
   a. Cessation of vaginal bleeding
   b. Increasing hematocrit
   c. Decreasing BHCG levels
   d. Negative Rh status

25. To detect cholecystitis in a child with sickle cell disease, the nurse should be alert for which assessment finding?
a. Localized abdominal tenderness
b. Generalized abdominal pain
c. Left upper quadrant pain
d. Rebound abdominal tenderness

26. The nurse is caring for a patient with a suspected ectopic pregnancy. The patient asks the nurse to explain how her smoking history is related to this condition. Which of the following statements correctly identifies the relationship between smoking and the development of an ectopic pregnancy?
a. Smoking decreases the oxygen saturation of the fetal circulation, which compromises the process of implantation.
b. Smoking alters progesterone levels, which interferes with the transfer of the fertilized ovum to the uterus.
c. Smoking alters the endometrial lining, making it an inhospitable environment for the fertilized ovum, thereby preventing implantation.
d. Smoking damages the cilia in the fallopian tube, which decreases motility and alters the movement of the fertilized ovum.

27. Which statement is typical of data collected on a patient with Grave's disease?
a. Female over age forty
b. Female under age forty
c. Male over age forty
d. Male under age forty

28. Which of the following is an indication for the placement of a vena cava filter to prevent pulmonary embolism (PE)?
a. Pregnancy
b. Documented recurrent PE
c. Active smoking history
d. Age > 65 years

29. Which phase of the nursing process provokes the nurse to prioritize diagnoses?
a. Assessment
b. Analysis
c. Planning
d. Implementation

30. The nurse is caring for a fifty-two-year-old female patient with metabolic syndrome. Which of the following is the nurse NOT likely to assess?
a. Low HDL cholesterol level
b. High triglyceride level
c. Fatty deposits on the upper back
d. History of a stroke

31. The nurse is developing a teaching plan for a patient with newly diagnosed type 2 diabetes. Which of the following symptoms of hyperglycemia would the nurse include?

a. Tremors, fatigue, dizziness
b. Excessive urination, excessive thirst, confusion
c. Anxiety, blurred vision, headache
d. Slurred speech, sweating, fainting

32. A patient with a known history of lupus presents to the emergency department complaining of chest pain. During the physical assessment, the nurse identifies a scratchy, squeaky sound at the end of exhalation. Which *next* action by the nurse indicates an understanding of the patient's presenting symptoms?

a. The nurse requests a breathing treatment for the patient.
b. The nurse auscultates at the left lower sternal border in the fourth intercostal space with the patient in the seated position.
c. The nurse establishes IV access.
d. The nurse auscultates at the left lower sternal border in the fourth intercostal space with the patient lying on his or her right side.

33. A twenty-five-year-old male presents to the Emergency Department (ED) after accidentally inhaling a dime. He can speak and recounts that the incident occurred eight hours ago. His only complaints are a cough and wheezing. Upon bronchoscopy, where would the ED physician likely find the dime?

a. Left lung
b. Trachea
c. Larynx
d. Right lung

34. A twenty-two-year-old male comes in with a gunshot wound to the right upper quadrant of his abdomen. The bleeding has been controlled, the wound was closed, and he has been hemodynamically stabilized. What solid organ of the abdomen does the nurse suspect might have been hit by the gunshot?

a. Stomach
b. Small intestine
c. Liver
d. Colon

35. The patient with decreased level of consciousness is brought to the emergency department by EMS. During the assessment, the nurse observes mottled extremities and distant heart sounds. The nurse demonstrates an understanding of the physician's diagnosis of cardiogenic shock by anticipating which of the following?

a. Arterial blood gas (ABG)
b. Chest x-ray
c. Angiogram
d. Doppler study of the lower extremities

36. Which interventions should the medical-surgical nurse include while implementing a plan of care for a patient experiencing a dysautonomic flare?
    a. Promote sustained increased activity
    b. Reduce sodium intake
    c. Eat 2-3 large meals per day
    d. Administer corticosteroid

37. While facilitating a unit-based in-service on the prevention of medication errors, what factor is identified to be the greatest cause of medication error?
    a. Illegible handwriting
    b. Poor staffing
    c. Systems failure
    d. Medication dispensing technology

38. The nurse is teaching a patient about modifiable risk factors for aneurysm formation. Which of the following risk factors would NOT be included in this teaching plan?
    a. Smoking
    b. Cocaine use
    c. Hypertension
    d. Age

39. The nurse is assessing an eighty-seven-year-old patient admitted with a urinary tract infection. The nurse notes that the patient is confused. The patient's daughter reports that prior to being admitted to the hospital, her mother lived alone and was able to manage her apartment and perform her own self-care. The nurse understands that this patient is most likely exhibiting manifestations of which of the following conditions?
    a. Delirium
    b. Dementia
    c. Alzheimer's disease
    d. Agitation

40. A thirty-three-year-old female presents to the emergency room complaining of vomiting blood. Which description of the hematemesis indicates an active upper GI bleed?
    a. Coffee ground
    b. Bright red
    c. Large amount
    d. Small amount

41. Which sound should be assessed using the bell of the stethoscope for proper detection?
    a. Bruit
    b. Inspiratory wheeze
    c. S2 heart sound
    d. Stridor

42. The medical-surgical nurse is caring for a 48-year-old patient assessed to have an elevated white blood cell count following anesthesia. What is the normal range for white blood cells in a healthy adult patient?
   a. 2,000-3,000/µL
   b. 4,000-11,000/µL
   c. 15,000-16,000/µL
   d. 21,000-36,000/µL

43. The nurse identifies a patient care safety risk while rounding on the unit at the start of shift. Which member of the care team should the nurse elevate this concern to?
   a. Director of nursing
   b. Charge nurse
   c. Chief nursing officer
   d. Nursing supervisor

44. Which nonpharmacologic intervention should the medical-surgical nurse include when caring for a patient with baroreflex failure?
   a. Stress management
   b. Bed rest
   c. Cool showers
   d. Spicy foods

45. The medical-surgical nurse is evaluating the patient's understanding of ways to reduce their risk of colon cancer post discharge. Which statement made by a patient supports a clear understanding of the plan for wellness?
   a. "I will have an annual endoscopy."
   b. "I will eat more produce from my garden."
   c. "I will go on daily jogs."
   d. "I will eat more red meat from my local butcher."

46. Tensilon has been administered to treat an acute relapse in a patient with myasthenia gravis. The attached tracing is consistent with the expected response in which form of crisis?

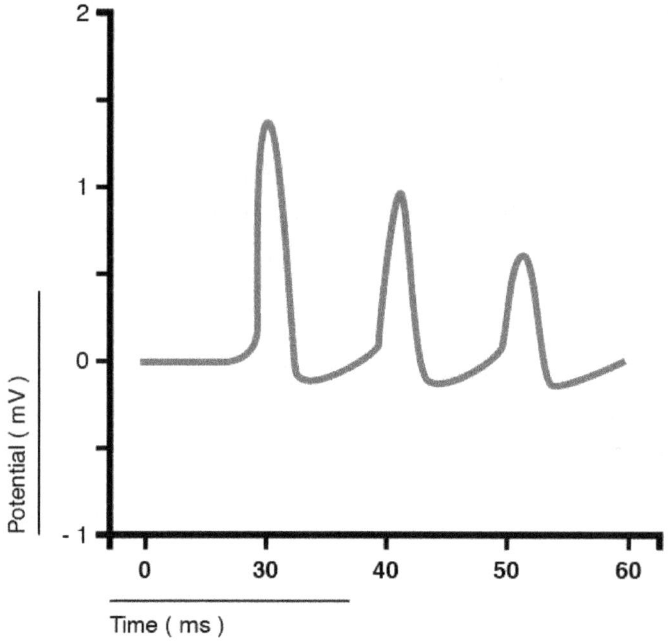

a. Tensilon is not an effective treatment for either form of crisis.
b. The tracing is consistent with the Tensilon response in a myasthenic crisis.
c. The tracing is consistent with the Tensilon response in a cholinergic crisis.
d. Tensilon will improve the muscle function in both forms of crises.

47. The nurse is caring for a patient from China who has HIV. The nurse would expect that this patient has which of the following subtypes of HIV?
a. Subtype A
b. Subtype B
c. Subtype C
d. Subtype D

48. A seven-year-old male presents with hypoxia, hoarseness, fever, agitation, dysphagia, drooling, and complaints of a sore throat. What is the most likely diagnosis for this patient?
a. Laryngotracheobronchitis
b. Acute tracheitis
c. Acute epiglottitis
d. Bronchiolitis

49. The nurse is caring for a patient with manifestations of peptic ulcer disease. Which of the following statements is correct?
a. Stomach pain begins 20 to 30 minutes after eating.
b. The condition is associated with an increased risk of malignancy.
c. Endoscopy is used to establish hemostasis.
d. Chronic NSAID use is the most common etiology.

50. Which intervention should the medical-surgical nurse implement in the plan of care for a 53-year-old patient with acromegaly?
   a. Explain that the bone enlargement is temporary and will reverse
   b. Monitor for signs of diabetes mellitus, such as polyuria and polydipsia
   c. Reschedule pituitary surgery for when acromegaly has subsided
   d. Provide family teaching regarding the expectation for the patient's hands and feet to shrink

51. A patient has had three separate blood pressure readings of 138/88, 132/80, and 135/89, respectively. The nurse anticipates the patient to be categorized by the physician as which of the following?
   a. Prehypertensive
   b. Normal
   c. Stage 1 hypertension
   d. Stage 2 hypertension

52. The nurse is caring for a nineteen-year-old woman who presents in the emergency department with manifestations of acute hepatitis. She tells the nurse that she thinks she might be pregnant and asks the nurse how this disease could affect her baby. The nurse understands that which of the following genotypes is associated with the most significant risk for perinatal transmission of the hepatitis virus?
   a. HAeAb negative
   b. HBeAg positive
   c. HCeAg negative
   d. HDeAb positive

53. The emergency care of the patient with temporal arteritis is complex due to the wide range of possible complications that are associated with this condition. Which of the following complications requires immediate intervention to prevent irreversible damage?
   a. Lower extremity claudication
   b. Vertebral body fracture
   c. Early onset of blindness
   d. Infection related to immunosuppression

54. The plan of care for a patient who is eleven weeks pregnant and diagnosed with hyperemesis gravidarum should include which of the following actions?
   a. Encouraging the patient to eat so her baby will grow
   b. Avoiding administering medications for relief of nausea and vomiting
   c. Assessing liver function tests
   d. Monitoring for fluid and electrolyte imbalances

55. Which psychosocial assessment findings does the medical-surgical nurse suspect will indicate a need for patient transfer to inpatient psychiatry once medically stable?
   a. Anhedonia
   b. Alcohol abuse
   c. Hopelessness
   d. Inability to care for self

56. The nurse is receiving reports at the beginning of the shift. One of the patients has been admitted to the hospital and is awaiting transfer to the ICU with an admitting diagnosis of obstructive shock. Which of the following findings are characteristic of obstructive shock?
a. Jugular vein distention, peripheral edema, and pulmonary congestion
b. Decreased urine output, increased BUN, and increased creatinine
c. Chest pain, fatigue, and lightheadedness
d. Problems with coordination, blurred vision, and partial paralysis

57. While evaluating a neurological plan of care, the medical-surgical nurse reviews the patient's cranial nerve function. Which cranial nerve is responsible for gag and swallow?
a. Glossopharyngeal
b. Hypoglossal
c. Facial
d. Trigeminal

58. The nurse is caring for a sixty-two-year-old woman with myalgia, fever, dyspnea, and decreased breath sounds. To assist with a more rapid diagnosis for possible viral pneumonia, the nurse should prepare the patient for which of the following tests?
a. Pulmonary function tests
b. Blood cultures
c. CT scan
d. Rapid antigen testing

59. During an ECG, the nurse observes an abnormally lengthened PR interval (greater than 0.3). The nurse recognizes this finding as a characteristic of which of the following?
a. Sinus rhythm
b. Junctional rhythm
c. Mobitz type I heart block
d. Mobitz type II heart block

60. Which of the following would the nurse expect to assess in a patient with Guillain-Barré syndrome who has cranial nerve involvement?
a. Core muscle weakness
b. Respiratory muscle weakness
c. Limb weakness
d. Eye muscle weakness

61. After a patient presents to the emergency department with a chief complaint of chest pain, which priority action should the nurse complete FIRST?
a. Assess vital signs
b. Ask questions regarding the radiation of pain
c. Start an IV with normal saline
d. Page the cardiologist

62. Which of the following statements is true?
a. As fluid levels decrease, electrolyte levels increase.
b. As fluid levels increase, electrolyte levels increase.
c. As fluid levels osmose, electrolyte levels diffuse.
d. As fluid levels homogenize, electrolyte levels dissipate.

63. The medical-surgical nurse percusses the patient's lungs during a focused assessment. Which sound aligns with a normal finding?
   a. Tympany
   b. Hyper-Resonance
   c. Dullness
   d. Resonance

64. The medical surgical nurse assesses the patient to have shortness of breath while in a recumbent position. How should the nurse document this finding?
   a. Orthopnea
   b. Dyspnea
   c. Tachypnea
   d. Bradypnea

65. During morning report, the oncoming nurse learns from the outgoing night nurse that a 38-year-old patient has been requesting discharge all night. Upon walking into the patient room to meet them after report, the patient exclaims, "I want to go home now!" Which action should the nurse implement FIRST?
   a. Page the physician for a consult for potential discharge
   b. Report suspected patient neglect to the nurse manager
   c. Administer a prn medication for anxiety
   d. Explore the patient's reasoning for requesting discharge

66. Which infection control precautions should the medical-surgical nurse implement to reduce the risk of transmission for a patient diagnosed with active tuberculosis?
   a. Standard
   b. Contact
   c. Droplet
   d. Airborne

67. All of the following ethnic groups are at increased risk for sickle cell anemia EXCEPT?
   a. African
   b. Asian
   c. Eastern European
   d. Middle Eastern

68. While completing an admission for a patient transferred from the intensive care unit, the medical-surgical nurse is concerned that a patient with a respiratory condition that requires isolation will be rooming with another patient. What action should the nurse take NEXT?
   a. Share this concern with the charge nurse
   b. Page the nursing supervisor
   c. Call the bed captain
   d. Contact the admitting physician

69. The nurse is caring for a twenty-four-year-old woman in her first trimester of pregnancy who has been experiencing moderate vaginal bleeding. The nurse understands that which of the following factors is true regarding first trimester spontaneous abortions?
    a. Young maternal age increases the risk
    b. Type 2 diabetes is a common cause
    c. Moderate exercise increases the risk
    d. Chromosomal abnormalities are the most common cause

70. Which test should the nurse anticipate in a patient who reports excessive fatigue, depression, and weight gain?
    a. Cortisol level
    b. T4 and TSH levels
    c. Blood glucose level
    d. Aldosterone level

71. Which focus represents a chief goal of the working phase of the nurse-patient relationship?
    a. Organize initial meeting
    b. Establish verbal contract
    c. Solidify trusting relationship
    d. Prepare for discharge

72. The emergency room nurse is caring for a female patient admitted with an ovarian cyst. Which manifestation would the nurse expect the patient to report?
    a. Recent weight gain
    b. A change in urination
    c. Increase in appetite
    d. Abdominal bloating

73. Nurses are responsible for which of the following elements of informed consent?
    a. Identification of alternatives to the planned procedure
    b. Description of associated risks and benefits
    c. Explanation of the planned procedure or diagnostic test
    d. Assessment of the patient's understanding of the information that is provided

74. The medical-surgical nurse is preparing a patient's treatment plan for the evening prior to an exercise stress test. The nurse is aware that much of what the 62-year-old patient typically consumes needs to be held. Which option is considered safe for the patient at this time?
    a. Beta Blockers
    b. Caffeine
    c. Calcium Channel Blockers
    d. Orange Juice

75. The medical-surgical nurse should implement all of the following acute care measures for a burn victim patient EXCEPT:
    a. NPO for 24 hours
    b. Monitor EKG for arrhythmias
    c. Low protein, low calorie diet
    d. Apply antimicrobial ointment

76. During breakfast, a patient with dysphagia states, “Well, I haven't choked yet,” then knocks on the wooden side-table. The nurse educates the unlicensed assistive personnel regarding this behavior. What is knocking on wood an example of?
  a. Cultural norm
  b. Undoing
  c. Repetitive behavior
  d. Compulsion

77. The nurse is caring for a patient with bacterial meningitis. Which classic findings of this disease should the nurse expect to find on assessment?
  a. Fever, nuchal rigidity, headache
  b. Fever, vomiting, photophobia
  c. Confusion, decreased level of consciousness, photophobia
  d. Fatigue, muscle aches, decreased appetite

78. When caring for a patient with autoimmune gastritis, the nurse should assess the patient for manifestations of which vitamin deficiency?
  a. Vitamin B-1
  b. Vitamin B-12
  c. Vitamin D
  d. Vitamin K

79. Which of the following statements is true?
  a. 95 percent of the patients diagnosed with multiple sclerosis will potentially advance to a non-remitting disease pattern.
  b. The clinically-isolated incident is a definitive precursor of active MS.
  c. The primary-progressive form of MS is the most common presenting form of the disease.
  d. Prednisone is the medication of choice to slow progression in all forms of MS.

80. Which action is considered a dependent nursing intervention?
  a. Bedbound care
  b. Infection control
  c. Health education
  d. Tube feeding

81. What flow rate should the nurse set for the nasal cannula of a patient with chronic obstructive pulmonary disease (COPD)?
  a. 1 L/min
  b. 3L/min
  c. 5 L/min
  d. 7 L/min

82. The nurse is caring for a patient who presents to the emergency department with an exacerbation of congestive heart failure (CHF). Which clinical manifestation should be most concerning to the nurse?
  a. An oxygenation level of 92 percent
  b. Dyspnea on exertion
  c. New onset of peripheral edema
  d. Elevated BNP levels

83. Which condition does the medical-surgical nurse attribute the patient's ascites to?
    a. Liver Failure
    b. Celiac disease
    c. Benign Prostatic Hypertrophy
    d. Diverticulitis

84. An eighteen-year-old female presents to the Emergency Department (ED) complaining of worsening wheezing, shortness of breath, and a cough over the past twelve hours. She has a history of asthma and has been using her albuterol metered-dose inhaler (MDI) every ten minutes for the past two hours. She's given supplemental oxygen, both albuterol and ipratropium (Combivent®) via nebulizer, and methylprednisolone IV in quick succession. Shortly afterwards, she complains of anxiety, develops hand tremors, and her pulse increases from 80 to 120 beats per minute (bpm). Which treatment is most likely responsible for her anxiety, tremors, and tachycardia?
    a. Supplemental oxygen
    b. Albuterol
    c. Ipratropium
    d. Methylprednisolone

85. A 32-year-old patient with scleroderma has developed severe sensations of cold in their fingers, nose, and nipples. Which condition does the nurse suspect is responsible for these symptoms?
    a. Hypertension
    b. Raynaud's phenomenon
    c. Grave's disease
    d. Asthma

86. After receiving opposing opinions from interdisciplinary team members regarding a patient's care, what should the medical-surgical nurse do NEXT to navigate this situation?
    a. Collect clinical data affecting the dilemma
    b. Phone Quality Assurance and establish a collaborative meeting
    c. Elevate this problem to the charge nurse
    d. Page the physician to request an ethics consult

87. While implementing a plan of care for a patient experiencing alcohol withdrawal, which supplement should the medical-surgical nurse include?
    a. Calcium
    b. Magnesium
    c. Vitamin D
    d. Thiamine

88. When examining a patient with a bulls-eye rash, which diagnosis does the medical-surgical nurse continue assessing for further symptoms of?
    a. Celiac disease
    b. Lyme disease
    c. Polycystic Kidney disease
    d. Alzheimer's disease

89. While explaining discharge instructions, the medical-surgical nurse finds that the Japanese-American patient frequently nods their head. How should the nurse understand this behavior?
   a. The patient agrees to the discharge plan.
   b. The patient is nervous and unsure of the plan.
   c. The patient is producing normal cultural conduct.
   d. The patient is encouraging the nurse to finish their sentence.

90. Which finding gathered in the patient's history is a risk factor for a cerebrovascular accident?
   a. Male gender
   b. Diabetes mellitus
   c. Caucasian race
   d. Hypotension

91. What is the therapeutic reference range for carbamazepine, an anti-epileptic agent?
   a. 1-3 mg/L
   b. 4-12 mg/L
   c. 18-22 mg/L
   d. 26-29 mg/L

92. Which position should the medical-surgical nurse help a patient into for pain management of acute appendicitis?
   a. High Fowler's position
   b. Fetal position
   c. Prone position
   d. Supine position

93. What ethical principle sets forth that the nurse must maintain truthful engagements with their patient?
   a. Justice
   b. Veracity
   c. Nonmaleficence
   d. Beneficence

94. The nurse is caring for a patient who is thirty-six weeks pregnant with manifestations of abruptio placenta. Which of the following statements is consistent with the use of the Kleihauer-Betke test?
   a. The test is a highly sensitive indicator of the onset of preterm in pregnant patients with trauma.
   b. The test measures the amount of fetal blood in the maternal bloodstream, which guides RhoGAM dosing.
   c. The test is only used in the assessment of Rh-negative patients who present with abruptio placenta during a second pregnancy.
   d. Based on the amount of fetal blood that is transferred to the maternal circulation, the test is predictive of the degree of separation of the placenta.

95. The Five Rights of Delegation include all of the following EXCEPT:
   a. Person
   b. Task
   c. Narrative
   d. Direction

96. The medical-surgical nurse is discussing patient care planning with the neurologist of a 62-year-old patient with liver failure after noting asterixis. How should the nurse communicate these findings?
   a. Explain that the patient had a flapping tremor.
   b. Describe the patient's proximal muscle weakness.
   c. Include a report of the patient's jerking arm muscles.
   d. Emphasize the patient's reeling, wide gait.

97. The nurse in the coronary care unit is assessing a patient's electrocardiogram. Which of the following statements by the nurse indicates that the nurse understands the significance of the P wave?
   a. "The P wave represents atrial depolarization."
   b. "The P wave represents repolarization of the ventricles."
   c. "The P wave represents the spread of impulses across the ventricles."
   d. "The P wave represents the end of ventricular depolarization."

98. Which intervention should the nurse include in a treatment plan for a patient with thrombophlebitis?
   a. Ambulate around the unit hourly
   b. Remain on bed rest
   c. Complete range of motion exercises every two hours
   d. Ambulate in isolated room only

99. The patient with primary hypertension is being treated with medications to reduce blood volume and lower systemic vascular resistance. Which of the following medication combinations should the nurse anticipate for the patient?
   a. A diuretic and a calcium channel blocker (CCB)
   b. A diuretic and an angiotensin-converting enzyme (ACE) inhibitor
   c. An angiotensin II receptor blocker (ARB) and morphine
   d. A diuretic and a beta-blocker

100. Which food item consumed by a patient taking phenelzine sulfate, a monoamine oxidase inhibitor, concerns the medical-surgical nurse because it is contraindicated and must be avoided with this treatment?
   a. Sausage
   b. Cottage Cheese
   c. Chicken
   d. Egg

101. While caring for a patient with impaired renal function, the medical surgical nurse assesses ascites and dependent edema. Which electrolyte imbalance does the nurse suspect may be present?
   a. Hyperkalemia
   b. Hypokalemia
   c. Hypernatremia
   d. Hyponatremia

102. While implementing a plan of care for a patient with heart failure, how should the nurse address activity?
   a. Increase activity and limit time in bed
   b. Remain on bed rest
   c. Alternate rest and activity
   d. Ambulate to the bathroom only

103. The nurse is caring for a patient after an emergency delivery in the ER. The newborn had an Apgar score of 8 at 1 minute and a score of 9 at 5 minutes after delivery. Which of the following statements is consistent with these scores?
   a. The scores are normal.
   b. The deficit is most likely due to decreased muscle tone.
   c. The newborn will require only short-term mechanical ventilatory support.
   d. The newborn is at risk for cardiac anomalies.

104. The nurse in the emergency department is providing discharge education for a sixty-six-year-old patient with type 2 diabetes who has had a TIA. Which of the following patient statements indicates that the teaching has been effective?
   a. "There is nothing I can do to change my risk for another episode."
   b. "The best thing I can do is to keep my A1C level below 6.5 like my doctor said."
   c. "I only have type 2 diabetes, so that doesn't affect my blood vessels."
   d. "I'm glad I don't have to take insulin to fix this."

105. Which of the following patients is NOT at increased risk for the development of an embolism?
   a. A twenty-four-year-old with a broken femur
   b. An eighty-five-year-old female with a history of a stroke
   c. A sixty-two-year-old male with first-degree heart block
   d. A nineteen-year-old female two weeks postpartum

106. The nurse understands that which of the following is the most concerning symptom associated with peripheral vascular disease (PVD)?
   a. Faint peripheral pulses
   b. Restricted mobility
   c. Critical limb ischemia
   d. Pale feet when elevated

107. A patient with heart failure tells the nurse that he spends most of his day sitting in a chair because this helps him to breathe better. He also reports shortness of breath walking the twenty feet, on a flat surface, from his chair to the bathroom. Using the New York Heart Association (NYHA) classification tool, this nurse documents that the patient is at which stage?
   a. Stage I
   b. Stage II
   c. Stage III
   d. Stage IV

108. During an integumentary assessment of the hand, the medical-surgical nurse notes the patient's fingernails resemble upside-down spoons. Which of the patient's conditions is most likely responsible for this finding?
   a. Chronic Obstructive Pulmonary Disease
   b. Lung Cancer
   c. Pneumonia
   d. Asthma

109. The medical-surgical nurse is caring for a 71-year-old patient with fecal impaction. Which position should the medical-surgical nurse assist the patient into for proper administration of an enema?
   a. Left-lying
   b. Prone
   c. Right-lying
   d. Supine

110. A 39-year-old Hispanic-American patient visits with her husband and her young child during unit visiting hours. The medical-surgical nurse ensures not to stare or overtly admire her young child as this could be interpreted as giving the "evil eye." Understanding cultural considerations to care, what may this belief lead the patient to feel?
   a. Her child will become weak and ill.
   b. Her child is unusually short in stature.
   c. Her child will become lucky.
   d. Her child is too attractive.

111. A fifty-five-year-old male is undergoing an endoscopy to discover the source of his hematemesis. The gastroenterologist encounters an active, bleeding lesion. What procedure using the application of heat to seal the lesion will probably be used next?
   a. Banding
   b. Biopsy
   c. Angioplasty
   d. Cauterization

112. A sixty-six-year-old female with type 2 diabetes mellitus presents with a nonproductive cough, nasal congestion, wheezing, and occasional shortness of breath for the last ten days. She reports that her symptoms are worse at night. A chest x-ray, complete blood count (CBC), and comprehensive metabolic panel (CMP) are all unremarkable, except for an elevated blood glucose level of 150 mg/dL. What is the most appropriate course of management?
   a. Bronchoscopy with bronchoalveolar lavage (BAL)
   b. Sputum gram stain and culture
   c. Arterial blood gas (ABG) analysis
   d. Doxycycline 100 mg BID for seven days

113. Which ethical principle guides the medical-surgical nurse's actions while guaranteeing that the patient with the most critical condition receives priority treatment?
   a. Hedonism
   b. Virtue ethics
   c. Act deontology
   d. Utilitarianism

114. The nurse is providing patient education regarding the pending procedure to further assess and diagnose a potential abdominal aortic aneurysm. Which procedure does the nurse explain will examine blood flow through the aorta?
   a. Doppler ultrasound
   b. Chest x-ray
   c. Computed tomography angiogram
   d. Abdominal radiograph

115. The nurse is caring for a fifty-two-year-old-man with Cushing's syndrome. When developing a plan of care for this patient, which of the following statements should the nurse keep in mind?
   a. This disease is caused by insufficient mineralocorticoid production.
   b. This disease is caused by excessive mineralocorticoid production
   c. This disease is caused by insufficient glucocorticoid production.
   d. This disease is caused by excessive glucocorticoid production.

116. The medical-surgical nurse is evaluating a patient for suspected Lyme disease after a tick is found and removed from their groin during a head-to-toe assessment. While educating a student-nurse, the nurse explains that the patient with early, localized disease may likely display all of the following symptoms EXCEPT:
   a. Fever
   b. Erythema migrans
   c. Facial palsy
   d. Headache

117. In planning care for a patient with acute renal failure, what imbalance does the medical-surgical nurse expect to manage?
   a. Elevated GFR
   b. Decreased BUN
   c. Elevated Calcium
   d. Decreased Sodium

118. The nurse is assessing the pulse oximetry for a full-term newborn. What action should the nurse take for a reading of 92 percent?
   a. Nothing, this result is normal
   b. Call the physician immediately
   c. Prepare for mechanical ventilation
   d. Administer supplemental oxygen

119. Which response should the nurse make when a patient with advanced pancreatic cancer and a poor prognosis asks why she is receiving chemotherapy?
   a. "Your chance of remission is increased with chemotherapy."
   b. "There is always the chance that chemotherapy can cure your cancer."
   c. "Chemotherapy will keep your cancer from advancing further."
   d. "Chemotherapy is being used to help manage your pain."

120. The medical-surgical nurse is caring for a patient with a partial duodenal obstruction. Which abdominal quadrant should the nurse reassess pain in to evaluate the effectiveness of the interventions?
   a. Right lower quadrant (RLQ)
   b. Left lower quadrant (LLQ)
   c. Right upper quadrant (RUQ)
   d. Left upper quadrant (LUQ)

121. Which action should the nurse delegate to the unlicensed assistive personnel (UAP)?
   a. Obtain sterile equipment
   b. Document early detection education
   c. Provide discharge teaching
   d. Prepare an incident report

122. A patient walks into the emergency department and collapses. The nurse identifies the condition as cardiopulmonary arrest, and resuscitation efforts are started. The nurse understands that, in addition to CPR, defibrillation, and the ACLS protocol, the most important factor for patient survival is which of the following?
   a. Administration of oxygen
   b. Establishing IV access
   c. Inserting a Foley catheter
   d. Time between the collapse and the start of resuscitation efforts

123. The medical-surgical nurse auscultates the patient's heart sounds and notes both an S3 and an S4 sound. Which rhythm aligns with this finding?
   a. Still's Murmur
   b. Regular Rhythm
   c. Summation Gallop
   d. Systolic Murmur

124. Which intervention is a PRIORITY in the plan of care for a patient who is confused?
   a. Place the call bell within reach and explain its use.
   b. Explain the daily schedule to the patient.
   c. Check on the patient every two hours.
   d. Provide a stable environment.

125. When assessing a patient's electrocardiogram (ECG), the nurse on the telemetry unit notes an atrial rate of 260 beats a minute, a ventricular rate of 130 beats a minute and a sawtooth pattern. The nurse calls the cardiologist and reports that the patient has which of the following dysrhythmias?
   a. Atrial fibrillation
   b. Atrial flutter
   c. Sinus tachycardia
   d. Ventricular tachycardia

126. The community health nurse understands that which child is most at risk for developing bronchiolitis?
   a. A six-month-old child
   b. A two-year-old child
   c. A child in kindergarten
   d. A high school student

127. The pediatric nurse is caring for a child who has had three seizures lasting five to eight minutes over a thirty-minute period. The nurse understands that the child is experiencing which of the following conditions?
   a. Generalized seizures
   b. Focal seizures
   c. Status epilepticus
   d. Postictal state

128. The nurse is caring for a thirty-eight-year-old male who presents with marked left-sided scrotal swelling and distention of the abdomen. The nurse understands that which of the following is an UNEXPECTED finding in this patient?
   a. Diarrhea
   b. Tachycardia
   c. Rebound tenderness
   d. BUN 27

129. Which intervention is appropriate for the medical-surgical nurse to delegate to the unlicensed assistive personnel (UAP)?
   a. Respond to patient call light
   b. Adjust oxygen flow
   c. Auscultate breath sounds
   d. Wound dressing change

130. Which of the following statements by a patient with type 2 diabetes indicates that more teaching is needed?
   a. "My pancreas produces insulin, but my body isn't able to use it effectively."
   b. "I need to maintain an ideal body weight."
   c. "I need to cut down on carbohydrates in my diet."
   d. "I will need to take insulin for the rest of my life."

131. When evaluating the teaching plan for a patient with diabetes, which patient statement indicates to the nurse that the patient understands the teaching?
   a. "High glucose levels can damage my organs."
   b. "I should monitor my blood glucose level after meals."
   c. "Insulin helps to transport glucose into the bloodstream."
   d. "Hyperglycemia occurs when my body secretes too much insulin."

132. The nurse in the emergency department is caring for a patient who is being evaluated for a small-bowel obstruction. The nurse understands that which of the following assessment findings is consistent with this condition?

a. pH 7.32, PCO_2 38, HCO_3 20
b. Serum osmolality 285 mosm/kg
c. Serum sodium 128 mmol/L
d. Lower abdominal distention

133. While undergoing warfarin anticoagulant therapy, a 71-year-old patient experiences an elevated INR and signs and symptoms of over-anticoagulation. Which antidote should the medical-surgical nurse administer?

a. Vitamin K
b. Protamine
c. Ethanol
d. Amyl nitrate

134. The medical-surgical nurse recognizes that a patient is having a severe reaction to Enoxaparin. What medication should be given to neutralize this medication and inhibit this reaction?

a. Pilocarpine
b. Romazicon
c. Naloxone
d. Protamine

135. Which abdominal quadrant does the nurse assess pain in the patient with cirrhosis of the liver?

a. Left Lower Quadrant
b. Right Lower Quadrant
c. Left Upper Quadrant
d. Right Upper Quadrant

136. When gathering narrative information regarding the patient's perceived outcome of an intervention, the medical-surgical nurse uses the communication technique known as back channeling. Which phrase is an example of this communication cue?

a. "Go on…"
b. "Can you clarify?"
c. "Slow down."
d. "Repeat that."

137. The nurse is answering an HIV-positive patient's questions about the differences between the HIV-1 and HIV-2 viruses. Which information would the nurse tell this patient?

a. HIV-2 is highly transmissible.
b. HIV-1 is the dominant strain worldwide.
c. HIV-2 is well studied and highly understood.
d. HIV-1 is the weaker virus strain.

138. Patients on the cusp of respiratory failure may exhibit which of the following early signs and symptoms?
   a. Decreased respiratory rate
   b. Unconsciousness
   c. Cyanosis
   d. Agitation

139. After teaching the patient how to properly apply their compression stockings, the nurse tests for understanding. Which phase of the nursing process is the nurse functioning within at this time?
   a. Analysis
   b. Planning
   c. Implementation
   d. Evaluation

140. The nurse in the intensive care unit is monitoring the intracranial pressure of a thirty-six-year-old patient who was in a motor vehicle accident resulting in trauma to the head. Which of the following measurements does the nurse recognize as a normal intracranial pressure reading of an adult in the supine position?
   a. 5 millimeters of mercury
   b. 10 millimeters of mercury
   c. 18 millimeters of mercury
   d. 22 millimeters of mercury

141. The nurse in the emergency department is caring for a diabetic patient who reports that he has been experiencing tremors, fatigue, and dizziness. Which blood glucose level would the nurse expect in this patient?
   a. 58 milligrams per deciliter
   b. 120 milligrams per deciliter
   c. 180 milligrams per deciliter
   d. 220 milligrams per deciliter

142. While establishing a treatment plan for a patient newly admitted to the medical-surgical floor from the emergency department, which understanding regarding discharge planning should the nurse consider?
   a. Discharge planning starts at admission.
   b. Discharge planning starts after all providers have met with the patient.
   c. Discharge planning starts once an official discharge diagnosis has been charted.
   d. Discharge planning starts after significant progress towards wellness has been established.

143. The nurse is caring for a woman with mitral valve regurgitation who experienced a postpartum hemorrhage following a full-term Cesarean section. The nurse understands that which of the following should guide the care of this patient?
   a. A blood loss of 500 milliliters or less should not affect hemodynamic status.
   b. A blood loss of 500 milliliters or less may cause hemodynamic instability.
   c. A blood loss of 500 milliliters or less is no cause for concern.
   d. A blood loss of 500 milliliters or less is only of concern after a vaginal delivery.

144. The nurse in the emergency department is caring for a patient who had a seizure today for the first time. The patient said that she noticed a strange odor just prior to "not feeling well." Vital signs are BP 120/74, HR 76, and an oral temperature 97.8°F. The patient has no complaints of pain and no recent history of viral or bacterial illness. A friend witnessed that seizure and stated that the muscular movement lasted about thirty seconds. The patient was incontinent during the seizure but did not suffer any injuries. The patient recovered without any further manifestations of seizure activity. The nurse understands that which of the following interventions is most appropriate for this patient?

a. Obtain laboratory analysis of recreational drug use.
b. Institute oral therapy of AEDs.
c. Prepare the patient for an immediate lumbar puncture for CSF analysis.
d. Obtain an EEG and an MRI.

145. Using the Revised Trauma Score assessment tool, the emergency department nurse is assessing a patient who sustained pelvic injury in a motor vehicle accident. Which of the following sets of data would the nurse collect using this assessment tool?

a. Heart rate, core body temperature, respiratory rate
b. Diastolic blood pressure, response to pain, level of consciousness
c. Core body temperature, eye reflexes, level of consciousness
d. Glasgow Coma Scale score, systolic blood pressure, respiratory rate

146. During morning rounds, the medical surgical nurse assesses early inspiratory and expiratory crackles in a focused respiratory assessment on a 51-year-old patient. Which clinical condition aligns with this finding?

a. Pneumonia
b. Chronic bronchitis
c. Congestive heart failure
d. Atelectasis

147. The nurse is caring for patient with myasthenia gravis. Altered transmission of which of the following neurotransmitters would the nurse understand guides the care of this patient?

a. Serotonin
b. Dopamine
c. Acetylcholine
d. Norepinephrine

148. The medical-surgical nurse is preparing written patient education for a patient with chronic otitis media. Which surgical treatment does the nurse print patient education on to include in their teaching?

a. Tympanoplasty
b. Septoplasty
c. Rhinoplasty
d. Myringoplasty

149. Which nursing diagnosis should the medical-surgical nurse include while establishing a treatment plan for a patient with parathyroid disease?

a. Ineffective airway clearance
b. Impaired gas exchange
c. Alteration of protective mechanisms
d. Risk for unstable blood pressure

150. Which statement made by the patient displays understanding of the self-administration of Advair-Diskus post discharge?
   a. "I will use my inhaler to relieve sudden, unprovoked breathing issues."
   b. "I will use my inhaler before and after exercise."
   c. "I will use my inhaler every morning and evening."
   d. "I will use my inhaler when I develop a tight chest and cough."

151. When assessing a pregnant woman at twenty-four weeks gestation, which early manifestation would alert the nurse to a possible diagnosis of preeclampsia?
   a. Hypertension on bedrest
   b. Facial edema
   c. Increasing liver enzymes
   d. Thrombocytopenia

152. A patient is being discharged from the emergency department with the diagnosis of peripheral vascular disease with intermittent claudication. Which of the following information should be discussed with the patient prior to discharge?
      I. Avoid tight clothing.
      II. Wear compression stockings.
      III. Avoid airplane travel.
      IV. Minimize exercise.
   a. I and II only
   b. I and III only
   c. I, II, and III only
   d. I, II, III, and IV

153. When assessing a patient with a primary spontaneous pneumothorax, the nurse would expect to assess which of the following findings?
   a. Tall, thin body type
   b. Age greater than 50 years
   c. History of COPD
   d. Nonsmoker

154. The nurse is taking a health history from a patient with the primary progressive form of multiple sclerosis. The nurse would expect the patient to report which of the following?
   a. Constantly active manifestations without remission
   b. A variable pattern of active and inactive disease
   c. Progression of a variable pattern to a permanently active disease
   d. An initial episode of neurological findings that last for at least 24 hours

155. A sixty-year-old ex-smoker presents with a complaint of increasing shortness of breath over the past 24 hours. He has a medical history conducive of chronic obstructive pulmonary disease (COPD). He is administered supplemental oxygen, albuterol via nebulizer, methylprednisolone IV, and a dose of azithromycin IV. Which of these therapies has been clinically proven to decrease the risk of treatment failure and death?
   a. Supplemental oxygen
   b. Albuterol
   c. Methylprednisolone
   d. Azithromycin

156. A 19-year-old patient was admitted to the medical-surgical floor with a fever of 104.1, sore throat, and small white spots inside their mouth. On the second day of hospitalization, a rash of flat red spots breaks out, and the patient is tested for measles. Which precautions should the medical-surgical nurse implement for this patient while awaiting the confirmation of illness?

a. Standard
b. Contact
c. Droplet
d. Airborne

157. Which physiologic function requires close monitoring by the medical-surgical nurse post diagnosis with tardive dyskinesia?

a. Urination
b. Ocular motor control
c. Bowel control
d. Breathing

158. Which serum laboratory result concerns the medical-surgical nurse and requires further investigation?

a. Creatinine 1.9 mg/dL
b. Thyroid-Stimulating Hormone 2.3 mIU/L
c. Chloride 102 mEq/L
d. Carbon Dioxide 27 mEq/L

159. The medical-surgical nurse is planning to provide patient education on thyroid disease. Which value from the laboratory results is considered inactive because it attaches to thyroid receptors but does not activate them?

a. Free T4
b. Reverse T3
c. Free T3
d. Total T4

160. A fifty-five-year-old male presents with dyspnea, cough, and chest pain. A chest x-ray reveals a large pleural effusion. Thoracentesis is performed and pleural fluid analysis reveals a ratio of pleural fluid to serum LDH > 0.6. What is the most likely diagnosis for this patient?

a. Malignancy
b. Congestive heart failure (CHF)
c. Cirrhosis
d. Nephrotic syndrome

161. A patient presents to the emergency department with the complaint of fever and shortness of breath. During the physical examination, the nurse observes a petechial rash on both hands and a recent nipple piercing on the right chest. The patient reports being on a corticosteroid for a respiratory infection. These findings alert the nurse to the possibility of which of the following?

a. Endocarditis
b. An autoimmune disease
c. Pneumonia
d. Heart failure

162. The nurse is assessing a forty-two-year-old female patient with a benign ovarian cyst. When taking a health history from this patient, the nurse would expect which of the following findings?

a. History of hypothyroidism
b. Positive family history
c. Early menarche
d. Nulliparity

163. A patient presents with severe impairment of functioning due to the malfunction of a variety of bodily processes. While inpatient on the medical-surgical floor for testing, the patient ultimately is diagnosed with celiac disease, an autoimmune disorder that attacks the small intestine and leads to symptoms that span multiple organ systems and requires strict adherence to a gluten free diet. In addition to gluten avoidance, what additional dietary item should the nurse encourage the patient to avoid, as it is unable to be broken down until the small intestinal villi regenerate?

a. Dairy
b. Soy
c. Nuts
d. Shellfish

Answer Explanations for Practice Test #1

1. B: One of the classic findings in a patient with appendicitis is periumbilical pain that may progress to the right lower quadrant. Because the patient with appendicitis may develop peritonitis, the nurse would expect to assess a rigid abdomen rather than a soft abdomen; therefore, Choice *A* is not correct. Choices *C* and *D* are not correct because they are not typical assessment findings in the patient with appendicitis.

2. A: Choice *A* is a significant concern when assessed in a patient with pneumonia and requires priority intervention post assessment. Choices *B*, *C*, and *D* are not causes for concern in a patient with this illness at this time. Choices *B* and *C* are within normal range. Choice *D*, while potentially concerning outside of pneumonia, is a normal finding for this illness and encouraged during active illness to support movement towards wellness and a resolution of symptoms.

3. C: Choice *C* should NOT be implemented for a patient with epilepsy. Side-rails should be up to discourage patient falls during seizure activity. Choice *A* provides additional protection from injury. Choices *B* and *D* include equipment that should be ready for use in case it is needed during a seizure. The nurse should support the patient into a side-lying position and maintain their airway.

4. B: The risk of brain herniation is higher in patients who are immunosuppressed, over sixty years old, have a history of recent seizure activity, or have a disease of the CNS. A CT scan may be done prior to the lumbar puncture in this patient population; however, instituting antibiotic therapy to prevent morbidity remains the priority intervention. Bacterial meningitis is associated with a characteristic erythematous rash. However, depending on the causative organism, rashes may also be present with viral meningitis; therefore, the presence or absence of the rash cannot differentiate between the two conditions, which means that Choice *A* is incorrect. The protein level of the CSF is elevated, not decreased, in bacterial meningitis. The inflammatory response resulting from the bacterial infection alters the blood-brain barrier, which allows the leakage of protein from the blood into the subarachnoid space, causing marked increase in the protein level of the CSF; therefore, Choice *C* is incorrect. The meningococcal vaccine, MCV 4, is effective against meningococcal meningitis and has decreased the incidence of the disease among college students and military personnel who typically reside in close quarters. Residents of long-term care facilities are protected against pneumococcal meningitis by the PPSV; therefore, Choice *D* is incorrect.

5. A: Choice *A* is a supportive intervention to establish effective communication with a withdrawn patient. Choice *B* should be avoided as it may encourage the patient's withdrawn behavior. Choice *C* should be avoided as it may produce heightened anxiety that induces further withdrawn behavior. Choice *D* should be avoided as it encourages the patient to withhold information about their symptoms, which impairs the communication process as well as treatment planning.

6. D: Choice *D* represents the patient's dress and behavior, as she mimics an idol. Choices *A*, *B*, and *C*, while all defense mechanisms, do not align with the patient's current presentation at this time.

7. A: Choice *A* provides an accurate explanation of the mechanism of action of immunosuppressive therapy agents and should be included in the nurse's patient education. Choices *B*, *C*, and *D* are not true to the basic principles of this therapy's action and should not be included in the education provided to a patient with myasthenia gravis.

8. D: There is evidence that patients who are diagnosed with diverticulosis before the age of fifty have a greater risk for episodes of diverticulitis, which may be due to an unidentified difference in the infective process, living longer, or delays in seeking care for the initial episode. The presence of diverticulosis is age-dependent, affecting less than 5 percent of individuals less than forty years old and up to 65 percent of individuals over eighty years old; therefore, Choice *A* is incorrect. Diverticulitis is caused by infection of the diverticula due to impacted fecaliths and other cellular debris, which results in overgrowth of normal colonic bacteria with progression to an inflammatory process that is responsible for the clinical manifestations of the acute attack. Therefore, Choice *B* is incorrect. Initial episodes of diverticulitis are treated with bowel rest, antibiotics, and IV fluids. Emergency surgical intervention of an initial attack is required only for severe manifestations, and an elective colectomy is recommended after three episodes of diverticulitis; therefore, Choice *C* is incorrect.

9. C: Placenta previa is the abnormal placement of the placenta over the internal cervical os or within 2 centimeters of the internal cervical os. The risk factors for placenta previa are previous C-section, maternal age greater than thirty-five years, and increased number of previous pregnancies, making Choices *A*, *B*, and *D* incorrect. Other risk factors include infertility treatments, multiple births, previous abortions, and smoking or cocaine use.

10. C: Choice *C*, a serious disorder of the skin and mucous membranes, aligns with the nurse's assessment of a painful, reddish-purple blistering rash. Choice A represents a possible butterfly-shaped rash on the face. Choice *B* represents a rash of lost pigment. Choice *D* represents a possible rash in a bull's-eye pattern secondary to a tick bite.

11. A: Abruptio placenta is the premature separation of the placenta from the wall of the uterus. Common risk factors for this condition are smoking, maternal hypertension, trauma (such as car accidents, falls, or assaults), cocaine or alcohol abuse, maternal age greater than thirty-five or less than twenty-years-old, and previous history of abruptio placenta. Therefore, *B*, *C*, and *D* are not correct.

12. C: Choice *C* is a supportive intervention that should be implemented in the plan of care for a patient with acute renal failure. Choices *A*, *B*, and *D* all should be avoided in this patient's treatment plan.

13. B: Choice *B* is a dye known to numb pain within the urinary tract and is administered as an analgesic for pain management for a patient experiencing a urinary tract infection. Choices *A* and *C* represent analgesics; however, neither fit this description or this need for a patient with a urinary tract infection. Choice *D* indicates a medication used for the treatment of urinary tract infection but does not provide pain management and is an antibiotic rather than an analgesic.

14. C: Choice *C* represents the length of time that the medical-surgical nurse must auscultate the apical heart rate while completing a focused assessment. Choices *A* and *B* are too short in length, thereby limiting the assessment. Choice *D* is longer than necessary and not typical. Auscultating longer than a minute would only be indicated if the nurse was unable to obtain a clear finding after auscultating for a full minute or if additional considerations warranted further review.

15. B: Choice *B* should be administered to the patient to counteract the effects of the acetaminophen overdose. Choices *A*, *C*, and *D*, while all antidotes for a variety of medications, would not prove effective in reversing the progression of acetaminophen poisoning.

16. C: Left bundle branch block is not assessed using the TIMI tool with a diagnosis of NSTEMI, although it is a category scored with a diagnosis of ST elevation myocardial infarction (STEMI). The TIMI tool for patients with NSTEMI provides a score in seven categories: age, risk factors, a prior coronary artery stenosis, ST deviation on ECG, prior aspirin intake, presence and number of angina episodes, and elevated creatinine kinase or troponins. As a result, Choices *A*, *B*, and *D* are not the correct answers.

17. B: Therapy with magnesium sulfate is recommended for preterm labor from twenty-four to thirty-three weeks' gestation. Since facial flushing is a side effect of therapy with magnesium sulfate, the nurse should notify the physician immediately. The physician may then order the rate of infusion to be reduced or stopped to reduce the risk of toxic effects, but the nurse's priority action is to notify the physician, making Choices *A* and *C* incorrect. While the nurse will continuously monitor the patient, the physician should be notified first to making treatment decisions, making Choice *D* an incorrect response.

18. C: Choice *C* is an expected side effect of long-term corticosteroid use and should be assessed by the medical-surgical nurse. Choices *A*, *B*, and *D* are not associated with the long-term use of this medication and would not cause the nurse to suspect these issues. Expected side effects of long-term use of this medication include hypertension, weight gain, and thinning of the skin.

19. D: Although electrical shock may not result in visible burns on the skin, extensive damage to skeletal muscle tissue can result in myonecrosis of the muscle cells. This damage leads to the release of large amounts of potassium from the cell, resulting in hyperkalemia. Potassium levels in excess of 8.5 mEq/L will cause lethal cardiac arrhythmias; therefore, Choice *D* is correct. Hypovolemic shock can potentially contribute to cardiac complications. However, there is no evidence of hypovolemia in this discussion; therefore, this is an unlikely cause of the cardiac arrest, and Choice *A* is incorrect. The patient's oxygenation is normal, and the patient is alert and oriented; therefore, hypoxia is an unlikely cause of the cardiac arrest, so Choice *B* is incorrect. Cardiac perforation is a possible consequence of electrical burns. However, in this discussion, more than five hours has elapsed since the injury, and this lethal consequence is most commonly evident immediately after the injury occurs; therefore, Choice *C* is incorrect.

20. D: Pulmonary edema can be of cardiogenic or non-cardiogenic origin. There is no single test to differentiate whether the cause of pulmonary edema is cardiac or noncardiac. Bilateral pulmonary infiltrates and hypoxemia are nonspecific symptoms and can occur in both. A pulmonary artery wedge pressure < 18 mmHg is consistent with pulmonary edema of non-cardiogenic origin.

21. C: Treatment of Alzheimer's disease, a chronic progressive form of dementia, is supportive; however, cholinesterase inhibitors and N Methyl D aspartate receptor antagonists have been demonstrated to slow the disease progression if they are started early in the course of the disease. Choices *A* and *B* are incorrect since early use of these medications will not cure the disease or cause it to enter remission. Choice *D* is incorrect because these medications have been shown to work for a limited time, if started early in the disease.

22. A: Choice *A* is responsible for the jugular vein distention as it induces bulging veins as the blood accumulates. Choices *B*, *C*, and *D* do not cause jugular vein distention as pressure is reduced in all of these choices. Jugular vein distention is a sign of increased central venous pressure and presents itself as a visible bulging vein in the neck.

23. C: Aldactone® (spironolactone), Choice *C*, is a potassium-sparing diuretic and supports the patient's concern regarding their potassium level at this time. This medication does not encourage the excretion of potassium via urine. Lasix® (furosemide) and Demadex® (torsemide) are loop diuretics and Aldactone® (spironolactone) is a thiazide diuretic. These medications do not specifically target conserving potassium in the body to address the patient's concern arising from their history. Therefore, Choices *A*, *B*, and *D* are incorrect.

24. C: Intramuscular methotrexate, administered intramuscularly as a single dose, is administered to a woman with ectopic pregnancy to impede DNA synthesis and prevent cellular replication. Evidence of the effectiveness of this treatment is evidenced by decreasing BHCG levels. *A*, *B*, and *D* are not indicative of the effectiveness of methotrexate administered in the woman with ectopic pregnancy.

25. B: Chronically ill children may not present with the typical manifestations of cholecystitis, such as colicky epigastric pain that radiates to the right upper quadrant. The chronically ill child with sickle cell disease may present with generalized abdominal pain. Therefore, Choices *A, C,* and *D* are not correct.

26. D: An ectopic pregnancy results from the abnormal implantation of the fertilized ovum at a site other than the uterus. The fallopian tube is the implantation site in 94 percent of ectopic pregnancies, which means that there is some impedance to the normal eight- to ten-day passage of the fertilized ovum from the fallopian tube to the uterus. The fallopian tube is lined by hair-like extensions, or cilia, which provide the motility that propels the ovum from the point of fertilization to the appropriate implantation site in the uterus. There is clear research evidence that one of the effects of smoking is the blunting or destruction of the cilia, which decreases the efficiency of this process, thereby contributing to the likelihood of faulty implantation. The process of implantation and initial development of the placenta is a hypoxic environment in the initial weeks of the first trimester due to "plugging" alterations in the vasculature of the endometrium that prevent maternal hemorrhage. Hypoxia from smoking is associated with fetal intrauterine growth delay later in the pregnancy. However, it does not directly affect implantation; therefore, Choice *A* is incorrect. Smoking affects the lining of the fallopian tube but has no identified effect on progesterone levels; therefore, Choice *B* is incorrect. Smoking directly affects the lining of the fallopian tubes. However, there is no evidence of any similar effect on the endometrium; therefore, Choice *C* is incorrect.

27. B: Hyperthyroidism occurs when there is an overproduction of T4 and/or T5 by the thyroid gland. Women under age 40 are most likely to be diagnosed with this disorder. This makes Choices *A*, *C*, and *D* incorrect.

28. B: Vena cava filters are also known as inferior vena cava (IVC) filters or Greenfield filters. They are used to prevent a pulmonary embolism (PE). Indications for the placement of a vena cava filter include:

- An absolute contraindication to anticoagulants
- Survival after a massive PE and a high probability that a recurrent PE will be fatal
- Documented recurrent PE

29. C: Choice *C* provokes the nurse to prioritize diagnoses while developing a nursing plan and setting goals. Choice *A* involves a review of subjective and objective data. Choice *B* involves interpreting signs and symptoms to identify the patient's needs. Choice *D* involves providing patient education and carrying out procedures.

30. C: Metabolic syndrome, also called Syndrome X, is the presence of comorbid cardiovascular and insulin-related conditions. Those with metabolic disease may have excess belly fat, not excess fat on the upper back. Choices *A* and *B* are incorrect since patients with metabolic syndrome must have three or more of the following conditions: hypertension, elevated fasting blood glucose levels, low HDL cholesterol, high triglycerides, and excess belly fat. Patients with this disorder are typically overweight or obese and are at an increased risk for organ failure, heart attack, and stroke, making Choice *D* incorrect.

31. B: Hyperglycemia occurs when the patient's blood sugar level is greater than 200 milligrams per deciliter. Common symptoms of hyperglycemia include polyuria (excessive urination), polydipsia (excessive thirst), nausea, abdominal pain, fruity-scented breath, and confusion. Choices *A*, *C*, and *D* describe symptoms of hypoglycemia.

32. B: A pericardial friction rub is a scratchy, squeaky sound heard at the end of exhalation. It is indicative of pericarditis. It is best heard at the left lower sternal border in the fourth intercostal space while the patient is seated. The best *next* action for the nurse to take is to reposition the patient and the stethoscope. A breathing treatment is needed when oxygen saturations are low and in the presence of wheezing. The nurse needs more information to confirm the suspicion of a pericarditis. Establishing IV access is important but not the next action to be taken. A pericardial friction rub is best heard when the patient is seated, not lying down.

33. D: This scenario depicts a foreign body aspiration in an adult. Since the patient can speak, it's a partial obstruction of the airways. The foreign body should be promptly extracted as the likelihood of complications increases after 24 to 48 hours. Bronchoscopy (rigid or flexible) can be diagnostic as well as therapeutic. Due to the acute angle of the right mainstem bronchus, aspirated foreign bodies in an adult are most commonly found in the right lung.

34. C: The liver is a solid organ located in the right upper quadrant of the abdomen. When a penetrating wound such as a gunshot has occurred to the abdomen, it is important to be mindful of organ damage underneath the point of penetration. The small intestine, stomach, and colon are all hollow organs located in different areas of the abdomen.

35. C: An angiogram to restore coronary blood flow is the priority treatment for cardiogenic shock. ABGs, a chest x-ray, and a Doppler study are not treatments; they are diagnostic tools.

36. D: Choice *D* is a supportive intervention for a patient experiencing a dysautonomic flare. This condition causes substantial drops in blood pressure, which can be controlled via corticosteroid use. Choice *A* causes risky blood pressure fluctuations and should be avoided. Choice *B* promotes further reduction in blood pressure; therefore, the nurse should encourage an increased intake of sodium. Choice *C* encourages postprandial syncopal episodes and should be avoided.

37. C: Choice *C* indicates the greatest cause of medication error. Systems failures are important to detect, no matter how small, as their consequences can result in significant harm or larger errors. Choices *A*, *B*, and *D* are factors in medication error; however, they are not the greatest cause of this error.

38. D: While individuals over forty years of age are at increased risk for aneurysm formation, age is a nonmodifiable risk factor and would not be included in the teaching plan for modifiable risk factors. Smoking, cocaine use, and hypertension are all modifiable risk factors for aneurysm formation, making Choices *A*, *B*, and *C* incorrect.

39. A: An acute situation, such as a urinary tract infection, may lead to delirium, a condition marked by confusion and agitation. Delirium is transient and resolves once the cause is eliminated, such as successfully treating a urinary tract infection. Choice *B* is not correct since dementia is a chronic condition in which the patient experiences reduced cognition over time. Choice *C* is not correct since Alzheimer's disease is a form of dementia and develops over time. Choice *D* is not correct since a patient who is agitated demonstrates acute anxiety and may be verbally abusive.

40. B: Bright red blood that is being vomited usually indicates an active upper GI bleed. Coffee ground blood indicates the blood has been sitting in the stomach for a while, indicating a slower bleed. The amount of blood, whether large or small, does not indicate active bleeding necessarily. It could be a small amount vomited, but a large bleed that has not fully manifested itself.

41. A: Choice *A* should be assessed using the bell of the stethoscope for detection. Choices *B*, *C*, and *D* should be auscultated with the diaphragm of the stethoscope. The bell supports auscultation of low frequency sounds, while the diaphragm filters low sounds out. The bell is helpful for detecting abnormal heart sounds and bruits.

42. B: Choice *B* represents the normal range for white blood cells in a healthy adult patient. Choices *A*, *C*, and *D* are outside of the normal range and would indicate a potential problem requiring further assessment by the medical-surgical nurse at this time. Choice *A* is below normal range. Choices *C* and *D* are above normal range.

43. B: Choice *B* indicates the appropriate team member for the nurse to elevate a patient care safety risk to. Choices *A*, *C*, and *D* fall higher in the nursing chain of command, therefore should not yet be prompted to handle this concern at this time.

44. A: Choice *A* is a nonpharmacologic intervention the nurse should support to aid in the management of baroreflex failure. This condition involves marked increases in blood pressure, which are aggravated by stress. Therefore, the nurse should encourage stress management techniques to be integrated in the plan of care. Choices *B*, *C*, and *D* do not directly influence the maintenance of this condition and should not be focuses of care at this time.

45. B: Choice *B* represents an understanding of ways to reduce colon cancer risk post discharge. Increasing fruits and vegetables in the diet is one way to support a reduction in risk. Choice *A* is incorrect because this invasive routine is not supported. Choice *C* is incorrect; exercise does not directly correlate to a reduction of risk. Choice *D* is incorrect, as red meat is associated with a heightened risk of colon cancer.

46. B: Tensilon is used in myasthenic crisis to improve muscle function affected by deficient cholinesterase inhibitor levels; however, the improvement is temporary. Tensilon administration results in improved muscle function in myasthenic crisis; therefore, Choice *A* is incorrect. Tensilon effectively treats a myasthenic crisis. However, it will not improve a cholinergic crisis and may worsen the symptoms; therefore, Choices *C* and *D* are incorrect.

47. C: HIV-1 consists of four groups: M, N, O, and P. Group M is the most common group globally, and it consists of nine subtypes: A, B, C, D, E, F, G, H, J, and K. Globally, subtype C is the most common; however, in the Western world, subtype B is the most common. Therefore, this patient from China, in East Asia, most likely has subtype C. As a result, Choices *A*, *B*, and *D* are not correct.

48. C: This scenario depicts the classic triad of symptoms of acute epiglottitis, including hypoxia, drooling and dysphagia. Acute epiglottitis is most often caused by *Haemophilus influenzae* type B. Direct visualization reveals that the epiglottis appears cherry red in color. Treatment includes antibiotic therapy, analgesic-antipyretic agents, and emergency airway management. Laryngotracheobronchitis (classic croup) is a common viral illness that primarily affects children and toddlers from six months to three years of age. The parainfluenza viruses (types 1, 2, and 3) account for 80% of all cases. Presenting symptoms include a barking cough, wheezing, tachypnea, and tachycardia. Treatment is symptomatic and includes corticosteroids, racemic epinephrine, and mechanical ventilation. Tracheitis is the inflammation of the trachea caused most commonly by *Staphylococcus aureus*. Children under the age of fifteen are most commonly affected. Antibiotic therapy and anti-pyretic medications are used.

Mechanical ventilation is rarely necessary. Bronchiolitis is an inflammation of the bronchioles caused by the respiratory syncytial virus. It most commonly affects children under the age of two. Its diagnosis is based on clinical examination and the disease is self-limiting.

49. C: Endoscopy is used to diagnose the condition and to cauterize hemorrhagic sites. The treatment algorithm for peptic ulcer disease recommends surgical intervention if two endoscopic attempts at hemostasis are unsuccessful. The pain related to peptic ulcer disease does not begin until the ingested food has reached the duodenum; therefore, the pain does not begin for 2 to 3 hours after a meal, while the onset of pain with gastric ulcers is 20 to 30 minutes after a meal. Choice *A* is incorrect. Gastric ulcers are associated with an increased incidence of malignancy, not peptic ulcers; therefore, Choice *B* is incorrect. NSAID use is a commonly-associated cause of peptic ulcer disease. However, even excluding patients who use NSAIDs, more than 60 percent of the cases of peptic ulcer disease are related to *H. pylori* infection; therefore, Choice *D* is incorrect.

50. B: Choice *B* is a likely condition associated with acromegaly. The medical-surgical nurse should be aware of this association and monitor for signs and symptoms of diabetes mellitus, such as polyuria and polydipsia. Choice *A* is incorrect, as the patient's bone enlargement is permanent. Choice *C* is incorrect, as the patient needs to engage in surgery as soon as possible. Choice *D* is incorrect, as the patient's hands and feet will grow larger.

51. A: Prehypertension is defined as systolic pressures ranging between 120 and 139 mmHg or diastolic pressures between 80 and 89 mmHg. Normal blood pressure is less than 120/80 mmHg. Stage 1 hypertension ranges from 140 to 159 mmHg systolic or 90 to 99 mmHg diastolic. Stage 2 hypertension is greater than or equal to 160 mmHg systolic or greater than or equal to 100 mmHg diastolic.

52. B: The greatest risk for perinatal virus transmission occurs with the antigen-positive hepatitis B virus. Hepatitis A virus spreads most commonly by the fecal-oral route, and perinatal transmission has not been established; therefore, Choice *A* is incorrect. Hepatitis C is rarely transmitted to the fetus, and the antigen-negative genotype would be less likely than the antigen-positive genotype to affect the fetus; therefore, Choice *C* is incorrect. Perinatal transmission of the hepatitis D virus is rare, and release of the hepatitis D virions requires coinfection with the hepatitis B virus; therefore, Choice *D* is incorrect.

53. C: If complete or partial blindness develops in a patient with temporal arteritis prior to therapeutic intervention, the deficit may progress and become irreversible, which constitutes an ophthalmologic emergency. Lower limb claudication due to vasculitis and ischemic changes may occur as the result of the inflammatory process, and the condition does require assessment and monitoring; however, visual alterations remain a higher priority for emergency care. Vertebral body fractures and infection are related to steroid therapy, which may occur during therapy, and both conditions will require assessment and intervention; however, the need to prevent irreversible blindness is a more urgent priority.

54. D: Hyperemesis gravidarum is an extreme form of morning sickness that can result in fluid and electrolyte depletion, ketosis, and weight loss; therefore, the nurse should monitor the patient's fluid and electrolyte status. *A* is incorrect because encouraging the patient to eat, before the nausea and vomiting are controlled, may trigger more vomiting. Once the nausea and vomiting are under control, the patient should be encouraged to eat. Antiemetics that have been shown to be safe during pregnancy may be administered to control nausea and vomiting, making Choice *B* incorrect. While monitoring liver function tests may be performed, they are not a priority action, making Choice *C* incorrect.

55. D: Choice *D* supports suspicion for the need to transfer the patient to inpatient psychiatry once medically stable. Reasons for acute inpatient psychiatric hospitalization include danger to self, danger to others, and gross inability to care for self. Psychosocial symptoms warrant the need for a psychiatric consult to evaluate continuation of care options. Choices *A*, *B*, and *C* may each be present symptoms of the patient's mental illness but not reason enough for inpatient care. Patient presentations outside of the needs listed here for acute inpatient stabilization can be referred for outpatient management.

56. A: Jugular vein distention, peripheral edema, and pulmonary congestion are characteristics of blood volume backing up due to an obstruction. Decreased urine output, increased BUN, and increased creatinine are signs of renal failure. Chest pain, fatigue, and lightheadedness are signs of an MI. Problems with coordination, blurred vision, and paralysis are symptomatic of a stroke.

57. A: Choice *A* represents the cranial nerve responsible for the patient's reflex to gag and swallow. Choice *B* is responsible for tongue movements. Choice *C* is responsible for taste. Choice *D* is responsible for jaw movements.

58. D: Viral pneumonia, commonly caused by RSV, parainfluenza virus, and adenovirus, may be diagnosed by chest x-ray and viral cultures. Rapid antigen testing is now also being used for diagnosis and has the advantage of shortening the time for diagnosing this infection. Choices *A*, *B*, and *C* are incorrect as these tests are not used to neither diagnose viral pneumonia nor shorten the diagnostic time.

59. C: In second-degree heart block, specifically Mobitz type I, the PR interval is lengthened and greater than 0.20. The PR interval for a normal sinus rhythm is 0.12–0.20. In a junctional rhythm, the impulse is starting at the AV node, so the P wave is absent. In Mobitz type II second-degree heart block, the P waves are not followed by the QRS complex. The atria and ventricles are asynchronously contracting.

60. D: The patient with Guillain-Barré syndrome with cranial nerve involvement may exhibit weakness or paralysis of the eye muscles, facial drooping, diplopia, dysphagia, and pupillary alterations. Therefore, Choices *A*, *B*, and *C* are not correct.

61. A: The nurse must first assess the patient's vital signs before continuing on with subsequent actions. Therefore, Choice *A* is correct. Choice *B*, Choice *C*, and Choice *D* are all relevant interventions, though lack the priority in the case of the patient complaining of chest pain upon presentation to the emergency department. Once the vital signs have been assessed, the nurse should follow the nursing process to proceed with further care options.

62. A: Since electrolytes need to be suspended in a certain amount of liquid to move optimally and carry out their intended function, fluid level in the body is important. As fluid levels increase beyond a state of fluid-electrolyte balance, electrolyte levels will decrease, since there is too much fluid present. If fluid levels are too low, such as in a state of dehydration, there will be too many electrolytes per unit of fluid, which also prevents the electrolytes from carrying out their intended function.

63. D: Choice *D* demonstrates a normal finding when auscultating the patient's lungs. Choice *A* is not a normal finding over the lungs, rather normal over the stomach. Choice *B* is not a normal finding, as it is indicative of air hyperinflation, such as with asthma. Choice *C* is not a normal finding over the lungs, rather normal over dense areas such as the liver.

64. A: Choice *A* is correct as this finding represents the shortness of breath that is present specifically in a recumbent position. Choice *B* identifies difficulty breathing. Choice *C* identifies elevated breathing rate. Choice *D* correlates with decreased breathing rate.

65. D: Choice *D* designates the applicable first action to be implemented by the nurse in response to the patient's request for discharge. Exploring the patient's reasoning for discharge is patient-centered and allows the nurse to gather additional information to formulate a clear understanding of the present issue(s) before deciding on next steps. Choice *A* may be an appropriate second step, depending on the patient's response to the original inquiry in step one. Choices *B* and *C*, while potential actions that may be necessary at some point, are not priorities in this situation.

66. D: Choice *D* indicates the appropriate level of infection control to reduce the risk of transmission for a patient diagnosed with active tuberculosis. Choices *A*, *B*, and *C* would not provide enough protection in reducing this risk. Tuberculosis is an airborne disease; therefore, transmission of the bacillus, mycobacterium tuberculosis, must be minimized.

67. C: Choice *C* does NOT represent an ethnic group at an increased risk for sickle cell anemia. Choices *A*, *C*, and *D* are all ethnic groups that have a heightened risk for developing this inherited red blood cell disorder.

68. A: Choice *A* represents the appropriate party for elevation of this concern. In following the nursing chain-of-command, the staff nurse should elevate the bed management issue to the charge nurse. Choices *B*, *C*, and *D*, while all potential influencers to a change, represent inappropriate reports for this issue by the staff nurse at this time. As the nurse works within a chain-of-command hierarchy, consideration to the appropriate party must be given when elevating concerns.

69. D: Chromosomal abnormalities of the fetus are the most common cause of early spontaneous abortions. Other factors that increase the risk include advanced maternal age, type 1 diabetes, renal disease, severe hypertension, thyroid dysfunction, anatomical defects of the uterus, illicit drug use, smoking, alcohol abuse, and non-ASA NSAID use; therefore, Choices *A* and *B* are not correct. Moderate exercise is not a risk factor for spontaneous abortion, making Choice *C* an incorrect answer.

70. B: Hypothyroidism occurs when there is an underproduction of T3 and/or T4 hormones. Low levels of these hormones may cause depression, excessive fatigue, chills, dry skin, lowered heart rate, constipation, and unexplained weight gain. Therefore, the nurse anticipates that the physician will order serum T4 levels. Cortisol, blood glucose, and aldosterone levels are not used in the diagnosis of hypothyroidism, making Choices *A*, *C*, and *D* incorrect.

71. C: Choice *C* indicates a chief goal of the working phase of the nurse-patient relationship. Choices *A* and *B* represent chief goals of the orientation phase. Choice *D* indicates a chief goal of the termination phase.

72. D: While the majority of cysts do not produce clinical manifestations, they may be associated with abdominal bloating as well as early satiety, change in bowel habits, weight loss, and, if ruptured, severe pain. Since the patient is likely to experience weight loss, *A* is not correct. A cyst may cause a change in bowel habits, but not urinary habits, so *B* is not correct. A patient with an ovarian cyst may experience early satiety, but not an increase in appetite, making *C* an incorrect answer.

73. D: While the physician is legally responsible for satisfying all elements of informed consent, nurses are ethically responsible for assessing the patient's ability to process and understand the implications of informed consent. Nurses protect the patient's autonomy by raising these questions and concerns. The remaining elements of informed consent are required of the physician, rather than the nurses.

74. D: Choice *D* is considered safe to consume by a patient scheduled for an exercise stress test the next day. Choices *A*, *B*, and *C* all must be held as they can interfere with the results of the test. Consuming these substances may inhibit the body's response to the exercise and can also interfere with medication that may be given during the test.

75. C: Choice *C* should be avoided in the plan of care for a patient with acute burns; instead, a high protein, high caloric diet would be appropriate. Choices *A*, *B*, and *D* indicate supportive measures that should be implemented for this patient to monitor for and reduce additional complications.

76. B: Choice *B* indicates the patient's behavior to undo something that they hope will not take place. Undoing involves a sense of magic. Choices *A*, *C*, and *D* are not present in the patient's actions.

77. A: The classic manifestations of bacterial meningitis include fever, nuchal rigidity, and headache. Other manifestations may include nausea, vomiting, photophobia, confusion, and a decreased level of consciousness; therefore, Choices *B* and *C* are incorrect. Manifestations of viral meningitis may include fatigue, muscle aches, and decreased appetite, making Choice *D* incorrect.

78. B: In autoimmune gastritis, there is a deficiency of intrinsic factor, which is responsible for the absorption of vitamin B-12. Therefore, the patient with autoimmune gastritis will have a vitamin B-12 deficiency. As a result, Choices *A, C,* and *D* are incorrect.

79. A: 10 percent of MS patients are initially diagnosed with the primary-progressive form of MS, which means that the disease is always active without periods of remission. The relapsing-remitting form of MS accounts for 85 percent of the patients diagnosed with MS, which means that they will eventually progress to the secondary-progressive form; this means that the disease is always active. The potential progression of an isolated incident to MS depends on the presence or absence of plaque formation on MRI scans. The presence of alterations in the myelin sheath is strongly predictive of eventual progression. However, the absence of those lesions does not rule out the possibility of subsequent progression to MS; therefore, Choice *B* is incorrect. Only 10 percent of MS patients present with the primary-progressive form; therefore, Choice *C* is incorrect. Disease-modifying drugs are the preferred agents to treat MS. However, prednisone may be used if a patient is unable to tolerate the DMDs; therefore, Choice *D* is incorrect.

80. D: Choice *D* is a dependent nursing intervention as it requires a provider's order to carry out. Choices *A*, *B*, and *C* are all within the nursing scope to initiate and are therefore considered independent nursing interventions. A third classification, interdependent intervention, involves nursing and collaborative specialties providing care measures.

81. A: Choice *A* is an appropriate flow rate for the nurse to set for the nasal cannula. Patients with chronic obstructive pulmonary disease (COPD) require oxygen at low flow rates to maintain the hypoxic stimulus to breathe. Choices *B*, *C*, and *D* are too high for a patient with COPD because these rates would suppress their stimulus to breathe.

82. C: New onset of peripheral edema may be signaling decompensation by the right side of the heart and progressive heart failure. Oxygenation levels for CHF patients are generally lower but tolerated well. Ninety-two percent is an acceptable oxygen saturation level for this patient. Dyspnea upon exertion is not an unusual finding during a CHF exacerbation. Elevated BNP levels, although abnormal, are anticipated with CHF.

83. A: Choice *A* is correct, as ascites is a condition that may develop secondary to liver failure. Choices *B*, *C*, and *D* do not directly cause ascites, the buildup of fluid in the abdomen.

84. B: The scenario depicts an episode of status asthmaticus. Common pharmacological agents used to treat this condition include albuterol (short-acting Beta-2 agonist), ipratropium (anticholinergic), and methylprednisolone (corticosteroid). Her new symptoms (anxiety, tremors, and tachycardia) are all common side effects which can be attributed to albuterol. Anticholinergics can induce side effects such as dry mouth, blurred vision, and constipation. Corticosteroids (if used for longer than two weeks) can have side effects such as weight gain, osteoporosis, thinning of skin, cataracts, easy bruising, and diabetes. She should be switched to the short-acting Beta-2 agonist levalbuterol because it's as effective as albuterol but without the alarming side effects.

85. B: Choice *B* is correct as this condition encourages the development of cold fingers, nose, and nipples. These areas become discolored due to impaired circulation and can feel numb. Raynaud's phenomenon differs from Raynaud's disease in this condition happens secondary to a primary illness, such as scleroderma in this patient's case. Choices *A*, *C*, and *D* do not encourage the development of these symptoms.

86. A: Choice *A* indicates the priority action in navigating a dilemma of opposing opinions within the interdisciplinary team. Choices *B*, *C*, and *D* are actions that may or may not need to happen depending on what is found when collecting clinical data.

87. D: Choice *D*, a vitamin found in food and supplements, is a key element of an alcohol withdrawal protocol. Thiamine is typically deficient in those with alcohol abuse and dependence and is replaced during treatment. Choices *A*, *B*, and *C*, while all potentially helpful supplements across a variety of conditions, are not specifically associated with the needs of the patient at this time.

88. B: Choice *B* represents a diagnosis with a hallmark symptom presentation of a bulls-eye rash. While not all patients with Lyme disease will experience the rash, symptoms of Lyme disease are further assessed by the nurse in patients who do. Choices *A*, *C*, and *D* do not match with the symptom presentation of a bulls-eye rash, as this is not an expected symptom of these diseases.

89. C: Choice *C* indicates a thorough understanding of cultural considerations to care as this behavior represents normal cultural conduct. Choices *A*, *B*, and *D* are inappropriate as this behavior does not insinuate anything more than cultural norms regarding the patient's level of understanding, agreement, or pace of discussion.

90. B: Choice *B* is correct as diabetes mellitus increases one's risk of a cerebrovascular accident due to pathologic changes in blood vessels. Choices *A*, *C*, and *D* are not considered risk factors for cerebrovascular accident.

91. B: Choice *B* indicates the therapeutic reference range for serum carbamazepine. Choices *A*, *C*, and *D* represent serum medication ranges outside of therapeutic limits. The therapeutic range is measured by fluorescence polarization immunoassay.

92. B: Choice *B* should be supported by the nurse, as it brings the knees to chest and typically encourages some pain relief in acute appendicitis. Choices *A*, *C*, and *D* represent positions that would likely exacerbate the patient's pain symptoms and should not be encouraged at this time.

93. B: Choice *B* aligns with the ethical principle to maintain truthful engagements. Choice *A* aligns with ethical fairness. Choice *C* aligns with refraining from harm. Choice *D* promotes doing right by the patient.

94. B: In the event of major trauma, there is an increased incidence of fetal-to-maternal hemorrhage, which can alter the amount of Rho(D) immune globulin (RhoGAM) that is required to protect the fetus. The Kleihauer-Betke test can be used to quantify the concentration of fetal hemoglobin in the maternal blood, which then is used to calculate the appropriate dose of Rho(D) immune globulin (RhoGAM) in Rh-negative mothers; therefore, Choice *B* is correct. Although some authors recommend the use of the test in all patients as an indicator of preterm labor, the research indicates that this test is not specific for, or sensitive to, the occurrence of preterm labor and is not a reliable indicator for preterm labor; therefore, Choice *A* is incorrect. The transfer of fetal hemoglobin to the maternal circulation must be addressed with the first pregnancy to avoid the formation of anti-D antibodies; therefore, Choice *C* is incorrect. The test can only measure the concentration of fetal hemoglobin in the maternal circulation. It is not sensitive or specific to the degree of the precipitating trauma; therefore, Choice *D* is incorrect.

95. C: Choice *C* is not involved in the Five Rights of Delegation, which include the right person, task, circumstance, direction, and supervision. Choices *A*, *B*, and *D* are all components of the Five Rights of Delegation and used by the medical-surgical nurse when assigning patient care.

96. A: Choice *A* accurately depicts the signs associated with asterixis, which also include liver failure. Choice *B* aligns with a positive Gower's sign. Choice *C* indicates cogwheel rigidity. Choice *D* describes ataxia.

97. A: The electrocardiogram (ECG) represents the electrical events of the cardiac cycle. An electrical impulse begins in the sinoatrial node and travels to the atrioventricular node. This is represented by the P wave on ECG and corresponds to atrial depolarization. Therefore, Choices *B*, *C*, and *D* are not correct.

98. B: Choice *B* should be included in the treatment plan for the patient with thrombophlebitis to inhibit dislodging the clot. Choices *A*, *C*, and *D* pose increased risk for complication and should be avoided for this patient at this time.

99. B: The diuretic reduces blood volume, and the ACE inhibitor reduces SVR by interfering with the RAAS. An ARB reduces systemic vascular resistance, but morphine is used to treat pain. The diuretic reduces blood volume, but a beta-blocker increases myocardial contractility. The diuretic reduces blood volume, but a CCB works by increasing myocardial contractility.

100. A: Choice *A* is correct as sausage is a high tyramine-containing food and must be avoided by the patient taking a monoamine oxidase inhibitor, such as phenelzine. Foods rich in tyramine need to be avoided in order to prevent tyramine levels in the blood from becoming critically high and leading to a hypertensive crisis. Choices *B*, *C*, and *D* are not considered high tyramine-containing foods and are not contraindicated for the patient at this time.

101. D: Choice *D* is correct as this imbalance can cause a build up of fluid in the form of edema and ascites for patients with impaired renal function. Low sodium levels alter the fluid balance of the body, encouraging the retention seen in these findings. Choices *A*, *B*, and *C*, while significant imbalances to measure, do not directly influence the development of ascites and dependent edema secondary to impaired renal function.

102. C: Choice *C* represents the appropriate level of activity for the patient with heart failure. Alternating rest with activity supports a reduced cardiac workload. Choice *A* would encourage a higher level of activity than the patient's condition can maintain. Choices *B* and *D* place unnecessary restrictions on the patient's activity.

103. A: Apgar scores of 8 and 9 are normal scores for a healthy newborn with acrocyanosis, which is a benign condition manifested by peripheral cyanosis of the hands and feet that usually resolves within the first few hours after birth. Decreased muscle tone or flexion is most often associated with other deficits that would result in a lower Apgar score; therefore, Choice *B* is incorrect. If the newborn required ventilatory support, there would also be deficits of muscle tone and heart rate, resulting in lower Apgar scores; therefore, Choice *C* is incorrect. The Apgar score is not predictive of specific anomalies, and the indicated scores are considered as normal; therefore, Choice *D* is incorrect.

104. B: The elevated glucose levels associated with both type 1 and type 2 diabetes result in atherosclerosis, or wall thickening of the small arterioles and capillaries, which alters the circulation in the brain, retina, peripheral nerves, and kidneys. These changes are cumulative and irreversible; however, long-term control of the serum glucose level as measured by the A1C can limit the progression of this process. Current research indicates that the optimum A1C level is patient-specific. In this discussion, the patient knows his personal A1C target and understands the association between the elevated glucose levels and the occurrence of the TIA; therefore, Choice *B* is correct. Two of the $ABCD^2$ score categories are modifiable risk factors. Maintaining the systolic and diastolic blood pressure and blood glucose level as defined by the A1C within normal limits may lower the risk of a repeated attack. The patient should be encouraged to make the necessary lifestyle changes, including smoking cessation, dietary modifications, exercise participation, and compliance with the medication regimen that may include antihypertensive and glucose-lowering agents. Choice *A* is incorrect. There are differences in the pathophysiology between type 1 and type 2 diabetes; however, the complications are similar. In type 2 diabetes, hyperglycemia and insulin resistance contribute to increased low-density lipoproteins and triglycerides and decreased levels of high-density lipoproteins and alterations in microvasculature; therefore, Choice *C* is incorrect. To prevent further damage to the vascular system and reduce the risk of recurrent TIAs, the use of insulin may be necessary to control hyperglycemia as evidenced by the A1C level; therefore, Choice *D* is incorrect.

105. C: A first-degree heart block is NOT a direct risk factor for the development of an embolus. Women during pregnancy and in the postpartum period, individuals with a history of a previous stroke, and patients with fractures that involve long bones are all at risk for the development of am embolus.

106. C: Critical limb ischemia (CLI) is the most concerning symptom of PVD. It is indicative of decreased circulation even at rest. Faint peripheral pulses may be a finding associated with PVD but are not the most concerning symptom. Restricted mobility may be a sequela to PVD, but it is also not the most concerning. Feet that become pale when elevated are a symptom of PVD, but this is not the most concerning symptom.

107. C: At Stage III of the NYSA classification tool, the patient with cardiac disease has marked limitations with physical activity but no symptoms at rest. The patient in this example is experiencing symptoms walking a short distance but not while at rest. Choice *A* is incorrect because Stage I is marked by no symptoms during physical activity. Choice *B* is incorrect because Stage II is marked by slight limitations on physical activity. Choice *D* is incorrect because in Stage IV, the patient is unable to perform physical activity and experiences symptoms at rest.

108. B: Choice *B* is correct, as the medical-surgical nurse would associate upside-down spoon nails, also known as nail clubbing, with the patient's diagnosis of lung cancer. The nurse would observe the nails to appear reddish in color and sponge-like in appearance. Choices *A*, *C*, and *D* do not cause this change in the structure of the fingernail.

109. A: Choice *A* involves the proper position for a patient receiving an enema as it promotes the flow of fluid into the rectum due to anatomy and gravity. Choices *B*, *C*, and *D* should be avoided as they do not facilitate the ease of passage necessary for effective enema treatment.

110. A: Choice *A* identifies the patient's potential fear regarding the consequence of the nurse's actions. Giving what is perceived to be the "evil eye" may induce significant worry that the patient's child will become weak and ill and can even lead to fears that the child may die. Choices *B*, *C*, and *D* represent concerns of staring outside of the definition of this cultural consideration.

111. D: The gastroenterologist will likely use cauterization, an application of heat, to seal the bleeding lesion. Banding is a procedure used to help stop bleeding in esophageal varices. Biopsy is where tissues are removed for histological analysis. Angioplasty is performed in cardiac catheterizations and involves balloon inflation and stent placement to open up occluded blood vessels.

112. D: This scenario depicts a case of acute bronchitis. The most common causes of acute bronchitis are respiratory viruses (such as influenza A and B), respiratory syncytial virus (RSV), parainfluenza, adenovirus, rhinovirus, and coronavirus. Acute bronchitis should not be routinely treated with antibiotics, but there are exceptions to this rule. It's reasonable to use antibiotics if an existing medical condition poses a risk of serious complications. Antibiotic treatment of acute bronchitis is also reasonable in individuals older than sixty-five years of age with a hospitalization in the past year, those being currently treated with a steroid, and those diagnosed with congestive heart failure or diabetes.

113. D: Choice *D* includes bringing about the greatest good for the greatest number of people, which is what the medical-surgical nurse does when prioritizing patient care. Choices *A*, *B*, and *C*, while all ethical considerations, do not align with the nurse's actions at this time.

114. A: Choice *A* indicates a technique used to examine the blood flow through the aorta to further assess and diagnose an abdominal aortic aneurysm. Choices *B*, *C*, and *D* do not align with the nurse's explanation of the pending procedure while providing patient education.

115. D: Cushing's disease is caused by excessive glucocorticoid production which, in turn, is responsible for producing steroids. Therefore, Choices *A*, *B*, and *C* are not correct.

116. C: Choice *C* is a later development of Lyme disease and is not associated with early, localized disease. Choices *A*, *C*, and *D* are all early symptoms. Lyme disease occurs in three stages: early localized, early disseminated, and late disseminated disease.

117. D: Choice *D* is a likely imbalance that presents in a patient with acute renal failure and will require diligent management. Choices *A*, *B*, and *C* are unlikely as the patient is at risk for a decreased GFR, increased BUN, and decreased calcium level. Acute renal failure involves poor filtering ability and a build up of waste in the blood.

118. A: The normal pulse oximetry for a full-term newborn is 92 to 96 percent. Therefore, this result is normal and no action by the nurse is needed. Therefore, Choices *B*, *C*, and *D* are not correct.

119. D: In advanced stages of cancer, even when the prognosis is poor, chemotherapy may be able to manage pain and suffering. Choices *A*, *B*, and *C* are not correct, because the chance of remission, cure, or halting the advance of cancer in advanced stages of cancer with a poor prognosis is low and the nurse should not give the patient false hope.

120. C: Choice *C* represents the quadrant the nurse should request the patient to report their pain in to evaluate the effectiveness of the interventions aimed at improving the duodenal obstruction. Choices *A*, *B*, and *D* are quadrants outside of the location of the blockage and are not involved in the focused nursing evaluation at this time.

121. A: Choice *A* indicates an action that aligns with the scope of practice of the unlicensed assistive personnel (UAP), which can safely be delegated by the nurse. Choices *B*, *C*, and *D* indicate actions that should be carried out by the nurse, as they align with the scope of practice of the nurse and not with the scope of the UAP.

122. D: Time between the collapse and the start of resuscitation efforts is the most important factor in patient survival. Administering supplemental oxygen is a component of resuscitation efforts. Establishing IV access is an essential component of resuscitation efforts. Inserting a Foley catheter to drain the urinary bladder is not related to survival.

123. C: Choice *C* is correct as audible S3 and S4 sounds upon cardiac auscultation indicate summation gallop. Choice *A* sounds musical or vibratory. Choice *B* contains two audible heart sounds, S1 and S2. Choice *D* is heard as a sound between the S1 and S2 heartbeat cycle.

124. C: Since the patient is confused, the intervention with the highest priority is to ensure safety by checking on the patient at least every two hours. At this time, the nurse can make sure all items are within reach, assist the patient to the toilet, and reinforce use of the call bell, all measures that can prevent falls. Choice *A* is an important intervention but is not a priority since the patient is confused and may not use the call bell. Explaining the daily schedule and providing a stable and calm environment are also helpful to the patient who is confused, but only after safety has been ensured, making Choices *B* and *D* incorrect answers.

125. B: Atrial flutter occurs when an ectopic atrial focus fires at a rate of 250 to 350 times a minute, producing a sawtooth pattern on the ECG. Because the atrioventricular node cannot transmit impulses that fast, only one out of every 2 impulses generally reaches the ventricles. Choice *A* is not correct because atrial fibrillation is marked by multiple foci in the atria firing randomly, producing an irregular atrial rhythm with a normal or rapid ventricular rate. Choice *C* is not correct because sinus tachycardia is caused by an SA node that fires at a regular rate of greater than 100 beats a minute. Choice *D* is not correct since ventricular tachycardia occurs when a singular ventricular focus fires at a rate of 150 to 250 times a minute.

126. A: Bronchiolitis, an inflammation of the small airways in the lung, most commonly affects children under the age of two, with the greatest incidence between 3 and 6 months old. Children age 2 and older, including children entering kindergarten or in high school, are less likely to be affected, making Choices *B*, *C*, and *D* inappropriate choices.

127. C: Status epilepticus is prolonged seizure activity involving multiple seizures, each lasting five minutes or more, over a thirty-minute period of time. A generalized seizure is a seizure that originates in two or more networks of the brain, making Choice *A* incorrect. A focal seizure is one that originates in a single area of the brain, making Choice *B* incorrect. The postictal state follows a seizure and is characterized by alterations in consciousness and awareness and increased oral secretions, making Choice *D* incorrect.

128. A: The patient's manifestations are consistent with an incarcerated or strangulated hernia that is progressing to a small-bowel obstruction as evidenced by the abdominal distention. This complication is associated with decreased peristalsis and eventual absence of bowel activity, which means that diarrhea would be an uncommon manifestation. Tachycardia and a BUN of 27 are related to fluid volume losses resulting from the accumulation of fluid proximal to the obstruction in the small bowel; therefore, Choices *B* and *D* are incorrect. Rebound tenderness is also an expected finding in a bowel obstruction due to the trapped gas and fluid proximal to the obstruction; therefore, Choice *C* is incorrect.

129. A: Choice *A* is within the scope of practice of the unlicensed assistive personnel (UAP) and can be delegated by the nurse. The UAP can respond to the patient call light to listen to a patient's concerns and form a plan for the next steps. If the patient requests assistance outside of the UAP's scope, the care concern is then elevated back up to the nurse. Choices *B*, *C*, and *D* involve actions outside of the UAP scope of practice and should not be delegated by the nurse at this time. The nurse should assist the patient with adjusting oxygen flow, auscultating breath sounds, and changing the wound dressing.

130. D: In type 2 diabetes, the pancreas produces insulin, but the body does not use it effectively. This type of diabetes may be treated with oral anti-diabetic medications and, in some cases, insulin. However, many people can control their type 2 diabetes through lifestyle changes, such as losing weight and eating less carbohydrate-rich and sugar-laden foods, making Choices *A*, *B*, and *C* incorrect.

131. A: In diabetes, a disorder in which the body's insulin response to blood glucose is compromised, high blood glucose levels occur that can damage the body's organ and tissue over time. Choice *B* is not correct because insulin levels should be monitored before meals. Choice *C* is not correct since the role of insulin is to help glucose be absorbed from the bloodstream into the cells of the body. Choice *D* is not correct because hyperglycemia occurs when the body has inadequate insulin, not too much insulin.

132. C: Small-bowel obstruction is associated with severe fluid and electrolyte losses. The normal serum sodium level is 135 to 145 mEq/L; therefore, Choice *C* is indicative of deficient serum sodium and severe alterations in fluid balance. Small-bowel obstruction is manifested by metabolic alkalosis due to the loss of acids with vomiting. Choice *A* is consistent with metabolic acidosis, not alkalosis, and is therefore incorrect. As noted, small-bowel obstruction is associated with fluid volume deficits; however, the reported serum osmolality at 285 mosm/kg is within the normal range for serum osmolality (275–295 mosm/kg); therefore, Choice *B* is incorrect. Abdominal distention in large-bowel obstruction most commonly occurs in the lower abdomen, while abdominal distention in the small bowel most commonly occurs in the epigastric or upper abdominal area; therefore, Choice *D* is incorrect.

133. A: Choice *A* is the antidote to be given to a patient experiencing over anticoagulation to halt the progression of this process. Choices *B*, *C*, and *D*, while antidotes for a variety of medications, will not work for this issue.

134. D: Choice *D* is the antidote given to counteract the effects of Enoxaparin. Choices *A*, *B*, and *D* represent medications used as antidotes for a wide variety of medications but will not neutralize this medication and inhibit the reaction.

135. D: Choice *D* is correct as cirrhosis of the liver should be assessed in the right upper quadrant by palpated for an enlarged liver under the lower edge of the patient's right rib cage. Typically, the liver is unable to be palpated; however, if it is enlarged, the nurse can examine this via a focused assessment. Choices *A*, *B*, and *C* represent quadrants outside of the direct location of this organ's focused assessment.

136. A: Choice *A* is a back channeling communication cue that signals to the patient that the nurse is actively listening and would like the patient to continue with their narrative. Choices *B*, *C*, and *D*, while all potentially useful communication cues, do not meet the description of back channeling.

137. B: Of the two types of human immunodeficiency virus (HIV), HIV-1 is the dominant strain among global cases. HIV-2 is not highly transmissible, so Choice *A* is not correct. Since HIV-2 is poorly understood, Choice *C* is not correct. HIV-1 is the more severe strain, making Choice *D* an incorrect choice.

138. D: An early sign of respiratory distress is agitation, along with confusion and oxygen hunger. Later signs of respiratory distress occur when the patient has become fatigued because of the respiratory effort they have put forth. These signs include decreased respiratory rate, unconsciousness, and cyanosis.

139. D: Choice *D* indicates the phase of the nursing process that the nurse is functioning within when testing the patient's understanding of properly applying compression stockings. Choices *A*, *B*, and *C* indicate phases of the nursing process that do not directly evaluate understanding or outcomes, therefore do not represent the nurse's phase of function at this time.

140. B: In an adult lying in the supine position, a normal intracranial pressure reading ranges from 7 to 15 millimeters of mercury. Therefore, Choices *A*, *C*, and *D* are incorrect.

141. A: Since tremors, fatigue, and dizziness are manifestations of hypoglycemia, the nurse would expect to see a low blood glucose level. Since a normal blood glucose level is 70 to 130 milligrams per deciliter, 58 milligrams per deciliter is consistent with hypoglycemia. Choice *B* is not correct since 120 milligrams per deciliter is a normal blood glucose level. Choice *C* is not correct since 180 milligrams per deciliter is above normal. Choice *D* is not correct since a blood glucose level greater than 200 milligrams per deciliter is considered hyperglycemic.

142. A: Choice *A* indicates an accurate understanding of the discharge process. Discharge planning starts upon admission to ensure that resources are allocated appropriately, interventions align with an established treatment plan, and an ultimate safe discharge outcome is recognized. Choices *B*, *C*, and *D* do not represent a clear understanding of treatment planning for the discharge process.

143. B: Postpartum hemorrhage occurs when there is a blood loss of more than 500 milliliters following a vaginal delivery or 1000 milliliters after a Cesarean section in a pregnancy that has progressed beyond twenty weeks. A blood loss of less than 500 milliliters may lead to hemodynamic instability in patients with comorbidities, such as this woman's mitral valve regurgitation. Other comorbidities that can cause hemodynamic instability with less substantial blood losses include anemia, other cardiac diseases, dehydration, or preeclampsia. Therefore *A*, *C*, and *D* are not correct.

144. D: The appropriate response to an initial unprovoked seizure episode—one that is not related to a specific cause such as head trauma—is to identify any abnormal electrical activity of the brain with an EEG and any anatomical lesions in the brain with MRI. There is no indication of substance abuse in the patient's history, which means that this assessment would not be a priority for this patient at this point; therefore, Choice *A* is incorrect. General guidelines indicate that AED therapy should be delayed until a second unprovoked seizure episode occurs and after the initial EEG and MRI studies are completed; therefore, Choice *B* is incorrect. The patient's history does not support the possibility of infection as the precipitating event for this seizure activity, which means performing the invasive lumbar puncture would not be indicated; therefore, Choice *C* is incorrect.

145. D: The patient with severe pelvic and other injuries from trauma may be assessed using the Revised Trauma Score assessment tool, which assesses the probability of survival in trauma patients. The parameters measured are the Glasgow Coma Scale score, systolic blood pressure, and respiratory rate. Therefore, *A*, *B*, and *C* are not correct.

146. B: Choice *B* is correct as a patient experiencing chronic bronchitis will often present with audible early inspiratory and expiratory crackles upon auscultation during a focused respiratory assessment. These lung sounds are consistent with this condition. Choices *A*, *C*, and *D* typically correlate with late inspiratory crackles.

147. C: Myasthenia gravis is an autoimmune disease caused by the altered transmission of the neurotransmitter acetylcholine at the neuromuscular junction due to antibody formation. Therefore, Choices *A*, *B*, and *D* are incorrect.

148. A: Choice *A* is a surgical procedure highly associated with chronic otitis media. This procedure, also known as eardrum repair, provides needed reconstruction. Choices *B*, *C*, and *D* represent Ear, Nose, and Throat (ENT) surgical procedures that are not typically associated with this diagnosis. The nurse would not need to print and share patient education on these options at this time.

149. D: Choice *D* is a concern for a patient with parathyroid disease, which is influenced by the levels of calcium and parathyroid hormone in the blood. High levels of calcium induce hypertension, while high levels of parathyroid hormone induces hypotension. Choices *A*, *B*, and *C* are not associated concerns for a patient with parathyroid disease.

150. C: Choice *C* is correct, as the patient should use their Advair-Diskus inhaler routinely, twice per day. The patient appropriately understands that this inhaler is not designed for rescue breathing relief when they share that they will use it every morning and evening. Choices *A*, *B*, and *D* represent responses that align with inhalers indicated for rescue relief and are not appropriate for this medication.

151. B: Early manifestations of preeclampsia include facial edema, visual disturbances, altered mental state, dyspnea, and possible right upper quadrant pain. Severe manifestations include hypertension on bedrest, increasing liver enzymes with increased pain, thrombocytopenia, progressive renal dysfunction, and pulmonary edema, making Choices *A*, *C*, and *D* incorrect answers.

152. A: Avoiding tight clothing and wearing compression stockings are appropriate. Although prolonged sitting should be avoided, airplane travel itself is not contraindicated. Exercise should be continued with frequent rest periods as needed. The occurrence and severity of claudication can be decreased with regular exercise.

153. A: A pneumothorax occurs when air is abnormally present in the pleural space. Primary spontaneous pneumothorax is more likely to occur in those who are tall and thin, between eighteen and forty years of age, have a history of smoking, and who have no history of lung disease. As a result, Choices *B*, *C*, and *D* are not correct.

154. A: The patient with primary progressive multiple sclerosis is likely to report disease that is constantly active without any periods of remission. Choice *B* is incorrect since it describes the relapsing-remitting form of multiple sclerosis. Choice *C* is not correct since it describes the secondary-progressive form of the disease. Choice *D* is not correct since it describes an isolated episode of the disease.

155. D: This scenario depicts a moderate to severe acute exacerbation of COPD. Azithromycin is a macrolide antibiotic. In clinical trials, the use of antibiotics in individuals with a moderate to severe exacerbation of COPD diminishes the risk of treatment failure and death. Oxygen and albuterol target dyspnea. In clinical trials, the administration of oral corticosteroids fairly early in the midst of a COPD exacerbation decreased the need for hospitalization.

156. D: Choice *D* involves the appropriate plan for reducing the spread of measles. It is important for the nurse to understand that measles requires airborne precautions and that proactive initiation is required once this illness is suspected. The nurse should NOT wait to start this precaution until the confirmation is received. Choices *A*, *B*, and *C* provide inadequate protection against the transmission of measles.

157. B: Choice *B* must be closely monitored in the patient with tardive dyskinesia, as the development of this physiologic dysfunction presents a medical emergency. Choices *A*, *C*, and *D* do not represent dysfunctions in physiologic processes that the patient with tardive dyskinesia would be at heightened risk of developing; therefore, they do not require close monitoring by the nurse at this time.

158. A: Choice *A* represents a creatinine level outside of the normal range, which is 0.5-1.2 mg/dl. The patient's level is elevated and requires further investigation. Choices *B*, *C*, and *D* are all within normal range and do not alert the nurse to the need for additional investigation at this time.

159. B: Choice *B* represents a biologically inactive metabolite of T4, which attaches to thyroid receptors but is unable to activate them. Choice *A* represents thyroxine, a thyroid hormone that enters and influences tissues. Choice *C* represents triiodothyronine, another thyroid hormone able to enter and affect bodily tissues. Choice *D* involves the free T4, along with the T4 that is bonded to protein.

160. A: This scenario depicts the diagnosis of pleural effusion. Pleural effusions can be categorized as transudates or exudates. The pleural effusion is exudative, which can be characterized by the following:

- Ratio of pleural fluid to serum protein > 0.5
- Ratio of pleural fluid to serum LDH > 0.6
- Pleural LDH > 2/3 of the upper limit of normal blood value

161. A: Fever and petechial rash are signs of endocarditis. Body piercings and corticosteroids are among the risk factors for developing endocarditis. Autoimmune conditions vary, but the most frequent presenting symptoms are fatigue and body aches. Pneumonia presents with fever, chills, and cough. Heart failure (HF) is not associated with a petechial rash or a fever.

162. A: Risk factors for benign ovarian cysts include hypothyroidism, infertility treatment, history of breast cancer, smoking, and tubal ligation. *B*, *C*, and *D* are not correct because risk factors for malignant cysts include a positive family history, early menarche, and nulliparity as well as advancing age, Caucasian ethnicity, infertility, delayed menopause, and a history of breast cancer.

163. A: Choice *A* represents a dietary item that the nurse should encourage the patient newly diagnosed with celiac disease to avoid. The tips of the villi in the small intestine contain lactase, the enzyme needed to process lactose found in dairy. Celiac disease blunts the villi, leading to dairy intolerance until they recover. Choices *B*, *C*, and *D* represent dietary items that are appropriate for this patient to consume and do not require education encouraging otherwise.

Med Surg Practice Test #2

1. The senior nurse of a unit has taken on an informal leadership role by functioning as a resource to meet the needs of the team. Leading by example, the nurse focuses on values and ethics, while continuously using foresight and empathy to advance the team. Which leadership style is this nurse displaying in their role?
   a. Servant
   b. Bureaucratic
   c. Laissez-faire
   d. Transactional

2. The nurse in the emergency department is caring for a twenty-six-year-old female patient with abnormal uterine bleeding. Which of the following tests does the nurse anticipate will be obtained first?
   a. Pap smear
   b. Uterine biopsy
   c. Pelvic ultrasonography
   d. Pregnancy test

3. An English-speaking medical-surgical nurse is completing a history and physical on a newly admitted patient. How should the nurse communicate with a Spanish-speaking patient?
   a. Speak loud and slowly
   b. Use a monotone voice to avoid inflection
   c. Phone the interpreter line for assistance
   d. Request that a family member translate the discussion

4. The nurse is caring for a patient with diabetic ketoacidosis. Which of the following statements is consistent with the cause of this disorder?
   a. This condition results from having excess insulin in the body.
   b. Poor management of diabetes can cause this disorder.
   c. Reduced glucose ingestion can lead to this disorder.
   d. Taking too much oral anti-diabetic medication can cause this disorder.

5. What is the specific pathology responsible for brain damage in Alzheimer's disease?
   a. Invasion of the cortex by infectious prions
   b. Multiple hemorrhagic strokes
   c. Deposition of amyloid-β plaques
   d. Formation of Lewy bodies

6. Which action should the nurse include in the evaluation stage of the nursing process?
   a. Assess patient separate from views of goals
   b. Revise plan as needed
   c. Avoid modifying goals
   d. Maintain locus of control

7. Which symptom clinically supports the nurse's review of laboratory values suspecting uremic syndrome post systemic infection?
   a. Constipation
   b. Bloody diarrhea
   c. Low body temperature
   d. Increased urination

8. Which action should the medical-surgical nurse omit from the treatment plan for a patient struggling with hemorrhoids?
   a. Witch hazel
   b. Hydrocortisone cream
   c. Stool softeners
   d. Low fiber diet

9. Which communication technique hinders the discussion between the medical-surgical nurse and the patient?
   a. Empathetic engagement
   b. Open-ended questions
   c. Nurse-focused answers
   d. Restating

10. The nurse is caring for the twenty-five-year-old male patient with an acute spinal cord injury at the C3 to C4 level. Which of the following manifestations is consistent with this injury?
   a. Vital capacity 45 percent of normal, hemoglobin 10.4 g/dL, heart rate 96 beats per minute
   b. Loss of somatic and reflex function, BP 160/90, effective cough effort
   c. Coarse and fine crackles bilaterally, heart rate 56 beats per minute, core temperature 96.7°F
   d. BP 104/60, urinary output 18 mL over the last 60 minutes, heart rate 120 beats per minute

11. A patient is admitted with a diagnosis of heart block. The nurse is aware that the pacemaker of the heart is which of the following?
   a. AV node
   b. Purkinje fibers
   c. SA node
   d. Bundle of His

12. A patient with iron deficiency anemia is unsure which foods to consume to support an improvement in health status. Which food option should the nurse explain would provide the LEAST support for this condition?
   a. Beans
   b. Spinach
   c. Cheese
   d. Raisins

13. Which of the following interventions delegated by the licensed practical nurse (LPN) to the unlicensed assistive personnel (UAP) alerts the registered nurse (RN) to provide education on safe delegation?
  a. Removal of compression stockings
  b. Transfer of wheelchair-bound patient using device
  c. Application of over-the-counter numbing cream
  d. Documentation of vital signs

14. Which of the following manifestations is the nurse likely to assess in the patient with diabetic ketoacidosis?
  a. Alkalotic pH
  b. Ketones in the blood
  c. Fluid volume overload
  d. Hypoglycemia

15. During the nursing assessment, which data concerns the nurse regarding the patient's understanding of medication storage?
  a. Humira stored in refrigerator
  b. Amoxicillin, reconstituted, stored on the bedroom dresser
  c. Furosemide stored in the hallway closet
  d. Insulin, unopened, stored in the bedroom closet

16. The nurse manager of a busy unit continuously incorporates a charismatic leadership style, despite the challenging work environment. Which description aligns with the manager's style of leadership?
  a. Follows rules closely and avoids flexibility in action.
  b. Incorporates eloquent communication that inspires junior staff to admire them.
  c. Commits to the growth of each team member through high emotional intelligence and advanced conflict-resolution skills.
  d. Judges team members on performance, while offering little support.

17. The nurse notices the site around the patient's peripheral IV has become puffy, cold, and tight. She suspects what has occurred?
  a. Infection
  b. IV infiltration
  c. Allergic reaction
  d. Nothing, this is a normal assessment of peripheral IV

18. A fifty-two-year-old male presents to the emergency department (ED) complaining of burning in his chest. He is a long-time pack-a-day smoker, suffers from hypertension, and is overweight. What diagnosis does the nurse suspect?
  a. CAD
  b. TIA
  c. GERD
  d. MI

19. The nurse is providing discharge teaching for a patient recently diagnosed with Crohn's disease. Which of the following patient statements indicates the need for additional instruction?
   a. "I understand that once I get through this surgery, my disease will be cured."
   b. "I know that I have a risk for the development of arthritis."
   c. "I know that vitamin B-12 is important for me."
   d. "I will tell my doc if my pain localizes to the right lower quadrant of my abdomen."

20. A forty-year-old policeman presents to the Emergency Department (ED) after being physically assaulted by a suspect. He complains of shortness of breath and right-sided rib pain. A chest x-ray reveals fractures of ribs 4, 5, and 6 on the left. Physical examination reveals paradoxical movement of the area while breathing. What is the most likely diagnosis for this patient?
   a. Ruptured diaphragm
   b. Flail chest
   c. Tracheal perforation
   d. Pulmonary embolism (PE)

21. A patient involved in a motor vehicle accident (MVA) has sustained blunt nonpenetrating trauma to the chest. Upon arrival in the emergency department, the nurse observes asymmetrical chest rise. Which action(s) by the nurse indicate(s) an understanding of the presenting symptom?
      I. Preparation for placement of a chest drain.
      II. Assessment of oxygenation.
      III. Administration of pain medication.
      IV. Collection of a detailed medical history.
   a. II and III only
   b. II, III, and IV only
   c. I and III only
   d. I and II only

22. When taking a history from patient with unstable angina, the nurse would expect the patient to report which of the following findings?
   a. "My chest pain goes away when I rest."
   b. "I sometimes experience chest pain at rest."
   c. "Nitroglycerine always relieves my chest pain."
   d. "The chest pain only occurs when I walk too fast."

23. A sixty-year-old male with a history of alcohol abuse and IV drug abuse presents to the emergency department with encephalopathy, ascites, and jaundice. Which organ of the abdomen does the nurse suspect is in failure?
   a. Kidney
   b. Liver
   c. Stomach
   d. Spleen

24. The medical-surgical nurse is preparing a patient's treatment plan prior to surgery. How many hours before surgery should the heparin drip be discontinued?
   a. 2 hours
   b. 6 hours
   c. 24 hours
   d. 48 hours

25. The medical-surgical nurse is preparing a patient's treatment plan prior to a colonoscopy. How many hours prior to the procedure should the patient be placed on total npo?

a. 2 hours
b. 6 hours
c. 8 hours
d. 12 hours

26. The nurses in the emergency department are reviewing the treatment protocol for the emergency resuscitation of the newborn. Which of the following statements correctly identifies the rationale for the use of intravenous 0.9 percent sodium chloride (normal saline) as the initial treatment of metabolic acidosis?

a. Normal saline can be administered intraosseously and is, therefore, more readily available.
b. Sodium bicarbonate ($NaHCO_3$) causes adverse fluid shifts due to its low osmolarity.
c. Normal saline does not generate additional CO_2, which can be harmful to cardiac and cerebral function.
d. Sodium bicarbonate is not as effective as normal saline for the treatment of hyperkalemia resulting from prolonged resuscitation of the newborn.

27. A nurse in the oncology unit is caring for a female patient receiving chemotherapy. When the patient develops a low neutrophil level, which of the following instructions is a PRIORITY for the nurse to give the patient?

a. Use a safety razor
b. Take iron supplements
c. Avoid crowds
d. Drink plenty of fluids

28. The nurse is caring for a patient with heart failure following a myocardial infarction and is assessing the cardiac output. Which of the following statements describes the parameter being measured?

a. Cardiac output is the vascular resistance in the pulmonary circulation.
b. Cardiac output is the amount of ventricular stretch at the end of diastole.
c. Cardiac output is the resistance the heart needs to overcome to pump blood to the body.
d. Cardiac output is the volume of blood pumped by the heart in one minute.

29. What is the purpose of conducting an interdisciplinary 5 Whys Analysis?

a. Report the near miss to the correct agency
b. Identify the person at fault for an issue
c. Understand the root cause of an incident
d. Develop a chain-of-command for the elevation of a concern

30. What patient condition would require the medical-surgical nurse to wear a surgical mask?

a. Severe Acute Respiratory Syndrome
b. Influenza B Virus
c. Asthma
d. Chronic Obstructive Pulmonary Disease

31. A forty-four-year-old male patient presents to the emergency department with a complaint of chest pain and shortness of breath. Examination by the nurse reveals distended neck veins and muffled heart sounds. The patient's blood pressure is 80/55. The nurse should suspect which of the following?

a. Cardiac tamponade
b. Abdominal aortic aneurysm (AAA)
c. Cardiopulmonary arrest
d. Cardiogenic shock

32. While providing patient and family education regarding nervous system functions, which function does the nurse include in their teaching when discussing the parasympathetic nervous system?

a. Bronchi dilation
b. Reduced gastrointestinal motility
c. Decreased heart rate
d. Increased cardiac conduction

33. Which member of the interdisciplinary team should the nurse consult with regarding patient dressing and hygiene aids?

a. Physical therapist
b. Social worker
c. Occupational therapist
d. Case manager

34. A 72-year old patient was administered an IV push of furosemide indicated to reduce the edema secondary to renal impairment. Which finding post furosemide administration is an emergent concern for the medical-surgical nurse?

a. Hypotension
b. Pruritis
c. Headache
d. Agranulocytosis

35. Which of the following drugs is often used for treatment of acute seizure activity?

a. Memantine HCl
b. Phenytoin
c. Pregabalin
d. Rifaximin

36. Which food item should the nurse encourage a patient to avoid because it would pose the greatest risk for someone with acquired immunodeficiency syndrome (AIDS)?

a. Bok choy
b. Rice
c. Wheat crackers
d. Blue cheese

37. Which intervention should the nurse include in a treatment plan for a patient with early dumping syndrome?

a. Drink more fluids with meals
b. Consume two larger meals per day
c. Maintain low Fowler's position for 30 minutes post meals
d. Decrease fiber intake

38. The nurse in the neonatal nursery is assessing a newborn in the first hour of life. Which pathophysiology concept should the nurse apply to the newborn assessment?

a. Blood passes through the foramen ovale, bypassing the lungs
b. Blood flows to the lungs as the foramen ovale closes
c. There is high pulmonary vascular resistance reducing blood flow to the lungs
d. A patent ductus arteriosus allows blood to flow from the pulmonary artery to the aorta

39. A patient recently admitted to the floor as a direct admit from her cardiologist office begins complaining of new onset chest pain. Which of the following actions should the nurse anticipate as part of the MONA protocol?

I. IV administration of magnesium sulfate
II. IV administration of morphine sulfate
III. IV administration of nitroglycerine
IV. IV administration of acetaminophen

a. I and II only
b. I, III, and IV only
c. II and III only
d. II, III, and IV only

40. Which intervention should the medical-surgical nurse avoid in the plan of care for a patient with acute Deep Vein Thrombosis (DVT)?

a. Administer enoxaparin sodium subcutaneously
b. Apply spontaneous compression devices
c. Evaluate aPTT levels
d. Provide continuous cardiac monitoring

41. While working with a patient with a poor swallowing reflex secondary to a neurological condition, the medical-surgical nurse is assessing the patient's ability to safely consume their breakfast. Which food item on the tray does the nurse recognize conflicts with this meal plan and should be removed?

a. Beets
b. Scrambled eggs
c. Vanilla pudding
d. Mashed potatoes

42. The nurse is assessing the five-minute Apgar score of a newborn. The newborn has pink skin, an apical pulse rate of 120 beats per minute, cries when stimulated, and strong muscle tone. Which Apgar score would the nurse assign to this newborn?

a. 4
b. 6
c. 8
d. 10

43. The nurse is caring for a patient with a fracture of the eighth rib on the right side of the chest. The nurse should assess the patient for possible injury to which underlying body structure?

a. Bronchus
b. Trachea
c. Spleen
d. Liver

44. Which intervention should the medical-surgical nurse include in the plan of care for a patient with Alzheimer's disease?
  a. Limit physical activity
  b. Provide caprylidene medical food
  c. Perform activities of daily living in the evening
  d. Administer diphenhydramine for sleep

45. What statement made by the patient verbalizes understanding the education regarding safety precautions to take at home after being discharged from the hospital on oxygen for respiratory management?
  a. "I should switch from aerosol deodorant to a stick."
  b. "My cigarettes are safe to smoke as long as I smoke one at a time."
  c. "I must use an oven mitt while cooking on my gas stove."
  d. "I should switch from electric candles to flame-based ones."

46. A patient who is silently aspirating may exhibit which of the following signs and symptoms?
  a. Flat, red rash on the thoracic region
  b. Constant clearing of the throat
  c. Swollen lymph nodes on the neck
  d. Trouble remembering person, place, and time

47. Goals of care conversations are used at the end of life to do which of the following?
  a. Collaborate with experts
  b. Keep the focus on what the patient wants
  c. Support families during a difficult time
  d. Get the patient into palliative care

48. Which action witnessed by the medical-surgical nurse prompts immediate education while working with an unlicensed assistive personnel (UAP)?
  a. The UAP took a blood sugar finger-stick reading.
  b. The UAP wore gloves while providing a bed bath.
  c. The UAP used sanitizer to clean hands after caring for a patient with Clostridium difficile.
  d. The UAP placed the connected Foley catheter bag below the patient's waist.

49. The nurse is caring for a patient with Cushing's disease. The nurse understands that dysfunction of which of the following glands causes this disorder?
  a. Thyroid gland
  b. Adrenal gland
  c. Pancreas
  d. Parathyroid gland

50. Which statement made by a woman with gestational diabetes indicates to the nurse that more teaching is needed?
  a. "I need to monitor my weight."
  b. "I need to watch what I eat."
  c. "I need to stay off my feet as much as possible."
  d. "I need to see my obstetrician regularly."

51. While facilitating nursing student education, which condition does the medical-surgical nurse discuss when describing post-renal causes of acute renal failure?
   a. Obstruction
   b. Rhabdomyolysis
   c. Acute pyelonephritis
   d. Systemic vasodilation

52. The nurse is caring for an eighty-two-year-old man with acute bronchitis. In evaluating the effectiveness of therapy with a beta-2 agonist, the nurse would expect which assessment finding?
   a. Reduced or absent cough
   b. Reduced in fever
   c. Improved breath sounds
   d. Decreased pain

53. A fifty-year-old male presents with a cough producing rust-colored sputum, a fever (102° F), and shortness of breath. A complete blood count (CBC) reveals an elevated white blood cell count with predominant neutrophils. A chest x-ray reveals consolidation of the left, lower lobe of the lung. Blood cultures reveal gram-positive diplococci. What is the most likely cause of this patient's pneumonia?
   a. *Haemophilus influenzae*
   b. *Moraxella catarrhalis*
   c. *Streptococcus pneumoniae*
   d. *Staphylococcus aureus*

54. A sixty-eight-year-old woman with a history of gallstones is in the same-day surgery unit today for a cholecystectomy. This procedure will likely be performed using which technique that involves small incisions and minimal invasion?
   a. Laparoscopic
   b. Endoscopic
   c. Bronchoscopic
   d. Laparotomy

55. The nurse is caring for a fifty-eight-year-old man who has an active upper gastrointestinal bleed. The nurse notes a 10-millimeter drop in diastolic blood pressure when the man stands to urinate. The nurse estimates that which of the following volumes of blood loss is associated with this drop in diastolic blood pressure?
   a. 250 milliliters
   b. 500 milliliters
   c. 750 milliliters
   d. 1,000 milliliters

56. The medical-surgical nurse is reviewing laboratory results to assess the patient's ability to clot before surgery. Which prothrombin time test (PTT) result aligns with a normal range?
   a. 2 seconds
   b. 12 seconds
   c. 22 seconds
   d. 32 seconds

57. The medical-surgical nurse preceptor is educating the new nurse regarding safe antimuscarinic administration. Which patient is unable to receive antimuscarinic medications due to contraindication with their diagnosis?

 a. Patient with a peptic ulcer
 b. Patient with urinary incontinence
 c. Patient with angle-closure glaucoma
 d. Patient with reflux esophagitis

58. A twenty-five-year-old male arrives at the Emergency Department (ED) after blunt chest trauma. On initial evaluation, he has absent breath sounds over the right lung and tracheal deviation to the left. A chest x-ray reveals mediastinal shift to the left and depression of the right hemidiaphragm. What is the most likely diagnosis?

 a. Secondary spontaneous pneumothorax
 b. Bronchiolitis
 c. Tension pneumothorax
 d. Acute respiratory distress syndrome (ARDS)

59. The nurse is providing discharge instruction to a patient with Barrett's esophagus. Which statement by the patient indicates that more teaching is needed?

 a. "I am not at an increased risk for cancer."
 b. "I will need to take my corticosteroids, as prescribed."
 c. "I need to look at my lifestyle and make some changes."
 d. "I should report any heartburn or difficulty swallowing to my doctor."

60. Which of the following manifestations is considered to be a late sign of increased ICP?

 a. Mental confusion related to time
 b. Blurred vision
 c. BP of 170/40
 d. HR of 94 bpm

61. After taking a nurse-to-nurse report in the beginning of their evening shift, the medical-surgical nurse is reviewing laboratory results and surgical notes regarding their patient's emergency procedure from this afternoon. Which diagnosis correlates with an infection of the tissue that lines the inner abdominal wall?

 a. Iritis
 b. Dermatitis
 c. Cystitis
 d. Peritonitis

62. Which manifestation would the nurse expect to find in a patient with severe glycogenosis?

 a. Liver failure
 b. Kidney failure
 c. Respiratory failure
 d. Congestive heart failure

63. The nurse is caring for a patient with diabetes who is sweating and confused. Using a handheld blood glucose monitoring device, the nurse determines that the patient's capillary blood glucose level is 55 milligrams per deciliter. Which of the following intervention would the nurse NOT perform?
   a. Administer oral glucose
   b. Administer subcutaneous insulin
   c. Administer IV dextrose
   d. Administer parenteral glucagon

64. The nurse is caring for a patient with endoscopic evidence of esophageal varices. Which of the following statements correctly identifies the interventions associated with primary prevention of hemorrhage for this condition?
   a. Sclerotherapy ablation of the esophageal arteries
   b. Vasopressors to maintain the hepatic venous pressure gradient above 20 mmHG
   c. Transjugular intrahepatic portosystemic shunt implantation
   d. Endoscopic band ligation

65. The nurse is completing a shift assessment of a patient who had an unwitnessed fall yesterday afternoon in his hospital room. The nurse notices changes in her assessment since yesterday. Which signs and symptoms does the nurse identify that directly support a diagnosis of increased intracranial pressure? Select all that apply.
   a. Nausea
   b. Vomiting
   c. Headache
   d. Blurred vision
   e. Lethargy

66. The nurse would expect a patient with urinary retention to report having experienced which of the following types of urinary incontinence?
   a. Stress incontinence
   b. Urge incontinence
   c. Overflow incontinence
   d. Functional incontinence

67. During nurse-to-nurse shift report, the oncoming medical-surgical nurse learns that the patient has a history of aggressive behavior. What action should the nurse prioritize in this patient's plan of care?
   a. Proactive seclusion
   b. Administer sedative medication
   c. Request that asocial worker meets with the patient before the nurse
   d. Establish patient trust

68. The nurse is caring for a sixty-six-year-old male patient with a history of warfarin therapy who presents with complaints of decreased sensation of the right lower and upper limbs, visual alterations, right hemiparesis, blurred vision, ataxia, nystagmus, and aphasia. The nurse expects to administer which of the following medications?
   a. Mannitol and vitamin K
   b. Warfarin and labetalol
   c. Alteplase and nitroprusside
   d. ASA and enalapril

69. The medical-surgical nurse is describing their professional role and function as defined by state law to their interdisciplinary peer. What term describes this set of guidelines?
   a. Nursing Process
   b. Scope of Practice
   c. Code of Ethics
   d. Nursing Care Plan

70. A patient who has been NPO (nothing by mouth) all morning for a procedure complains of nausea and "just not feeling right." The nurse notices that he is sweating. What condition should the nurse suspect and investigate right away?
   a. Hypochondria
   b. Hypoglycemia
   c. Hypotension
   d. Hypothyroidism

71. The nurse is preparing a teaching plan for a patient with metabolic syndrome. Which statement by the patient indicated that the patient needs more instruction?
   a. "I will follow a low cholesterol diet."
   b. "I am going to get a gym membership and start to exercise."
   c. "I need to gain weight to reach my ideal body weight."
   d. "Lowering my sodium intake will help my blood pressure."

72. Which desired outcome is most appropriate for a patient with marfan syndrome?
   a. Patient maintained adequate tissue perfusion
   b. Patient remained free from self-harm
   c. Patient maintained optimal gas exchange
   d. Patient remained free from signs of infection

73. The 36-year old patient's current orders include levothyroxine 88 μg PO daily. Which assessment by the nurse prompts patient education regarding levothyroxine administration?
   a. The patient reports that they take their medication in the afternoon, 30 minutes after consuming lunch.
   b. The patient reports that they take their medication at night, at least four hours after their last meal.
   c. The patient reports that they take their medication in the morning, 30 minutes before their first meal.
   d. The patient reports that they take their medication in the morning, 2 hours before consuming their first meal.

74. The medical-surgical nurse is evaluating the patient's progress related to pain reduction secondary to appendicitis. Which abdominal quadrant does the nurse ask the patient to rate their pain in?
   a. Right lower quadrant (RLQ)
   b. Left lower quadrant (LLQ)
   c. Right upper quadrant (RUQ)
   d. Left upper quadrant (LUQ)

75. During a focused assessment of the abdomen, which examination technique should the medical-surgical nurse perform second?
   a. Percussion
   b. Palpation
   c. Auscultation
   d. Inspection

76. The medical-surgical nurse discovers a change in their 81-year old patient's level of consciousness and notes increased confusion, agitation, and poor motor skills. Which diagnosis does the nurse suspect may be responsible for these findings and warrants further examination?
   a. Urinary Tract Infection
   b. Diverticulitis
   c. Rectal Polyps
   d. Benign Prostatic Hypertrophy

77. The nurse is formulating a plan of care for an eighty-two-year-old patient with gastroenteritis who has been vomiting and experiencing frequent diarrhea. The nurse should give PRIORITY to which of the following interventions?
   a. Providing adequate nutrition
   b. Turning and positioning
   c. Restoring fluid volume
   d. Teaching proper handwashing

78. After attempting to support and deescalate an aggressive patient with a comorbid diagnosis of schizophrenia, the medical-surgical nurse calls the provider and discusses the situation using the SBAR technique. How should the nurse communicate their report?
   a. "I think we should provide the patient a sedative."
   b. "Should we call a behavioral code?"
   c. "Please share what you already know of this patient's background."
   d. "How should we proceed with the patient's care?"

79. The nurse in the emergency department is assessing a patient who was the driver in a car involved in a motor vehicle accident. Which assessment finding alerts the nurse that the patient may have a flail chest?
   a. Paradoxical chest wall motion
   b. Chest pain on inspiration
   c. Shortness of breath
   d. Tenderness on palpation

80. Which type of angina does the medical-surgical nurse attribute the patient's chest pain from coronary vasospasms to?
   a. Chronic Stable Angina
   b. Unstable Angina
   c. Prinzmetal's Angina
   d. Variant Angina

81. When taking a health history on a female patient with metabolic syndrome, the nurse would also expect to find a history of which of the following disorders?
    a. Diabetes insipidus
    b. Glomerulonephritis
    c. Hypoparathyroidism
    d. Polycystic ovary syndrome

82. The nurse is preparing a teaching plan for a patient with diabetes. Which of the following teaching points would the nurse include when teaching about the causes of hyperglycemia?
    a. Hyperglycemia may be caused by administering too much insulin.
    b. Skipping a meal can cause hyperglycemia.
    c. Taking too much anti-diabetic medication can cause hyperglycemia.
    d. Illness can lead to the development of hyperglycemia.

83. Which condition alerts the nurse to reconsider the provider's order to administer dextrose 5% in water?
    a. Hypoglycemia
    b. Dehydration
    c. Increased intracranial pressure
    d. Insulin shock

84. The nurse is assessing a woman in the emergency department with a possible ectopic pregnancy. Of the following symptoms, which would the nurse NOT expect to assess in this patient?
    a. Pain
    b. Amenorrhea
    c. Vaginal bleeding
    d. Foul-smelling vaginal discharge

85. Which of the following statements is typical of a patient with hyperthyroidism?
    a. "I have been experiencing diarrhea."
    b. "I am always cold."
    c. "I have been gaining weight."
    d. "I am always tired."

86. The nurse is assessing a twenty-two-year-old patient with asthma. Which manifestation would alert the nurse of impending respiratory failure?
    a. Tachycardia
    b. Cyanosis
    c. No audible wheezes
    d. Hypoxemia

87. Which diet would a patient with Meniere's disease likely benefit from?
    a. Low carbohydrate
    b. High fat
    c. Low sodium
    d. High protein

88. The emergency care provider is developing a care plan for the patient with increased ICP. Which of the following statements is INCORRECT?

a. Barbiturate coma decreases the cerebral metabolic rate and the cerebral blood volume.
b. The head of the bed should be elevated to 30 degrees to facilitate venous drainage.
c. Intravenous mannitol decreases blood viscosity and cerebral parenchymal fluid.
d. Hyperventilation decreases the $PaCO_2$, leading to arterial vasodilation.

89. A patient who has sustained multiple trauma has arrived at the emergency department. Which of the following are the first two priority assessments, in the correct order?

I. Respiratory rate and breath sounds
II. Level of consciousness
III. Airway patency

a. I, then II
b. I, then III
c. III, then I
d. III, then II

90. The medical-surgical nurse is caring for a patient two-days post colonoscopy. Which finding indicates the patient may be experiencing a perforated bowel?

a. Flatulence
b. Streaks of blood in stool for past two days
c. Bloated abdomen
d. Rigidity of the abdomen accompanied by tachycardia

91. Which of the following is a contraindication for thrombolytic therapy?

a. Current anticoagulant therapy
b. Over age seventy-five
c. Severe hepatic disease
d. INR of 3.5

92. After delivering unexpected news, the nurse states, "Don't worry, everyone feels that way." Which block to communication is the nurse committing during this engagement?

a. Judging
b. Falsely reassuring
c. Defending
d. Belittling

93. The medical-surgical nurse is planning to provide patient education on anemia and seeks to ensure a complete understanding of the patient's condition prior to the discussion. Which type of anemia should the nurse explain is characterized by a lack of intrinsic factor?

a. Pernicious anemia
b. Aplastic anemia
c. Hemolytic anemia
d. Sickle cell anemia

94. The nurse is caring for a patient with cirrhosis who arrives in the emergency room complaining of increasing abdominal distention. The nurse assesses the presence of ascites. Which of the following statements correctly describes the pathogenesis of ascites?
a. Epinephrine and norepinephrine levels are decreased.
b. Plasma albumin levels are decreased.
c. Portal hypotension is the initial defect.
d. Plasma oncotic levels are increased.

95. The nurse is taking a history from a thirty-eight-year-old male patient with high-flow priapism. Which of the following conditions would the nurse expect the patient to report?
a. A recent groin injury
b. A history of bladder cancer
c. Recreational cocaine use
d. A history of sickle cell disease

96. The nurse is preparing a teaching plan for a twenty-eight-year-old woman with hyperthyroidism, who is being treated with radioactive iodine. Which of the following instructions should the nurse include?
a. Take the medication for one week.
b. Use birth control while taking this medication.
c. Only one dose of the medication is needed.
d. Do not exercise while taking this medication.

97. Which precautions should the medical-surgical nurse engage in while caring for a patient with pertussis?
a. Standard
b. Contact
c. Droplet
d. Airborne

98. Which assessment findings should the nurse expect in a patient with Addison's disease?
a. Excessive body hair
b. Hypertension
c. Excessive energy
d. Fluid and electrolyte imbalances

99. Which of the following is the best antibiotic treatment for pneumonia caused by community-acquired methicillin-resistant Staphylococcus aureus (CA-MRSA)?
a. Azithromycin
b. Doxycycline
c. Vancomycin
d. Levofloxacin

100. The nurse is developing a teaching plan for a patient newly diagnosed with myasthenia gravis. To prevent relapses, which of the following instructions would NOT be included in the teaching plan?
a. Stay away from people who are sick
b. Take hot baths when feeling stressed
c. Consider a yoga class to reduce stress
d. Stay in air conditioning when the weather is hot

101. When must the discharge planning process start for each patient?
   a. The day before discharge is scheduled to occur
   b. The morning of the planned discharge
   c. After the discharge order has been written
   d. As soon as admission begins

102. The medical-surgical nurse is examining the effectiveness of the lactulose treatment for a patient with liver failure. Which condition, commonly treated with this medication, should the nurse assess for signs and symptoms of at this time?
   a. Hepatic encephalopathy
   b. Cardiac insufficiency
   c. Renal failure
   d. Macular degeneration

103. Which form of consent for treatment does the patient give by presenting for care and voluntarily moving forward with admission?
   a. Explicit
   b. Implied
   c. Expressed
   d. Surrogate

104. The nurse is teaching a female patient about treatment for pelvic inflammatory disease. Which of the following indicates that more teaching is needed?
   a. "I can take an over-the-counter analgesic for the pain."
   b. "Once I finish the antibiotics, I can have unprotected intercourse."
   c. "I understand that this infection may affect my fertility."
   d. "I should report any unusual vaginal discharge to my health care provider."

105. While completing an assessment on a patient with a gastrointestinal illness that has caused several days of diarrhea, which acid-base imbalance secondary to changes in electrolyte status does the medical-surgical nurse expect to note on the laboratory results?
   a. Metabolic Alkalosis
   b. Metabolic Acidosis
   c. Respiratory Alkalosis
   d. Respiratory Acidosis

106. Which diagnosis aligns with a symptom presentation that includes abnormal movements of the jaw, lips, and tongue?
   a. Akinesia
   b. Paresthesia
   c. Akathisia
   d. Tardive Dyskinesia

107. A patient arrives in the emergency department complaining of pain, tingling, and weakness in both feet and ankles. Which of the following assessment questions is of the highest priority for this patient?
   a. "When did you first notice the weakness in your feet and ankles?"
   b. "Which activities make the pain better or worse?"
   c. "Have you had a viral or bacterial infection in the last few weeks?"
   d. "Have you ever previously experienced these symptoms?"

108. The nurse is preparing a discharge plan for a patient with risk factors for acute pancreatitis. Which of the following information should be included in this plan?

a. Endoscopic retrograde cholangiopancreatography (ERCP) imaging is required to confirm the diagnosis.
b. Ultrasonography is the most useful imaging study when significant abdominal distention is present.
c. Current research confirms the efficacy of rectal administration of indomethacin to reduce the incidence of pancreatitis due to the ERCP procedure.
d. There is no scientific rationale to explain why some individuals with chronic ETOH abuse develop acute pancreatitis, while others do not develop pancreatitis.

109. The public health nurse is planning a screening program for detection of chlamydial infections. Which of the following U.S. Preventative Services Task Force principles should guide the nurse's planning of this program?

a. All sexually active women should be screened, regardless of age.
b. Women with multiple sex partners over age twenty-four should be screened.
c. Women age fifteen to twenty-four who use a condom during sexual intercourse should be screened.
d. All women age twelve to twenty-four should be screened.

110. The outgoing nurse is providing a report to the oncoming nurse regarding a patient fall during the shift. What information collected using the PQRST method of pain assessment should the nurse include in their report of a 42-year-old patient with vertigo who fell in the shower?

a. Pain, Quadrant, Radiate, Sensation, Timing
b. Provoke, Quality, Region, Severity, Timing
c. Pain, Quality, Radiate, Severity, Task
d. Provoke, Quadrant, Region, Sensation, Tension

111. The intensive care nurse would expect which of the following findings in a patient with Guillain-Barré syndrome?

a. Acute progressive muscle weakness on one side of the body
b. Acute progressive muscle weakness that starts distally and moves proximally
c. Slow progressive muscle weakness that moves proximally to distally
d. Slow progressive muscle weakness that starts at the head and moves down the body

112. The patient is admitted with a diagnosis of heart failure. Which assessment finding supports the diagnosis of left-sided heart failure?

a. Pitting edema
b. Ascites
c. Fatigue
d. Tachycardia

113. During a focused respiratory assessment, which position should the nurse assist the patient to assume to assess posterior lung sounds?

a. Sims' Position
b. Prone Position
c. High Fowler's Position
d. Lateral Position

114. The nurse is caring for a patient with an emerging ischemic stroke. The nurse prepares to administer which of the following fibrinolytic agents?
   a. Urokinase
   b. Streptokinase
   c. Alteplase
   d. Tenecteplase

115. All EXCEPT which of the following are components of Virchow's triad?
   a. Heart disease
   b. Hypercoagulability
   c. Endothelial injury/dysfunction
   d. Hemodynamic changes such as stasis or turbulence

116. While caring for a 31-year-old patient with major depression and posttraumatic stress disorder who was admitted last night following a diagnosis of pneumonia, the medical-surgical nurse evaluates a myriad of symptoms to decipher their etiologies and plan care. After narrowing down some symptoms that can be attributed to the patient's prazosin regimen, which finding prompts the nurse to page the physician, as this is an unlikely finding and warrants additional testing?
   a. Nausea
   b. Hypertension
   c. Headache
   d. Elevated pulse rate

117. Which statement by a patient going home on warfarin (Coumadin) for treatment of a pulmonary embolism alerts the nurse that more teaching is needed?
   a. "I will take this medication orally."
   b. "Any bleeding or bruising needs to be reported to my doctor right away."
   c. "I will seek medical attention if I develop chest pain or shortness of breath."
   d. "Blood monitoring is not needed."

118. A patient brought in to the emergency department by the paramedics is complaining of chest pain. Which of the following actions should the nurse anticipate as part of the MONA protocol?
      I. IV administration of magnesium sulfate
      II. IV administration of morphine sulfate
      III. IV administration of nitroglycerine
      IV. IV administration of acetaminophen
   a. I and II only
   b. I, III, and IV only
   c. II and III only
   d. II, III, and IV only

119. Which intervention patient education should the nurse include in the plan of care for a patient with carbon monoxide poisoning?
   a. Demonstrate how to care for burn dressings.
   b. Describe the indications and adverse effects of N-acetylcysteine.
   c. Teach what to expect during hyperbaric oxygen therapy.
   d. Explain how hydroxocobalamin will be administered.

120. The medical-surgical nurse is reviewing dietary orders prior to breakfast. Which diet should be implemented for a patient with gout?
   a. Low-Purine
   b. High-Fructose
   c. Low-Caffeine
   d. High-Fat

121. The medical-surgical nurse is reviewing dietary orders prior to dinner. Which diet should the patient with dermatitis herpetiformis adhere to?
   a. Dairy-Free
   b. Gluten-Free
   c. Soy-Free
   d. Shellfish-Free

122. Which action performed by the licensed practical nurse is a cause for concern and alerts the registered nurse to the need for further education regarding the care of acute appendicitis?
   a. Placed the patient in a semi-Fowler's position
   b. Applied heat to the abdomen
   c. Discussed the plan to refrain from enema use
   d. Maintained patient bed rest

123. The nurse is administering a blood transfusion to a patient with liver disease. Which signs and symptoms encourage the nurse to stop the transfusion due to a transfusion reaction? Select all that apply.
   a. Back pain
   b. Shortness of breath
   c. Skin flushing
   d. Hematoma at needle insertion site
   e. Damp IV dressing

124. Which of the following is/are true regarding advance directives?
   a. They are an expression of the patient's preferences.
   b. They are based on a person's values and beliefs.
   c. They include identification of a surrogate.
   d. All of the above

125. The nurse has been teaching a patient with HIV-1 about his condition. Which patient statement indicates that the patient understands the course of his disease?
   a. "I do not need to start treatment until I develop symptoms."
   b. "I am going to die young."
   c. "With treatment, I cannot transmit the virus."
   d. "With treatment, it's possible to have a healthy life."

126. The nurse is preparing a teaching plan for a patient with temporal arteritis who noticed a gradual loss of vision in the right eye over the past three weeks. When the patient saw her ophthalmologist earlier in the day, she was sent to the hospital for treatment. Which of the following would the nurse include in this patient's teaching?

a. The loss of vision in the right eye will return to normal with treatment.
b. Vision in the left eye will be affected since treatment was delayed.
c. Vision in the left eye will not be affected once treatment is started.
d. Some vision in the right eye may return since treatment was started early.

127. In order to support the patient in choosing the focus of a conversation, which therapeutic communication technique should the nurse use?

a. Broad opening
b. Use of silence
c. Reflection
d. Clarification

128. Which of the patient's comorbidities does the medical-surgical nurse consider to be responsible for their paralytic ileus?

a. Pyelonephritis
b. Parkinson's disease
c. Gout
d. Raynaud's syndrome

129. The nurse is caring for a patient with Conn's syndrome. Which hormone does the nurse explain to the patient is elevated in this disorder?

a. DHEA
b. Androstenedione
c. Aldosterone
d. Cortisol

130. A twenty-five-year-old male presents to the Emergency Department (ED) complaining of shortness of breath, coughing, and wheezing for two days. His cough is productive, and he reports seeing black material mixed in with his phlegm. Visual examination reveals carbonaceous sputum. At this point in the examination, he develops severe respiratory distress and is subsequently intubated and placed on mechanical ventilation. What is the mostly likely diagnosis for this patient?

a. Acute bronchitis
b. Inhalation injury
c. Community-acquired pneumonia
d. Hemothorax

131. Which of the following statements correctly identifies the difference between the forgetfulness that is common to the normal aging process and the memory alterations associated with Alzheimer's disease?

a. The processes are the same; however, memory alterations associated with Alzheimer's disease include only short-term memory loss.
b. Forgetfulness is progressive and eventually results in the individual's inability to perform ADLs independently.
c. Memory lapses associated with Alzheimer's disease improve with frequent cueing.
d. The end stage of memory impairment in Alzheimer's disease is the inability to recognize family members.

132. Which finding alerts the nurse to the effectiveness of corticosteroids in a two-year-old with acute laryngotracheobronchitis?

a. Afebrile
b. Clear chest x-ray
c. Feelings of hunger
d. Lack of stridor

133. An eighteen-year-old female comes in with a gunshot wound to the abdomen. Which of the following takes highest priority when caring for this patient?

a. Fluid resuscitation
b. Stopping the bleeding
c. Monitoring for infection
d. Assessing internal damage

134. The medical-surgical nurse assesses the results of the patient's blood work and reports antibodies to varicella, commonly known as chickenpox, which aligns with the patient's positive history of the childhood disease. The patient asks how their body still maintains immunity to an illness they had 30 years ago. How should the nurse respond to this inquiry?

a. "You have passive acquired immunity."
b. "You are not still immune to this disease but will gain immunity if you acquire the disease again."
c. "You have active acquired immunity resulting from your body's production of antibodies in response to antigen exposure."
d. "You are not still immune to this disease, so you may want to consider receiving the varicella vaccine."

135. The medical-surgical nurse becomes concerned after witnessing the provider use language that negatively impacts a patient's ability to make their own decision regarding their care without provider influence. Which ethical principle may the provider be violating at this time?

a. Nonmaleficence
b. Veracity
c. Beneficence
d. Autonomy

136. The nurse is preparing a community program on sexually transmitted diseases. Which of the following would the nurse explain is the most common sexually transmitted infection?

a. Chlamydia
b. Gonorrhea
c. Human papilloma virus
d. Herpes simplex virus-2

137. The nurse in the emergency department is caring for a thirty-year-old male patient with a ventriculoperitoneal shunt who is being assessed for shunt failure. The shunt was inserted four years ago when the patient developed hydrocephalus after a severe closed-head injury, and the patient has exhibited satisfactory control of ICP until twelve hours ago, when the patient complained of a headache, nausea, and tiredness. The patient's vital signs are BP 130/70, HR 82, RR 24, T 98.6°F, PaO_2 97 percent. Which of the following complications is most likely responsible for the patient's condition?

a. Choroid ingrowth of the proximal catheter
b. Migration of the distal catheter to an area that impedes absorption of the CSF
c. Disconnection of the distal reservoir from the distal catheter tip
d. Infection of the proximal catheter

138. The medical-surgical nurse is evaluating the patient's response to bupropion, which was prescribed for smoking cessation. Which finding does the nurse attribute to the use of this medication?

a. Bradycardia
b. Hypersalivation
c. Suicidal ideation
d. Increased sleep

139. Which precautions should the medical-surgical nurse engage in while caring for a patient with herpes zoster that is classified as disseminated inflection?

a. Standard
b. Reverse isolation
c. Contact
d. Airborne and contact

140. While using the SBAR method of communication, which term aligns with the patient's laboratory findings?

a. Situation
b. Background
c. Assessment
d. Recommendations

141. The medical-surgical nurse is establishing patient-centered goals in the nursing care plan. What do these measurable targets reflect?

a. Greatest improvement in individual health outcome
b. Interest in specific nursing interventions
c. Aims for care designated by the provider
d. Normalized behavior for specified illness

142. A 52-year-old male is admitted with symptoms of severe abdominal pain centered around the epigastric region of the abdomen and has a history of alcohol abuse and cigarette smoking. The nurse suspects which of the following conditions will be diagnosed?
  a. Gastritis
  b. Hepatitis
  c. Pancreatitis
  d. Kidney failure

143. Which imbalance does the nurse expect to observe as a complication of total parenteral nutrition (TPN)?
  a. Metabolic acidosis
  b. Respiratory acidosis
  c. Metabolic alkalosis
  d. Respiratory alkalosis

144. While caring for a 52-year-old patient with Broca's aphasia, which action should the medical-surgical nurse implement during verbal communication?
  a. Request assistance from a linguistic interpreter
  b. Speak loudly
  c. Use typical verbal expression, without significant change
  d. Provide only short, simple sentences of 3-4 words

145. The nurse is caring for a patient with pneumonia that she believes may be starting to show symptoms of septic shock. What findings support a septic shock diagnosis? Select all that apply.
  a. Metabolic acidosis
  b. Respiratory alkalosis
  c. Narrowing pulse pressure
  d. Increased cardiac output
  e. Hypertension

146. The medical-surgical nurse ensures the patient is fully supported to make their own decisions, without coercion, regarding their care. What ethical principle guides this practice?
  a. Autonomy
  b. Utility
  c. Fidelity
  d. Conflict of interest

147. During medication reconciliation, the medical-surgical nurse notes that a patient with dementia is struggling to recall how many times per day their gabapentin is ordered for. Which action should the medical-surgical nurse take next to best support a thorough history collection of patient data?
  a. Obtain a release of information to contact the outpatient pharmacy.
  b. Wait to complete the medication reconciliation until the patient's son arrives.
  c. Delegate completion of the medication reconciliation to the patient's physician.
  d. Check the discharge paperwork from last admission and record the finding.

148. The nurse is developing a teaching plan for a patient with a renal stone composed of calcium. Which statement should the nurse include in the teaching plan?

a. Increase intake of milk products
b. Drink plenty of fluids
c. Avoid high purine foods
d. Increase intake of antacids

149. The nurse is teaching a female patient with uncomplicated chlamydia of the lower tract about treatment. Which of the following statements by the patient indicates understanding of the nurse's teaching?

a. "I will take azithromycin twice a day for seven days."
b. "I will take azithromycin until all my symptoms are gone."
c. "I will take azithromycin once a day, for fourteen days."
d. "I need one dose of azithromycin that I will take before I leave the office."

150. After learning that a patient received an order for a medication they previously reported to be ineffective, which action should the nurse take next to navigate this clinical care issue?

a. Administer the medication
b. Call the prescriber
c. Elevate issue to charge nurse
d. Report finding to hospital board of ethics

151. Which of the following statements made by the patient would cause the nurse to suspect an abdominal aortic aneurysm (AAA)?

a. "I have indigestion when I lie down."
b. "I often have a pulsating sensation in my abdomen."
c. "I get fatigued and short of breath on exertion."
d. "I have extreme pain radiating down my left arm."

152. While receiving nurse-to-nurse report from the emergency department on a pending transfer, the medical-surgical nurse learns that an incoming 43-year-old patient is struggling with delusional thinking. What understanding is necessary to ensure effective communication is used upon receiving this patient?

a. The patient experiences insistent false beliefs despite invalidating evidence.
b. The patient experiences perceptions irrelevant to actual external stimuli.
c. The patient experiences acute, short-lasting confusion and disorientation.
d. The patient experiences a gradual impairment in cognitive functioning.

153. The nurse is teaching a patient with HIV about his disease. The nurse explains that acquired immunodeficiency syndrome (AIDS) is diagnosed when CD4/T cells drop to which of the following levels?

a. Less than 200 cells per cubic millimeter
b. Less than 400 cells per cubic millimeter
c. Less than 600 cells per cubic millimeter
d. Less than 800 cells per cubic millimeter

154. The medical-surgical nurse is planning care for a patient with a traumatic brain injury affecting the cerebellum. Which action does the nurse expect the patient to require extra support with?
   a. Visual recognition
   b. Balance
   c. Respirations
   d. Language recognition

155. While greeting a patient at the start of the evening shift, the nurse questions, "How are things going today?" Which communication technique is the nurse utilizing at this time?
   a. Acknowledgment
   b. Empathy
   c. Broad opening
   d. Clarification

156. Which action does the medical-surgical nurse engage in during the assessment phase of the nursing process?
   a. Perform nursing intervention
   b. Obtain a nursing health history
   c. Develop nursing care plan
   d. Establish physical and psychosocial outcomes

157. The effectiveness of antiretroviral therapy in the patient with HIV can be evaluated with which finding?
   a. A low viral load in the blood
   b. Therapeutic drug levels
   c. The degree of side effects
   d. No detection of HIV in semen

158. The nurse is providing discharge instructions to a male patient diagnosed with a urinary tract infection (UTI). Which should the nurse tell the patient is the most COMMON finding in a UTI?
   a. Penile discharge
   b. Flank pain
   c. Painful urination
   d. Fever

159. In planning care for a patient with acute glomerulonephritis, what should be the main goal for treatment?
   a. Maintain fluid balance
   b. Raise blood pressure
   c. Elevate serum potassium levels
   d. Increase consumption of protein

160. All EXCEPT which of the following help define acute respiratory distress syndrome (ARDS)?
   a. Timing
   b. Origin of edema
   c. Pulmonary artery wedge pressure
   d. Severity of hypoxemia

161. The medical-surgical nurse is assessing pedal pulses for a 67-year-old patient with congestive heart failure and notes that they are not palpable in either foot. Which action should the medical-surgical nurse engage in next?

a. Call a rapid response for assistance
b. Document absent pedal pulses in physical assessment
c. Locate a hand-held Doppler to reassess pedal pulses
d. Page the cardiologist to report this finding

162. Where does the medical-surgical nurse evaluate the effects of the Koebner phenomenon while caring for a 36-year-old patient with psoriasis?

a. Around the oral cavity
b. The perimeter of the rectum
c. Anywhere minor trauma has occurred
d. Spanning the chest

163. The nurse is caring for a patient who has a complete placenta previa and is twenty-two weeks pregnant. She asks the nurse to explain the action of betamethasone. Which of the following statements is consistent with the action of this medication?

a. The medication reduces newborn infections if the membranes rupture prematurely due to the placenta previa.
b. Prolonged gestation is more effective than treatment with betamethasone for lung maturation.
c. The therapy eliminates the occurrence of respiratory distress syndrome in the newborn.
d. Betamethasone is a tocolytic agent that can be used long-term to stop preterm labor.

164. A thirty-year-old female presents to the Emergency Department (ED) after penetrating chest trauma. She complains of chest pain and shortness of breath. On examination, she's found to have tachypnea, tachycardia, and hypotension. A chest x-ray reveals blunting of the left costophrenic angle. What's the most likely diagnosis for this patient?

a. Flail chest
b. Myocardial contusion
c. Inhalation injury
d. Hemothorax

Answer Explanations for Practice Test #2

1. A: Choice *A* represents the type of leadership style that involves the nurse taking on an informal leadership role by functioning as a resource to meet the needs of the team. Servant leadership also involves leading by example, focusing on values and ethics, and continuously using foresight and empathy to advance the team. While often engaged by informal leaders, formal leaders may also adopt this style. Choice *B* involves ensuring team members follow direction precisely, with little to no support of innovation or creativity. Choice *C* indicates leadership that involves tremendous leeway in work specifics with greater focus on the end-result rather than the process, while lending support only when requested. Choice *D* indicates leadership that involves expected output with reward and consequence.

2. D: A pregnancy test is performed first to determine if the patient is pregnant. A Pap smear, uterine biopsy, and pelvic ultrasound may be performed, based on the patient's history and physical findings, but they would not be the first test performed, making *A*, *B*, and *C* incorrect answers.

3. C: Choice *C* indicates the appropriate professional response by the medical-surgical nurse to address the present language barrier. Choices *A* and *B* would not directly support communication that is free from misunderstanding and should be omitted. Choice *D* would not rely on a professional, non-biased party for translation and should be avoided if possible.

4. B: Diabetic ketoacidosis is an acidotic metabolic state that can be caused by poor diabetic management, leading to hyperglycemia. Diabetic management involves regular visits to the health care provider, taking insulin or oral anti-diabetic agents as ordered, following a healthy diet, exercising regularly, and monitoring blood glucose levels at home. Hyperglycemia can occur when the patient does not have enough insulin in the body, making Choice *A* an incorrect answer. Since ingesting high glucose levels leads to hyperglycemia, not reduced glucose levels, Choice *C* is not the correct answer. It can also occur when the oral anti-diabetic management is not sufficient to control high blood glucose levels, making Choice *D* an incorrect answer.

5. C: The destruction of brain tissue in Alzheimer's disease is the result of amyloid-β plaque formation in the cerebral cortex. Creutzfeldt-Jakob disease is a rare form of dementia that results from tissue damage caused by infectious prions; therefore, Choice *A* is incorrect. Multiple hemorrhagic strokes may be a trigger for the deposition of amyloid-β plaque formation; however, this form of damage can exist without causing Alzheimer's disease. It is not the specific causative process for the disease; therefore, Choice *B* is incorrect. The formation of Lewy bodies is responsible for the damage associated with Parkinson's disease, not Alzheimer's disease; therefore, Choice *D* is incorrect.

6. B: Choice *B* involves the nurse revising the plan as needed to meet individualized patient-centered goals of treatment. The evaluation phase also involves comparing actual outcomes with expected outcomes. Choice *A* should be avoided, as the patient should be assessed in relation to established goals. Choice *C* should be avoided, as the goals should be modified as care priorities change. Choice *D* should be avoided, as the nurse should maintain flexibility, not rigid control.

7. B: Choice *B* is a common symptom found within uremic syndrome post systemic infection. Choices *A*, *C*, and *D* do not correlate with uremic syndrome and would not relate to a clinical presentation of this condition.

8. D: Choice *D* should be omitted from the plan of care for a patient struggling with hemorrhoids because this patient would benefit from a high fiber diet. Choices *A*, *B*, and *C* all provide symptom relief and encourage the management or resolution of hemorrhoids; therefore, these measures should be included in the treatment plan.

9. C: Choice *C* represents a hindrance to the development of a therapeutic nurse-to-patient discussion and should be avoided. Choice *A* displays understanding, Choice *B* encourages deeper dialogue, and Choice *D* shows comprehension of what the patient communicated.

10. C: Injuries above the T6 level are associated with neurogenic shock, due to alterations of the autonomic nervous system, resulting in the loss of vagal tone. This manifests as decreased vascular resistance and vasodilation. Injury at this level is also associated with alterations in respiratory function, which results in symptoms such as decreased vital capacity and the presence of adventitious breath sounds. In addition, hypothermia is common; therefore, Choice *C* is correct. A vital capacity level that equals 45 percent of normal is associated with injuries at the T1 level or below and is an indication of hemorrhagic shock rather than neurogenic shock. A hemoglobin level of 10.4 g/dL in a male patient is also associated with acute or occult blood loss rather than loss of vagal tone and is indicative of hemorrhagic shock. The patient's level of injury is consistent with neurogenic shock, which is manifested by bradycardia, not tachycardia; therefore, Choice *A* is incorrect. Loss of somatic and reflex function is associated with spinal shock, and hypertension and an effective cough effort are inconsistent with the level of the patient's injury; therefore, Choice *B* is incorrect. The collective manifestations of hypotension, oliguria, and tachycardia are associated with hypovolemic shock rather than neurogenic shock; therefore, Choice *D* is incorrect.

11. C: The SA, or sinoatrial, node is the heart's natural pacemaker. The AV node, which is positioned between the atria and ventricle, receives the impulse from the SA node. The Purkinje fibers are the end point of the conduction system. These fibers spread out across the ventricles after receiving the impulse through the Bundle of His. The Bundle of His receives the impulse from the AV node.

12. B: Of the two types of human immunodeficiency virus (HIV), HIV-1 is the dominant strain among global cases. HIV-2 is not highly transmissible, so Choice *A* is not correct. Since HIV-2 is poorly understood, Choice *C* is not correct. HIV-1 is the more severe strain, making Choice *D* an incorrect choice.

13. C: Choice *C* indicates a delegated role outside of the scope of the unlicensed assistive personnel (UAP), which alerts the registered nurse (RN) to provide education to the licensed practical nurse (LPN) regarding safe delegation. UAPs cannot administer medication of any kind, including over-the-counter medicated creams. Choices *A*, *B*, and *D* represent appropriate delegation, as all actions are within the scope of the UAP.

14. B: Diabetic ketoacidosis is an acute complication of type I diabetes due to a lack of adequate insulin. When this occurs, there is not enough insulin to break down nutrients into glucose. The body begins to break down fatty acids into ketones for energy, leading to ketones in the blood and an acidic body pH level; therefore, Choice *A* is not the correct response. Choices *C* and *D* are not correct since clinical manifestations include dehydration, hyperglycemia, nausea, sweet-smelling breath, confusion, and fatigue.

15. B: Choice *B* is a cause for concern regarding the patient's knowledge deficit on medication storage. The patient should not store reconstituted amoxicillin on the bedroom dresser. While this location would be appropriate prior to reconstituting, this medication must be stored in the refrigerator once reconstituted. Choices *A*, *C*, and *D* demonstrate proper storage of the medications and do not need to be addressed by the nurse at this time.

16. B: Choice *B* incorporates the characteristics witnessed within the charismatic leadership style. Choice *A* incorporates characteristics of the bureaucratic leadership style. Choice *C* incorporates characteristics of the transformational leadership style. Choice *D* incorporates characteristics of the transactional leadership style.

17. B: The nurse suspects that the IV has infiltrated, meaning the catheter tip has become dislodged and IV medication and/or fluids are leaking into the surrounding tissues. The nurse should stop the infusion, remove the IV, and dress the site. An allergic reaction or infection would be warm, not cold, due to the inflammatory response present in such conditions. This is not a normal assessment of a peripheral IV.

18. C: The nurse suspects a diagnosis of gastroesophageal reflux disease based on the burning sensation the patient complains of and the risk factors he has (hypertension, obesity, and cigarette smoking). A myocardial infarction (MI) can sometimes be confused with GERD in symptomology as the heart and esophagus are in close proximity to each other. However, an MI usually presents as a heavy, crushing weight rather than a burning sensation. Coronary artery disease (CAD) usually is found after the patient has had an MI and involves blockages in the coronary arteries caused by atherosclerosis. Transient ischemic attack would present with stroke-like symptoms, not a burning sensation in the chest.

19. A: Crohn's disease is recurrent. Surgery may be necessary to excise a segment of the intestine that has been damaged by the transmural effects of the disease process; however, progression to additional areas is common because Crohn's disease can affect the entire length of the GI tract. This is in contrast to ulcerative colitis, which may be cured by a total colectomy because the disease can only affect the colon. Therefore, Choice *A* reflects the need for additional teaching and is the correct answer. Crohn's disease is an autoimmune-mediated disease and is associated with an increased risk for other immune diseases such as arthritis; therefore, Choice *B* does not reflect the need for additional teaching. Crohn's disease commonly affects the terminal ileum, which is the site of vitamin B-12 absorption. Deficiency of this vitamin can result in decreased red cell production and anemia; therefore, Choice *C* does not reflect the need for additional teaching. Crohn's disease is often complicated by fistulae formation between bowel segments, which results in localized pain in the right lower quadrant of the abdomen. Early recognition and treatment are necessary to prevent systemic effects including sepsis; therefore, Choice *D* does not reflect the need for additional teaching.

20. B: This scenario depicts a case of flail chest, which is clinically defined as the paradoxical movement of a segment of the chest wall caused by at least two fractures per rib (usually anteriorly and posteriorly) in three or more ribs while breathing. Flail chest requires a tremendous amount of blunt force trauma to the thorax in order to fracture multiple ribs in multiple places. This type of trauma can be produced by motor vehicle accidents, serious falls, crush injuries, rollover injuries, and physical assaults.

21. D: Hypoventilation and hypoxia are the primary causes of death in chest trauma. Assessing oxygenation and preparing for placement of a chest drain to alleviate a possible hemothorax or pneumothorax are the correct first actions. Pain medication is secondary to ensuring airway, breathing, and circulation. A medical history is important, but it is secondary to the lifesaving interventions.

22. B: Unstable angina, caused by an unstable atherosclerotic plaque, is not predictable and may occur at rest. The pain may worsen over a brief time period, last up to 20 minutes, and is not responsive to nitroglycerine. Choices *A*, *C*, and *D* are descriptive of stable angina.

23. B: The patient is in hepatic (liver) failure based on the symptomology and the presentation. Kidney failure would present with electrolyte and fluid abnormalities and their symptoms. Diseases of the stomach would present with GI symptoms such as nausea, vomiting, and abdominal pain in the left upper quadrant. Diseases of the spleen would manifest as blood disorders and would not be similar to symptoms of liver failure.

24. B: Choice *B* is an appropriate length of time prior to surgery to discontinue the patient's heparin drip. Choice *A* is too close to surgery, which poses a risk for bleeding complications. Choices *C* and *D* would discontinue a needed therapy too far in advance of the scheduled surgery time and should be avoided.

25. A: Choice *C* is the appropriate length of time for the patient to be total npo, which involves nothing by mouth, before their scheduled colonoscopy. Choice *B* represents the length of time before a procedure where the patient is supported to continue consuming clear liquids. Choices *C* and *D* represent times that are too early prior to procedure to encourage the patient to refrain from all food and drink.

26. C: Normal saline is preferred for the treatment of metabolic acidosis in the event of a brief episode of cardiopulmonary resuscitation because sodium bicarbonate (bicarb) generates additional carbon dioxide, which is potentially harmful to the heart and brain. Normal saline can be administered intraosseously. However, that has no bearing on the use of normal saline versus bicarb for the treatment of metabolic acidosis; therefore, Choice *A* is incorrect. Bicarb exhibits hyperosmolarity; therefore, Choice *B* is incorrect. Bicarb is effective in the treatment of hyperkalemia, but its use is not recommended except in the case of prolonged resuscitation and must be administered only after effective ventilation and circulation have been restored; therefore, Choice *D* is incorrect.

27. C: Since chemotherapy may affect the bone marrow, the patient receiving chemotherapy may have low red blood cell, white blood cell, and platelet counts. This patient has a low neutrophil count, which means the patient does not have enough white blood cells in her body. Since white blood cells help the body fight infection, the patient is at risk for infection and should avoid being in crowds, especially during influenza season. Choice *A* is not correct; using a safety razor reduces the risk of bleeding due to a low platelet count. Choice *B* is not correct; iron supplements help in the production of red blood cells, not white blood cells. Although the patient may benefit from drinking fluids, this instruction will not reduce the risk of infection, making Choice *D* incorrect.

28. D: Cardiac output is the volume of blood that the heart pumps in one minute. It is measured by multiplying the heart rate by stroke volume. Choice *A* is the incorrect choice since it describes pulmonary vascular resistance. Choice *B* is not the answer since it describes preload. Choice *C* is incorrect because it describes afterload.

29. C: Choice *C* describes the chief reason for conducting a 5 Whys Analysis, which is to understand the root cause of an incident. Choices *A* and *D* represent potential gains from conducting this analysis but not the main purpose. Choice *B* may be deduced from this analysis but is not the main goal. The focus is on understanding and planning rather than on punitive consequences.

30. B: Choice *B* requires the medical-surgical nurse to don a surgical mask while interacting with the patient. Choice *A* requires the nurse to don an N95 respirator while working with the patient. Choices *C* and *D* do not require respiratory shielding.

31. A: Beck's triad of muffled heart sounds, distended neck veins, and hypotension are cardinal signs of cardiac tamponade. Chest pain and back pain are the most common presenting symptoms with the AAA. Heart function, breathing, and consciousness are not evident in cardiopulmonary arrest. Cardiogenic shock includes ashen, cyanotic, or mottled extremities; distant heart sounds; and rapid and faint peripheral pulses.

32. C: Choice *C* is a function of the parasympathetic nervous system, along with such functions as bronchi constriction and increased gastrointestinal motility. Choices *A*, *B*, and *D* are all functions of the sympathetic nervous system.

33. C: Choice *C* represents the member of the interdisciplinary team that the nurse should consult with regarding patient dressing and hygiene aids, as such aids are required for daily functioning and within the role of the occupational therapist. Choice *A* supports strength in movement. Choice *B* aligns services for quality of life and overall functioning. Choice *D* manages care coordination between disciplines.

34. D: Choice *D* indicates an emergent concern post furosemide administration. The medical-surgical nurse is aware that this patient is suffering from a significantly reduced white blood cell count and likely from a critically low neutrophil count in the blood. Choices *A*, *B*, and *C*, while potentially uncomfortable side effects of furosemide administration, are all expected and not emergent concerns at this time.

35. B: Phenytoin is FDA approved for most types of seizures. Memantine is a neurological drug used to treat dementia. Pregabalin is a drug used to treat diabetic neuropathy. Rifaximin is a drug used to treat hepatic encephalopathy.

36. D: Choice *D* indicates a food item that is risky for the patient with acquired immunodeficiency syndrome (AIDS) to consume. Blue cheese is an unpasteurized food item and should be omitted from the therapeutic diet, along with unpasteurized drinks, meats, and raw or undercooked animal products. Choices *A*, *B*, and *D* are considered safe to consume as they do not pose any direct risks to the health of a patient with AIDS.

37. C: Choice *C* is an intervention that is appropriate for the nurse to engage in to support the patient with early dumping syndrome. Choice *A* should be avoided; fluids should be consumed outside of mealtimes. Choice *B* should be avoided, as the patient should consume several small meals per day. Choice *D* should be avoided; the patient should increase fiber intake.

38. B: After birth, the foramen ovale closes, directing blood from the heart to the lungs. In the fetal circulation, the foramen ovale allows blood to bypass the lungs, so Choice *A* is not correct. After birth, pulmonary vascular resistance falls, increasing blood flow to the lungs. Therefore, Choice *C* is not correct. A patent ductus arteriosus allows blood to flow from the pulmonary artery to the aorta in the fetus, not the newborn. So, Choice *D* is not the correct answer.

39. C: Morphine is part of the MONA protocol given for pain relief, while nitroglycerine is a vasodilator that reduces preload in the presence of chest pain. Magnesium sulfate is administered for the Torsade de pointes dysrhythmia and is not part of the MONA protocol.

40. B: Choice *B* should be avoided in the plan of care for a patient with acute Deep Vein Thrombosis (DVT) as spontaneous compression devices may dislodge a pre existing thrombus and lead to a pulmonary embolism, a blockage in a lung artery. Choice *A* is an appropriate intervention as this medication is an anticoagulant. Choice *C* should be included in the plan of care to characterize the coagulation of blood. Choice *D* is necessary to monitor for irregular heartbeat including preventricular contractions that the patient may feel as palpitations, along with other cardiac signs and symptoms that may come from a dislodged blood clot.

41. A: Choice *A* is correct as the dysphagia diet places this food item at a level 3, proving challenging for a patient with difficulty swallowing to consume. Choice *B* is considered a level-2 item and is appropriate for this patient. Choices *C* and *D* are considered level-1 food items and are appropriate for this patient to consume. Soft solid foods should be avoided for this patient, while they are struggling to move food and liquid from their mouth to their stomach. The consumption of beets poses a safety risk.

42. D: When performing a newborn Apgar assessment, the highest score that may be assigned is 10. This score indicates that the newborn has pink skin without evidence of cyanosis, an apical heart rate greater than 100 beats per minute, cries or pulls away when stimulated, firm muscle tone, and a strong cry. Therefore, Choices *A*, *B*, and *C* are incorrect.

43. D: A fracture to the eighth rib on the right side of the chest may cause injury to the liver, which lies beneath this rib. Choices *A* and *B* are not correct since injury to the bronchus or trachea is likely to be caused by fractures to the first or second ribs. Choice *C* is incorrect since the spleen is likely to be injured with a fracture to the eighth rib or greater on the left side of the chest.

44. B: Choice *B* influences ketone bodies, which provide some symptom relief regarding cognition and memory for the patient with Alzheimer's disease. Choices *A*, *C*, and *D* should be avoided with this patient, as symptoms tend to be aggravated by these actions.

45. A: The patient utilizing oxygen for respiratory management should switch from aerosol to stick deodorant, as aerosol cans present a fire risk. To promote safe discharge, the nurse must assess for understanding of proper use of new equipment in the home. Choices *B*, *C*, and *D* do not show safe handling to prevent fire.

46. B: Constant clearing of the throat is a sign that a patient is silently aspirating. Integument symptoms such as rash are not associated with this condition. Swollen lymph nodes on the neck indicate possible upper respiratory infection. Neurological deficits such as memory and orientation loss are not associated with silent aspiration, but may occur because of stroke, which is a precursor to difficulty swallowing in some cases.

47. B: Goals of care are held to keep the focus on what the dying patient wants at their end time.

48. C: Choice *C* represents a risk to infection control and warrants further education. The unlicensed assistive personnel (UAP) should wash their hands with soap and water after caring for a patient with Clostridium difficile because hand sanitizers kill bacteria but do not kill the spores. Choice *A* is within the scope of the UAP and does not warrant education. Choice B is an appropriate care measure and does not warrant education. Choice *D* represents the correct placement of the Foley catheter bag to avoid urine collection in the bladder.

49. B: Cushing's disease is caused by a dysfunction of the adrenal glands, which are on top of the kidneys, leading to excess glucocorticoid production. As a result, Choices *A*, *C*, and *D* are incorrect.

50. C: Pregnant women with gestational diabetes need to exercise regularly, avoid excessive weight gain, and monitor food intake. They also need to seek regular prenatal care since gestational diabetes can affect fetal growth and increase the baby's risk of obesity. Therefore, Choices *A*, *B*, and *D* are not correct.

51. A: Choice *A* indicates a post-renal cause of acute renal failure. Sources of obstruction include stones, strictures, and tumors. Choices *B* and *C* are direct renal causes, while Choice *D* is a prerenal cause of acute renal failure.

52. C: Acute bronchitis, an inflammation of the bronchial tubes, can cause wheezing, coughing fever, myalgia, and chest pain. Other manifestations include sore throat, headache, nasal congestion, rhinorrhea, dyspnea, and fatigue. While treatment is generally supportive, a beta-2 agonist, such as albuterol, may be administered to reduce wheezing. Since this medication does not act as a cough suppressant, fever-reducing agent, or analgesic, *A*, *B*, and *D* are incorrect.

53. C: This scenario depicts a case of community-acquired pneumonia (CAP), specifically pneumococcal pneumonia. The most common cause of CAP is Streptococcus pneumoniae, or pneumococcus. It's a gram-positive bacterium, usually occurring in pairs (diplococci). The other bacteria (Haemophilus influenzae, Moraxella catarrhalis, and Staphylococcus aureus) are less common causes of CAP.

54. A: A laparoscopic procedure is minimally invasive and makes very small incisions for the surgeon to enter the abdominal cavity and remove the gall bladder. Laparotomy involves the surgeon making a large incision to completely open up the abdominal cavity. Bronchoscopy is a scope of the airways and lungs. Endoscopy is a scope of the upper GI tract.

55. D: The patient with an upper gastrointestinal bleed may be covertly bleeding superiorly to the junction of the duodenum and jejunum. Because the nurse cannot directly observe the bleeding, the amount of blood loss must be estimated. A patient with a gastrointestinal bleed who experiences a 10-millimeter drop in diastolic blood pressure when moving from a lying to a standing position is estimated to have lost 1,000 milliliters of blood. Therefore, Choices *A, B,* and *C* are not correct.

56. B: Choice *B* is correct, as a normal prothrombin time test (PTT) falls within a 10-14 second range. Choice *A* is below normal. Choices *C* and *D* are both above the normal range. The medical-surgical nurse is responsible for reviewing this laboratory result to ensure proper clotting ability prior to surgery.

57. C: Choice *C* represents a patient condition that is in direct conflict with the administration of antimuscarinic medications; therefore, the patient with this condition is unable to receive this treatment. Antimuscarinics can lead to pupillary blockage due to their effect on nerve impulses. Choices *A*, *B*, and *D* do not pose risks for contraindication and do not prevent the patient from engaging in this treatment option.

58. C: This scenario depicts the diagnosis of a right-sided tension pneumothorax. The triad of tracheal deviation (to opposite side), mediastinal shift (to opposite side), and depression of the hemidiaphragm (on affected side) is pathognomonic for tension pneumothorax. Medical professionals must be quick and decisive in their treatment of tension pneumothorax. The condition is life-threatening and valuable time is often wasted waiting around for the results of imaging studies. Definitive treatment of a tension pneumothorax is emergent needle thoracostomy.

59. A: Patients with Barrett's esophagus are at an increased risk for developing esophageal adenocarcinoma. When a patient has reflux disease, the cells of the esophagus become irritated and go through a metastatic transformation, thus increasing the risk for cancer. Therefore, the statement that the patient is not at an increased risk for cancer needs to be corrected by the nurse. Choice *B* is not correct since corticosteroids are used to treat Barrett's esophagus. Choice *C* is not the correct answer since the patient does need to make healthy lifestyle choices to reduce the risk of reflux disease. Choice

D is not correct since the patient should be taught signs and symptoms of reflux disease to report to the physician, including heartburn and difficulty swallowing.

60. C: Cushing's triad of manifestations are late signs of increased ICP. Choice *C* is an example of widening pulse pressure. Normal pulse pressure = 40 mmHg. Choice *C* pulse pressure = 130 mmHg. Choices *A, B,* and *D* are all early signs of increased ICP, and therefore are incorrect.

61. D: Choice *D* represents an infection of the tissue lining the inner abdominal wall. Choice *A* manifests as inflammation of the iris of the eye. Choice *B* involves an inflammation and the potential for infection of the skin. Choice *C* aligns with inflammation and the potential of infection of the bladder.

62. B: In glycogenosis, the patient's body is not able to convert stored glycogen to glucose when the body needs glucose. In severe cases, the patient can experience chronic gout, seizures, coma, intestinal sores, and kidney failure. Choices *A, C,* and *D* are not correct since liver failure, respiratory failure, and congestive heart failure are not common findings in severe glycogenosis.

63. B: Both the patient's symptoms and blood glucose level indicate that the patient is experiencing hypoglycemia. Manifestations of hypoglycemia include a decreased level of consciousness, tremors, fatigue, excessive sweating, dizziness, and syncope. A blood glucose level below 70 milligrams per deciliter confirms this diagnosis. Insulin would not be given to a patient with hypoglycemia, as this would further lower the blood glucose level. Choices *A, C,* and *D* are incorrect because it would be appropriate to administer oral glucose, IV dextrose, or parenteral glucagon to the patient with hypoglycemia.

64. D: Endoscopic band ligation should be implemented for all varices that are 5 millimeters or more in diameter and/or associated with red wales, because these characteristics are associated with a greater risk for hemorrhage. Band ligation decreases this potential but may be associated with stricture formation and obstruction of the esophageal lumen. This procedure may need to be repeated as the liver failure progresses. Therefore, Choice *D* is correct. Sclerotherapy of the esophageal veins is considered as a form of secondary prevention by many because beta-blocker therapy is readily available, well tolerated, and equally effective as compared to sclerotherapy. In the event of hemorrhage due to ruptured esophageal varices, sclerotherapy can be used to decrease the blood loss; therefore, Choice *A* is incorrect.

65. B, C, D, E: Choices *B, C, D,* and *E* all represent early warning signs of increased intracranial pressure which could be found in a patient suffering from a head injury. Nausea, Choice *A,* is not a typical finding, as a key assessment notation for this diagnosis is vomiting in the absence of nausea.

66. C: Urinary retention occurs when a patient has cessation of urination or incomplete emptying of the bladder. This may lead to overflow incontinence as the bladder becomes overfilled with urine, which then is involuntarily released from the overfull bladder. Therefore, *A, B,* and *D* are not correct.

67. D: Choice *D* is the priority action for the nurse to rank in the plan of care for a patient with a history of aggressive behavior. Choices *A, B,* and *C* are not yet necessary; these actions represent potential interventions that may come later in the treatment plan if warranted. The nurse should focus on the least restrictive measures first.

68. A: The patient's manifestations are consistent with a diagnosis of hemorrhagic stroke. Although there is no single therapeutic agent that is specific to the treatment of hemorrhagic stroke, aggressive treatment of hypertension and the use of agents to counteract the anticoagulative effect of warfarin are common interventions. Mannitol is an osmotic diuretic used to decrease intracranial pressure that results from the hematoma formation at the hemorrhagic site. Vitamin K is used to counteract warfarin therapy, and the dose will be titrated to the results of the coagulation studies; therefore, Choice *A* is correct. Warfarin is an anticoagulant that is not recommended for use in hemorrhagic stroke. Labetalol is an antihypertensive agent that might be used for hemorrhagic stroke. However, it would not be ordered with warfarin therapy; therefore, Choice *B* is incorrect. Alteplase is a fibrinolytic agent, and nitroprusside is a potent vasoconstricting agent. Neither of these medications is appropriate in the care of hemorrhagic stroke; therefore, Choice *C* is incorrect. Enalapril is an antihypertensive agent that might be used for hemorrhagic stroke. However, it would not be ordered with ASA, which is an antiplatelet agent; therefore, Choice *D* is incorrect.

69. B: Choice *B* represents the nurse's focus while discussing the professional role and function of the registered professional nurse with an interdisciplinary colleague. Choices *A*, *C*, and *D* do not rely on state law to define the description of scope witnessed in this engagement.

70. B: The nurse should suspect hypoglycemia based on the circumstances and symptoms being experienced by the patient. Hypoglycemia may occur when a patient receiving insulin therapy, as may be the case here if the patient is diabetic, has been NPO for a procedure. Fasting in addition to insulin therapy, if not carefully monitored and tweaked, will likely cause hypoglycemia. Sweating, nausea, and malaise are all hypoglycemic symptoms. A blood sugar reading should be immediately obtained to determine if hypoglycemia is the cause and, if so, treated with oral glucagon. Hypochondria is always possible but should be a diagnosis made by a psychiatrist. Hypotension is a less likely option given the circumstances, though not completely improbable. Hypothyroidism is unlikely and not a condition that the nurse would be able to independently diagnose without proper lab work and clinical workup.

71. C: A patient is diagnosed with metabolic syndrome if they have three or more of the following conditions: hypertension, elevated fasting blood glucose levels, low HDL cholesterol, high triglycerides, and excess belly fat. Since the patient has excess belly fat, it is important to engage in behaviors that lead to weight loss. Choices *A*, *B*, and *D* are not correct because the patient with metabolic syndrome does need to follow a low cholesterol diet, exercise regularly, and take measures to reduce blood pressure (such as following a low sodium diet).

72. A: Choice *A* is a significant outcome focus for a patient with marfan syndrome as this genetic disorder affects the cardiac system and leads to challenges with maintaining adequate tissue perfusion. Choices *B*, *C*, and *D* are not concerns associated with this disorder.

73. A: Choice *A* is a concerning response by the patient regarding their daily levothyroxine administration. This medication should be taken once daily on an empty stomach, at least 30 minutes before and four hours after meals. Choices *B*, *C*, and *D* all meet these administration guidelines and do not necessitate patient education at this time.

74. A: Choice *A* involves the quadrant where the appendix is located and where pain is typically felt. The nurse should ask the patient to rate their pain level in the right lower quadrant in order to provide effective pain management at this time. Choices *B*, *C*, and *D* represent quadrants outside of the appendix location.

75. C: Choice *C* should be performed second when completing a focused abdominal assessment. Choice *A* should be third; Choice *B* should be fourth, while Choice *D* happens first when engaging in a focused abdominal assessment. Other body systems retain the typical order of inspection, percussion, palpation, and auscultation, however with the abdomen, the medical-surgical nurse must auscultate prior to percussion to avoid altering the bowel sounds.

76. A: Choice *A* is often the cause of increased confusion, agitation, and poor motor skills in the geriatric patient population. These symptoms can present suddenly and alert the medical-surgical nurse to a notable change in the patient's level of consciousness. Further assessment is warranted. Choices *B*, *C*, and *D* are not associated with this symptom presentation and should not be considered for further assessment at this time.

77. C: The characteristic manifestation of gastroenteritis is diarrhea, which can be prolonged and accompanied by vomiting. As a result, the patient requires prompt administration of fluids to prevent fluid volume deficit and its resultant complications. Choices *A, B,* and *D* are all appropriate interventions, after the nurse has first addressed the fluid volume deficit.

78. A: Choice *A* includes language that aligns with the SBAR format of communication. This statement provides a direct recommendation. The SBAR technique calls for a report that includes situation, background, assessment, and recommendation. Choices *B*, *C*, and *D* request information or direction from the provider rather than offering a clear recommendation for treatment.

79. A: Flail chest is caused by blunt force, such as that experienced when a driver's chest comes in contact with the steering wheel in a motor vehicle accident, causing a minimum of two fractures in three or more ribs. The key assessment finding in flail chest is the paradoxical movement of a section of the chest when the patient breathes. Choices *B*, *C*, and *D* commonly occur in pulmonary disorders, including flail chest, but are not specific to flail chest.

80. C: Choice *C* represents a type of angina that is instigated by coronary vasospasms. Choice *A* occurs when the heart is chronically working harder than usual due to a lack of oxygen. Choice *B* is due to a lack of blood flow and oxygen from a blood clot, potentially leading to a myocardial infarction. Choice *D* is due to coronary artery spasms.

81. D: A history of polycystic ovary syndrome increases a woman's risk of developing metabolic syndrome. The risk of developing metabolic syndrome is not increased in patients with diabetes insipidus, glomerulonephritis, and hypoparathyroid disease, making Choices *A*, *B*, and *C* incorrect.

82. D: Hyperglycemia may occur in a patient who does not have enough insulin or anti-diabetic medication, ingests too much glucose, experiences an illness that disrupts the normal routine, or experiences a crisis that causes emotional stress. Therefore, Choices *A*, *B*, and *C* are not correct.

83. C: Choice *C* is a cause for concern and should influence the nurse to reconsider this intervention. Patients with increased intracranial pressure should not be given dextrose 5% in water. This solution increases brain water, which further increases intracranial pressure. The nurse should hold this treatment and contact the prescriber regarding this concern. Choices *A*, *B*, and *D* are all appropriate conditions to treat with this solution.

84. D: The three classic symptoms of ectopic pregnancy are pain, amenorrhea, and vaginal bleeding. Therefore, *D* is the correct answer.

85. A: Typical findings in a patient with hyperthyroidism include feelings of anxiety, trouble focusing, feeling overheated, gastrointestinal problems such as diarrhea, insomnia, elevated heart rate, and unexplained weight loss. Choices *B*, *C*, and *D* are not correct because experiencing cold or chills, weight gain, and excessive fatigue are manifestations of hypothyroidism.

86. C: The typical manifestations of status asthmaticus are wheezing, coughing, and dyspnea. With severe airway obstruction, auscultation of the chest may reveal a "silent chest" and a lack of audible wheezing. Tachycardia, cyanosis, and hypoxemia are all manifestations of the patient with status asthmaticus but are not signs of impending respiratory failure; therefore, Choices *A*, *B*, and *D* are incorrect.

87. C: Choice *C* should be limited in the diet of a patient with Meniere's disease. Sodium leads to a buildup of water, which can contribute to an increase in inner-ear fluid and exacerbation of symptoms. Choices *A*, *B*, and *D* do not directly lead to an improvement in symptoms of this condition.

88. D: Choice *D* states that decreasing the $PaCO_2$ results in arterial vasodilation, which is incorrect because vasodilation would increase, not decrease, ICP. Decreasing the $PaCO_2$ results in arterial vasoconstriction; therefore, Choice *D* is the correct answer. Choices *A, B,* and *C* all identify appropriate interventions for increased ICP; therefore, they are incorrect.

89. C: For the ABCD of primary survey, airway and breathing are the first two priority assessments. Assessing the level of consciousness is secondary to establishing and maintaining a patent's airway.

90. D: Choice *D* is a significant cause for concern in the patient post colonoscopy because it may signify a perforated bowel. While rare, this complication can happen during or after this procedure and may take place days later. A perforated bowel involves a tear in the lining that may be life threatening and requires prompt medical attention with subsequent surgical repair in most cases. Choice *A* is a normal finding. Choice *B* is a normal finding and should resolve within a few days. Choice *C* is a normal finding secondary to the residual air in the colon from the procedure.

91. D: An INR of 3.5 is elevated and will cause bleeding complications if thrombolytic therapy is initiated before the INR returns to the normal level of less than or equal to 1.1.

92. D: Choice *D* aligns with the nurse's statement, "Don't worry, everyone feels that way." and demonstrates a poor example of therapeutic communication, which hinders the nurse-patient relationship. Choice *A* projects the nurse's opinion. Choice *B* provides comfort in a misleading outcome. Choice *C* guards a party, such as a provider. All communication blocks reviewed in this question encourage misunderstandings and failure to listen, which should be avoided in patient care environments.

93. A: Choice *A* represents the type of anemia that is characterized by a lack of an intrinsic factor, which leaves the patient unable to use B12 consumed by mouth. Patients with pernicious anemia engage in B12 injections to increase serum levels and decrease symptoms. Choice *B* involves the body's lack of new blood cell production. Choice *C* involves the rapid destruction of red blood cells. Choice *D*, an inherited condition, causes red blood cells to be misshapen and degrade.

94. B: Hypoalbuminemia is an essential element in the development of ascites. Decreased oncotic pressure resulting from deficient plasma proteins allows the movement of fluid from the vasculature into the extracellular fluid where it accumulates as ascites. Cirrhosis can result in increased levels of nitric oxide, which leads to vasodilation. The renal response to this abnormal condition is sodium retention and the secretion of increased epinephrine and norepinephrine due to stimulation of the sympathetic nervous system. Therefore, Choice *A* is incorrect. The development of ascites is a complication of portal hypertension, not hypotension. Portal hypertension is defined as the blockage of blood flow through the vasculature of the liver due to fibrotic changes resulting from cirrhosis or hepatitis; therefore, Choice *C* is incorrect. Plasma oncotic levels are decreased, rather than increased, because the diseased liver is not able to synthesize albumin; therefore, Choice *D* is incorrect.

95. A: High-flow priapism is due to a straddle injury that causes trauma to the groin area. Low-flow priapism may be idiopathic, but other causes include dialysis, vasculitis, spinal cord stenosis, bladder and renal cancer, and some medications, such as heparin, cocaine, and omeprazole. Therefore, *B* and *C* are not correct. In children, low-flow priapism may be caused by sickle cell disease, making *D* an incorrect answer in this thirty-eight-year-old patient.

96. B: Since radioactive iodine should not be taken by pregnant women, the nurse should instruct this woman of child-bearing age to use a reliable form of birth control. Radioactive iodine is taken in a repeat-dose solution over the long-term, so Choices *A* and *C* are not correct. Since the patient with hyperthyroidism should be instructed to exercise regularly, Choice *D* is not correct.

97. C: Choice *C* involves appropriate precautions for the management of infection control in the patient with pertussis. This illness, also known as whooping cough, produces droplets that can spread when talking, coughing, and sneezing. Choice *A* and Choice *B* would provide inadequate protection with vulnerabilities in disease transmission. Choice *D* represents a higher level of precaution, which is not required for this patient at this time.

98. D: Addison's disease, also called adrenal insufficiency, occurs when the adrenal glands do not produce enough glucocorticoids and mineralocorticoids. Since mineralocorticoids are involved in fluid and electrolyte balance, the patient with Addison's disease is likely to have fluid and electrolyte imbalances. Choice *A* is not correct since the excessive body hair growth in Cushing's syndrome is caused by an excess of glucocorticoid production. Choice *B* is not correct since hypertension does not typically occur in Addison's disease, but it may occur in Cushing's syndrome and Conn's syndrome. Choice *C* is not correct since patients with Addison's disease typically have fatigue.

99. C: Community-associated, methicillin-resistant Staphylococcus aureus (CA-MRSA) is notoriously resistant to most antibiotics, except the vancomycin and linezolid, with linezolid quickly becoming the agent of choice for the treatment of CA-MRSA pneumonia.

100. B: Relapses are common in the patient with myasthenia gravis. To reduce the risk of relapse, the nurse should teach the patient to avoid infection, increases in body temperature, stress, and pregnancy. Therefore, Choices *A*, *C*, and *D* should be included in the plan of care.

101. D: The discharge planning process starts right away at admission for every patient. Each aspect of care is provided with an end-goal in mind. When the patient comes into the care of a healthcare organization, the treatment plan involves interventions with an ultimate anticipated outcome of safe discharge.

102. A: Choice *A* is correct as assessing that the body has effectively processed out excessive ammonia, the chief mechanism of the lactulose treatment in this patient population, supports evaluating treatment effectiveness. If the lactulose was not effective, the patient may display signs and symptoms of hepatic encephalopathy. Choices *B*, *C*, and *D* are not priority assessment areas for the medical-surgical nurse regarding evaluating the effectiveness of the lactulose regimen. Lactulose reduces circulating blood levels of ammonia via promoting excretion for patients with liver disease.

103. B: Choice *B* represents the form of consent for treatment that the patient gives by presenting for care and voluntarily moving forward with admission; implied consent is inferred by the patient's actions. Choices *A* and *C* involve the patient's direct agreement to move forward with treatment by giving either verbal or written permission to receive care. Choice *D* involves consent given by a third party acting on behalf of the patient's interest.

104. B: Pelvic inflammatory disease may be caused by any of the sexually transmitted organisms. To reduce the risk of receiving or transmitting these organisms, the patient should not engage in unprotected intercourse. Choices *A*, *C*, and *D* do not indicate a need for more teaching because over-the-counter analgesics may be taken for pain relief, pelvic inflammatory disease can affect fertility, and any unusual discharge should be reported to the health care provider.

105. B: Choice *B* is often assessed in the patient who has been experiencing diarrhea. Metabolic Acidosis can also be witnessed in renal failure, diabetic ketoacidosis, and aspirin overdose. Choice *A* is seen with vomiting and the overuse of antacids. Choice *C* is observed with hypoxia, fever, and hyperventilation. Choice *D* is witnessed secondary to airway obstruction and pulmonary edema.

106. D: Choice *D* aligns with tardive dyskinesia, an involuntary movement disorder that includes movements of the jaw, lips, and tongue, often seen as an adverse reaction to antipsychotic medication use. Choice *A* identifies the lack of movement, as the patient is unable to engage their muscles. Choice *B* involves an abnormal sensation of the skin, often described as pins and needles. Choice *C* involves restlessness with the urge to keep moving.

107. C: All of the assessment questions are appropriate for this patient; however, if the patient reports a recent infection, the emergency care providers understand that there is potential for the rapid onset of respiratory failure, which potentially alters the plan of care. Therefore, Choices *A, B*, and *D* are incorrect.

108. D: Chronic alcohol abuse and biliary tract dysfunction are the most frequent causes of acute pancreatitis; however, there are no identified criteria that explain why some individuals will experience pancreatitis while others do not. Acute pancreatitis is most often diagnosed by the presenting history and physical examination. ECRP is only indicated in patients with acute pancreatitis and concomitant biliary disease; therefore, Choice *A* is incorrect. Ultrasonography is generally less useful than CT imaging for pancreatitis, and its efficacy is significantly decreased in the presence of abdominal distention, which distorts the images; therefore, Choice *B* is incorrect. Although rectal indomethacin is used commonly to treat acute pancreatitis resulting from ERCP imaging, controversy remains regarding the efficacy of the therapy; therefore, Choice *C* is incorrect.

109. B: Since chlamydial infections may be asymptomatic, the U.S. Preventative Services Task Force recommends routine screening of all women fifteen to twenty-four years old and all females older than twenty-four who have a risk factor for chlamydia. Since having multiple sexual partners is a risk factor for all sexually transmitted diseases, Choice *B* is correct. *A* is not correct because the Task Force does not recommend screening for all women regardless of age. *C* is not correct since having protected intercourse is not a risk factor. *D* is not correct since the Task Force recommends screening start at age fifteen, not age twelve.

110. B: Choice *B* sets forth that when using the PQRST method the nurse should include information regarding the patient's pain that includes the following characteristics: provoke, quality, region, severity, and timing. Choices *A*, *C*, and *D* are incorrect as they do not provide accurate details of a PQRST method pain assessment for a nurse-to-nurse report. This method is exclusive to a focused pain assessment and includes specific characteristics.

111. B: Guillain-Barré syndrome, an acute immune-mediated demyelinating polyneuropathy, has an acute onset of progressive, bilateral muscle weakness of the arms and legs that starts distally and moves proximally. Therefore, Choices *A*, *C*, and *D* are not correct.

112. D: Symptoms of left-sided heart failure are tachycardia, shortness of breath, and the expectoration of frothy pink sputum. Pitting edema is symptomatic of right-sided heart failure and increased venous pressure that backs up into the tissues, causing edema. Ascites is a result of diffuse congestion in the liver caused by the increased venous pressure that characterizes right-sided heart failure. Fatigue is a generalized symptom not associated with the diagnosis of either right- or left-sided heart failure.

113. C: Choice *C* supports the patient into the position that allows for thorough assessment of lung sounds. Choices *A*, *B*, and *D* would inhibit the nurse from properly auscultating all lobes of the lungs and would alter the patient's ability to equally and bilaterally breathe during the focused assessment.

114. C: Alteplase is the single fibrinolytic agent approved for the treatment of ischemic stroke because it is associated with fewer adverse effects than the remaining agents. Streptokinase and tenecteplase have been used effectively to treat patients with acute myocardial infarction; however, in patients with ischemic stroke, streptokinase has been associated with an increased risk of intracranial hemorrhage and death. Current evidence for the efficacy and safety of urokinase and tenecteplase does not support their use for the treatment of ischemic stroke. Therefore, Choices *A*, *B*, and *D* are incorrect.

115. A: Virchow's triad identifies factors that contribute to the thrombotic process associated with deep venous thrombosis (DVT) and pulmonary embolism (PE). The triad consists of hypercoagulability, endothelial injury/dysfunction, and hemodynamic changes such as stasis and turbulence. Heart disease is a risk factor for DVT and PE, but it is not part of Virchow's triad.

116. B: Choice *B* is cause for concern, as prazosin typically causes hypotension, not hypertension; therefore, the nurse would page the physician to explore additional testing for this patient to understand the basis of this finding. Choices *A*, *C*, and *D* are expected findings with the use of prazosin and would not alert the nurse to additional complications at this time.

117. D: The patient who has had a pulmonary embolism may require warfarin (Coumadin) after discharge from the hospital to prevent blood clot formation leading to pulmonary embolism. With warfarin, frequent blood monitoring is needed to maintain INR between 2-3. Choice *A* does not require more teaching since warfarin is taken orally. Choice *B* does not require more teaching since bleeding is a risk with this drug and should be reported to the physician, if it occurs. Choice *C* does not require more teaching since chest pain and shortness of breath are possible manifestations of pulmonary embolism.

118. C: Morphine is part of the MONA protocol given for pain relief, while nitroglycerine is a vasodilator that reduces preload in the presence of chest pain. Magnesium sulfate is administrated for the Torsade de pointes dysrhythmia and is not part of the MONA protocol.

119. C: Carbon monoxide poisoning, occurring when this gas is inhaled through the lungs and builds up in the bloodstream, can be treated with hyperbaric oxygen therapy. The patient undergoing this treatment should be taught what to expect before, during, and after the procedure. Choice *A* is incorrect since carbon monoxide poisoning does not cause burns. Choice *B* is not correct since N-acetylcysteine is a mucolytic agent and does not treat carbon monoxide poisoning. Hydroxocobalamin (Cyanokit) is administered for hydrogen cyanide poisoning, making Choice *D* incorrect.

120. A: Choice *A* represents the diet that should be implemented for the patient with gout. Choices *B* and *C* should be avoided as they may exacerbate symptoms. Choice *D* is not necessary for this patient at this time. Purines can cause gout attacks and should be avoided. Some examples of high-purine foods include red meat, seafood, organ meat, and alcohol.

121. B: Choice *B* indicates the diet that should be maintained by the patient with dermatitis herpetiformis, which is aggravated by the consumption of gluten and requires strict dietary adherence. Choices *A*, *C*, and *D* represent dietary restrictions that are not necessary for this patient's condition and should not be encouraged.

122. B: Choice *B* represents a significant cause for concern that warrants further education at this time. A patient with acute appendicitis should not engage in heat on the abdomen, as this can exacerbate symptoms and lead to further complications. Choices *A*, *C*, and *D* are all supportive measures that the licensed practical nurse should implement.

123. A, B, C: Back pain, shortness of breath, and skin flushing (Choices *A*, *B*, and *C*) encourage the nurse to stop the transfusion due to a transfusion reaction. If the nurse suspects that the patient may be experiencing a transfusion reaction, the priority intervention is to stop the transfusion immediately. Blurred vision and lethargy (Choices *D* and *E*), while problematic, do not correlate with a transfusion reaction; rather, these signs indicate infiltration or vein injury.

124. D: The patient's preferences, values, and beliefs, as well as indication of a surrogate decision maker, are all included in advance directives.

125. D: With medical therapy, many people with HIV are able to live normal, healthy lives. The patient should not wait until symptoms are present to seek medical care, since the earlier HIV is treated, the better the viral load can be managed; therefore, Choice *A* is not correct. Choice *B* is also incorrect since early medical care can enable a person with HIV to lead a normal life. Choice *C* is not correct, because not all treatment leads to undetectable viral loads.

126. B: If the patient with temporal arteritis delays treatment for more than two weeks after the vision loss started, vision loss will also occur in the unaffected eye. Therefore, Choice *C* is not the correct answer. Any loss of vision that occurs before treatment is started will be permanent. Therefore, Choices *A* and *D* are incorrect.

127. A: Choice *A* involves the nurse enabling the patient to choose the focus of the conversation. With broad openings, the patient is supported to lead the dialogue in a direction that they value. Choices *B*, *C*, and *D* represent therapeutic communication techniques, but they do not directly align with the process the nurse is seeking to use.

128. B: Choice *B* can lead the patient to paralytic ileus, which includes symptoms such as pain, vomiting, and distention. Choices *A*, *C*, and *D* are not likely triggers of paralytic ileus.

129. C: Conn's syndrome is characterized by hypersecretion of the mineralocorticoid hormone aldosterone by the adrenal glands. Choices *A* and *B* are not correct since DHEA and androstenedione are sex hormones secreted by the adrenal glands and do not cause Conn's syndrome. Choice *D* is not correct since cortisol is a glucocorticoid hormone secreted by the adrenal glands but does not cause Conn's disease.

130. B: This scenario depicts an inhalation injury. Although the patient's history is limited, the fact that he produced carbonaceous sputum makes an inhalation injury the most likely diagnosis (specifically smoke inhalation). This scenario emphasizes the point that medical professionals should maintain a high level of suspicion when it comes to inhalation injuries. Treatment of inhalation injuries is largely supportive with an excellent prognosis for complete recovery.

131. D: Early manifestations of memory impairment in Alzheimer's disease are associated with short-term memory loss and the inability to assimilate new knowledge, with progressive impairment that affects long-term memory, mood, and independent functioning. The end stage of this process is the inability to recognize family members. The processes are not the same. Memory lapses associated with forgetfulness improve with cueing and do not progress to the inability to recognize family members. Therefore, Choices *A*, *B*, and *C* are incorrect.

132. D: Acute laryngotracheobronchitis, or croup, causes an inflammation of the airways in children. If the inflammation causes partial or complete airway obstruction, the child develops stridor, a high-pitched breath sound. Corticosteroids may be administered to reduce airway inflammation, resulting in reduced or absent stridor. Choice *A* is not correct since corticosteroids are not administered to reduce fever. *B* is not correct since the chest x-ray may not be affected in the child with croup. While hunger is a sign that the child is feeling better, it is not due to corticosteroid administration, making Choice *C* incorrect.

133. B: The highest priority in this patient is stopping the flow of blood out of her body. Nothing else can be addressed until this is performed. Fluid resuscitation is highly important, but useless if the bleeding continues. Monitoring for infection will happen later. Assessing for organ damage is ongoing, but ultimately secondary to stopping active bleeding.

134. C: Choice *C* successfully explains the patient's active acquired immunity represented via their history and laboratory findings. Choice *C* is not applicable because this immunity is found in those who were vaccinated against this illness, not in those who acquired it. Choices *B* and *D* are not correct because the patient's laboratory findings that indicate the presence of antibodies to varicella align with current immunity.

135. D: Choice *D* supports the patient's right to engage in independent, self-directed decision-making. The provider must avoid language that impedes this right. Choice *A* involves avoiding patient harm. Choice *B* represents truthfulness. Choice *C* includes the moral essential of doing right by the patient.

136. A: The most common sexually transmitted disease in the United States is chlamydia. Therefore, *B*, *C*, and *D* are not correct.

137. A: The most common complication associated with shunts is the obstruction of the proximal catheter. Over a period, the proximal tip of the catheter can become embedded in the choroid, obstructing the catheter and delaying the drainage of the CSF. The shunt valve on the proximal end can also become obstructed with blood cells and other cellular debris. Obstruction of the distal catheter is less common than proximal obstruction but occurs more frequently than infection or dislocation. Migration of the catheter tip is most commonly related to the growth of the patient, which means that this complication occurs in younger children most often. The patient referenced in this scenario was an adult at the time of insertion of the catheter; therefore, this is not a likely cause for his current problem, and Choice *B* is incorrect. Disconnection of the segments of the shunt system is a rare occurrence that is due to a manufacturer's defect or improper installation of the device. When this malfunction does occur, it is readily discovered in the postoperative period; therefore, Choice *C* is incorrect. Infection most commonly occurs during the initial two to four months after the catheter is inserted. Infection is most often associated with overt signs of infection such as erythema, purulent drainage, peritonitis, and abdominal pain; however, fever may or may not be present. The patient included in the scenario has had the shunt in place for four years, which exceeds the common timeline for site infection, and the assessment does not provide any support for a diagnosis of infection; therefore, Choice *D* is incorrect.

138. C: Choice *C* is a significant concern and must be closely monitored during treatment with bupropion. Patients can experience thoughts of self-harm and suicide while taking this drug. Choice *A* is not of concern because patients on this drug typically experience tachycardia as a side effect. Choice *B* is not a typical reaction associated with this drug. Choice *D* is not characteristically associated with this drug; instead, difficulty starting and staying asleep may be witnessed.

139. D: Choice *D* represents the proper infection control practices to reduce the transmission of herpes zoster for the patient with classified disseminated infection. Both airborne and contact precautions are necessary during this phase of illness. Choices *A*, *B*, and *D* would provide improper infection control and increased risk.

140. C: Choice *C* aligns with the patient's laboratory findings when utilizing the SBAR as a method of communication. SBAR stands for situation, background, assessment, and recommendations. Laboratory findings are a form of assessment data; therefore, they align with the assessment aspect of reports. Choice *A* includes the current condition. Choice *B* includes the context of the circumstance. Choice *D* includes the nurse's suggestions to respond to the situation.

141. A: Choice *A* reflects patient-centered goals to be included in the nursing care plan. These goals encourage the greatest improvement in individual health outcomes, encompassing physical and mental wellbeing and the ability to care for self. Choice *B* does not align, as patient-centered goals do not revolve around the interest of any specific nursing interventions. Choice *C* is provider-centered, not patient-centered. Choice *D* is not appropriate, as "normalized" is subjective and does not focus on this specific patient's individualized health improvement.

142. C: Pancreatitis is the likely diagnosis based on the location of the abdominal pain and the patient's history. The hallmark symptom of pancreatitis is abdominal pain, and that is the focus of treatment. Hepatitis presents with symptoms of liver dysfunction such as jaundice, ascites, enlargement of liver, and encephalopathy. Gastritis, an inflammation of the lining of the stomach, will present with nausea and vomiting. Kidney failure will present with oliguria and fluid and electrolyte imbalances.

143. A: Choice *A* is correct because the patient is at risk for developing metabolic acidosis while on total parenteral nutrition (TPN). The medical-surgical nurse should be aware of this risk and routinely assess for the development of this complication. Choices *B*, *C*, and *D*, while all significant imbalances that would profoundly affect the patient's health status, are not typically observed with this treatment and not expected responses at this time.

144. C: Choice *C* indicates the action that the nurse should implement at this time. The nurse understands that Broca's aphasia influences the patient's ability to produce verbal expression but does not limit their ability to understand incoming verbal responses. Choices *A*, *B*, and *C* are unnecessary as these actions would not provide care that is diagnosis-specific and supportive. Multiple types of aphasia exist; knowing the differences between them promotes sensitive care.

145. A, B: During septic shock, metabolic acidosis and respiratory alkalosis are expected findings, along with a symptom presentation of shortness of breath, temperature changes, confusion, and diaphoresis.

Thus, Choices *A* and *B* are correct. Choice *C* is incorrect, as the patient would likely experience a widening pulse pressure, not one that is narrowing. Choice *D* is incorrect, as the patient would display a decreased cardiac output. Choice *E* is incorrect, as the patient would typically present with hypotension in this case.

146. A: Choice *A* involves the patient's determination to self-directed decisions that are free from coercion. Choice *B* sets forth that actions are right or wrong depending on the level of pleasure they promote. Choice *C* endorses that the nurse will remain true to their professional commitments. Choice *D* involves conflicting concerns of multiple parties.

147. A: Choice *A* is the appropriate response by the nurse because it supports accurate medication reconciliation with continued management of care. Choices *B*, *C*, and *D* should all be avoided, as they would delay treatment and potentially provide inaccurate information. The medical-surgical nurse should obtain a written release of information from the patient, and then proceed to contact the outpatient pharmacy to discuss the patient's current prescription for gabapentin. If the patient is prescribed additional medication by other outpatient providers, it would also be appropriate for the nurse to gather that data as well to support a thorough medication reconciliation process.

148. B: The most common cause of a renal stone is insufficient fluid intake. Therefore, the teaching plan for this patient should include the instruction to drink plenty of fluids. *A* is incorrect since this patient has a stone composed of calcium and should avoid high calcium foods. *C* is not correct; since this patient has a stone composed of calcium, avoiding purines in the diet will have no effect. *D* is not correct since antacids are associated with renal stone formation.

149. D: An uncomplicated chlamydial infection of the lower tract is treated with a single dose of azithromycin that is witnessed and confirmed by a health care provider. Therefore, *A*, *B*, and *C* are incorrect.

150. B: Choice *B* represents the safe response to the finding of an order for a medication that the patient previously expressed was not effective for them. The nurse should deliver information regarding this finding and ensure that the provider is aware of the patient's history with the medication. Choice *A* does not represent best practice, as it fails to advocate for the patient's needs to ensure individualized, safe, and effective treatment. While the nurse may ultimately administer the medication, this should only be done after conferring with the prescriber and patient. Choices *C* and *D* are not appropriate parties to relay this concern to at this time, as they fall outside of the immediate task of safe patient care.

151. B: An abdominal aneurysm may present or be found on examination as a pulsating mass in the abdomen. Indigestion when lying down is associated with gastrointestinal reflux disease (GERD) and is not indicative of an AAA. Fatigue and shortness of breath on exertion may be indicative of coronary artery or pulmonary disease. It is not directly associated with an AAA. Pain radiating down the left arm is a classic sign of a myocardial infarction (MI).

152. A: Choice *A* describes the patient's thought process when experiencing delusional thinking. The medical-surgical nurse must understand how delusional thinking impairs beliefs, as well as understanding and cooperation, to ensure the establishment of effective communication and a holistic plan of care. Choice *B* describes hallucinations. Choice *C* describes delirium. Choice *D* describes dementia.

153. A: Acquired immunodeficiency syndrome (AIDS) is diagnosed when CD4/T cell levels drop below two hundred cells per cubic millimeter; therefore, Choices *B*, *C*, and *D* are incorrect. After patients are diagnosed with AIDS, they are vulnerable to serious chronic diseases such as cancer.

154. B: Choice *B* represents a function of the cerebellum. The nurse should also expect to support the patient to "fine-tune" their movement post brain injury when the cerebellum is affected. Choice *A* is a function of the occipital lobe. Choice *C* is a function of the brain stem. Choice *D* is a function of the temporal lobe.

155. C: Choice *C* aligns with the nurse's question, "How are things going today?" and demonstrates a positive example of therapeutic communication. Choice *A* recognizes the patient's outward expression. Choice *B* connects through understanding. Choice *D* explores a clear foundation of the patient's intended meaning of response. All communication techniques reviewed in this question signify therapeutic engagement.

156. B: Choice *B* is an activity that takes place during the assessment phase of the nursing process. Choice *A* aligns with the implementation phase. Choice *C* correlates with the planning phase. Choice *D* represents an activity in the evaluation phase.

157. A: Effective antiretroviral therapy (ART) reduces the viral load or how much HIV is present in the patient's blood. With ART, many HIV patients can achieve viral suppression or an undetectable viral load. Therapeutic drug levels measure how much drug is the bloodstream, but they do not indicate the effectiveness of the therapy; therefore, Choice *B* is not correct. Choice *C* is an incorrect answer since the presence of side effects does not determine drug effectiveness. Since the viral load may still be present in semen even if the virus cannot be detected, Choice *D* is not the correct answer.

158. C: Painful urination (dysuria) is the most common presenting manifestation in the patient with UTI. Dysuria, along with urinary frequency and urgency, is 75 percent predictive of UTI. Other findings in the male patient include fever, tachycardia, flank pain, suprapubic pain, penile discharge, scrotal masses and tenderness, and enlarged inguinal lymph nodes.

159. A: Choice *A* is significant, as a patient with acute glomerulonephritis struggles to maintain fluid balance and requires substantial assistance with this process. The medical-surgical nurse should monitor this balance and intervene as necessary. Choices *B*, *C*, and *D* are not goals for treatment. On the contrary, the patient should be supported to lower blood pressure, reduce serum potassium levels, and decrease consumption of protein in the diet.

160. C: Acute respiratory distress syndrome (ARDS) is defined by the timing, a chest x-ray, the origin of the edema, and the severity of hypoxemia. In terms of timing, the onset of symptoms in ARDS is within one week of inciting incident. A chest x-ray should reveal bilateral lung infiltrates not explained by consolidation, atelectasis, or effusions. The edema origin is not explained by heart failure or fluid overload, and the severity of hypoxemia is based on the PaO_2/FiO_2 ratio while on 5 cm of continuous positive airway pressure (CPAP).

161. C: Choice *C* represents the appropriate response by the nurse in support of continued assessment of pedal pulses in the patient with congestive heart failure. The nurse should locate a hand-held Doppler and obtain an accurate reading. Choice *A* would be inappropriate, as a non-palpable pedal pulse is a non-emergent expected finding for this patient. Choice *B* is an inappropriate response by the nurse because continued assessment should happen before determination, with later charting, that the pedal pulses couldn't be detected. Choice *D* is also inappropriate due to the non-emergent nature of this finding.

162. C: Choice *C* accurately indicates that the Koebner phenomenon can occur anywhere that minor trauma is noted; therefore, the medical-surgical nurse should evaluate its effect in those areas. Choices *A*, *B*, and *D* are targeted areas that would be appropriate focuses should the patient experience trauma to those areas; however, the Koebner phenomenon is not specific to those locations only.

163. B: Betamethasone therapy can improve the maturity of the fetal lungs by increasing the amount of available surfactant, which allows adaptation of the respiratory system immediately after birth. However, prolonged gestation, which permits additional time for the lungs to mature naturally, is more effective than administration of additional corticosteroids; therefore, Choice *B* is correct. Research indicates that the administration of steroids such as betamethasone in the presence of the premature rupture of membranes (PROM) increases the incidence of infection; therefore, Choice *A* is incorrect. Successful treatment with betamethasone may reduce the incidence of respiratory distress syndrome in the newborn. However, there is no evidence that the risk is eliminated by betamethasone; therefore, Choice *C* is incorrect. Betamethasone is only used to mature the fetal lungs by increasing the amount of surfactant that is available to facilitate the expansion of the newborn lungs. It is not a tocolytic agent (an agent that decreases uterine contractions in preterm labor), and in addition, tocolytic agents cannot be used for longer than 48 hours; therefore, Choice *D* is incorrect.

164. D: This scenario depicts the presentation of hemothorax, which is usually a consequence of a blunt or penetrating chest trauma. Blunting of the costophrenic angle on the affected side is pathognomonic for hemothorax. Chest tube drainage is the mainstay of treatment for hemothorax.

Dear Test Taker,

We would like to start by thanking you for purchasing this study guide for your exam. We hope that we exceeded your expectations.

Our goal in creating this study guide was to cover all of the topics that you will see on the test. We also strove to make our practice questions as similar as possible to what you will encounter on test day. With that being said, if you found something that you feel was not up to your standards, please send us an email and let us know.

We have study guides in a wide variety of fields. If you're interested in one, try searching for it on Amazon or send us an email.

Thanks Again and Happy Testing!
Product Development Team
info@studyguideteam.com

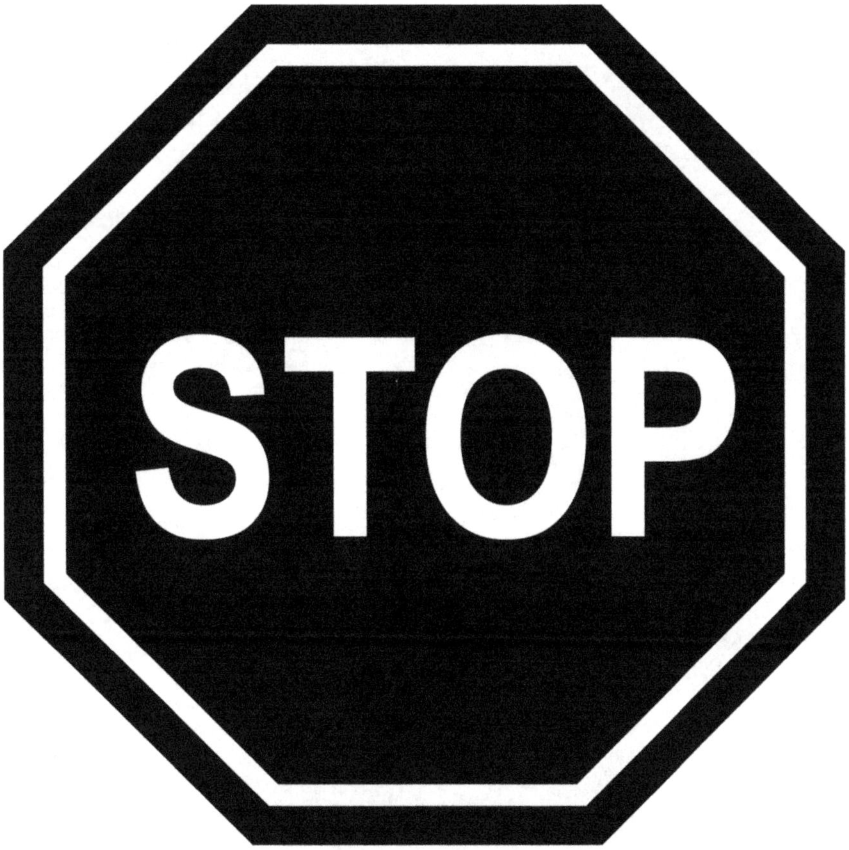

FREE Test Taking Tips DVD Offer

To help us better serve you, we have developed a Test Taking Tips DVD that we would like to give you for FREE. **This DVD covers world-class test taking tips that you can use to be even more successful when you are taking your test.**

All that we ask is that you email us your feedback about your study guide. Please let us know what you thought about it – whether that is good, bad or indifferent.

To get your **FREE Test Taking Tips DVD**, email freedvd@studyguideteam.com with "FREE DVD" in the subject line and the following information in the body of the email:

a. The title of your study guide.

b. Your product rating on a scale of 1-5, with 5 being the highest rating.

c. Your feedback about the study guide. What did you think of it?

d. Your full name and shipping address to send your free DVD.

If you have any questions or concerns, please don't hesitate to contact us at freedvd@studyguideteam.com.

Thanks again!

CPSIA information can be obtained
at www.ICGtesting.com
Printed in the USA
LVHW060918150321
681580LV00015B/526

9 781628 456684